Magnetic Resonance Imaging with Nonlinear Gradient Fields

Gerrit Schultz

Magnetic Resonance Imaging with Nonlinear Gradient Fields

Signal Encoding and Image Reconstruction

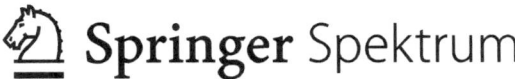 Springer Spektrum

Dr. Gerrit Schultz
Medical Physics
Department of Radiology
University Medical Center
Freiburg, Germany

Accepted as PhD thesis at the University of Freiburg, Germany.
With financial support of the Wissenschaftliche Gesellschaft Freiburg.

ISBN 978-3-658-01133-8   ISBN 978-3-658-01134-5 (eBook)
DOI 10.1007/978-3-658-01134-5

The Deutsche Nationalbibliothek lists this publication in the Deutsche Nationalbibliografie;
detailed bibliographic data are available in the Internet at http://dnb.d-nb.de.

Library of Congress Control Number: 2013934730

Springer Spektrum

Printed on acid-free paper

Springer Spektrum is a brand of Springer DE.
Springer DE is part of Springer Science+Business Media.
www.springer-spektrum.de

Preface

This work was accepted as a PhD thesis by the Faculty of Mathematics and Physics of the University of Freiburg, Germany. It spans five years of research conducted from April 2007 until March 2012.

In particular researchers and engineers who work in the field of biomedical engineering might profit from reading this text. A new approach of image encoding in magnetic resonance imaging is described: The fundamental principle of gradient linearity is challenged by investigating the possibilities of acquiring anatomical images with the help of nonlinear gradient fields. Besides a thorough theoretical analysis with a focus on signal encoding and image reconstruction, initial hardware implementations are tested using phantom as well as in-vivo measurements. Several applications are presented that give an impression about the implications that this technological advancement may have for future medical diagnostics.

Without the help of a great number of people, it would not have been possible to accomplish this piece of work.

Prof. Dr. Jürgen Hennig has given me the opportunity to become part of the amazing Medical Physics Group in Freiburg. It was his idea to combine parallel reception with nonlinear encoding fields, and I feel very fortunate that I could base my thesis on this intriguing and inspiring idea. He has given guidance and gave me abundant freedom to follow my own research interests, which he has always supported and promoted. Creativity at work and a vivid social life, most of what I have learned about science and many of the new friendships that I have found I owe to this unique working atmosphere. Thank you.

I deeply thank Dr. Maxim Zaitsev for his extensive support. I was very lucky to have him as teacher and advisor; he has contributed to this thesis with uncountable ideas and he has invested many hours in closely reviewing abstracts, papers and this dissertation, thereby helping me to get more and more familiar with scientific working. It is amazing how hard it is to confront him with problems he wouldn't understand; even harder to see him say "no!", no matter how many emails are waiting to be answered...

It was a pleasure working on a team project together with Anna Masako Welz, Hans Weber, Chris Cocosco, Dr. Daniel Gallichan, Dr. Walter Witschey, Sebastian Littin and lately also Dr. Feng Jia. I could fill pages here, but I force myself to be brief. We have achieved a lot together. It has been fantastic with you guys!

I could also always rely on the support of my other colleagues, be it on scientific, work-related or personal issues. Jakob Assländer, Sébastien Bär, Dr. Simon Bauer, Stefanie Buchenau, Dr. Martin Büchert, Dr. Peter Gall, Daniel Giese, Dr. Martin Haas, Dr. Matthias Honal, Dr. Jan-Bernd Hövener, Dr. Thimo Hugger, Dr. Valerij Kiselev, Dr. Thomas Lange, Dr. Julian Maclaren, Matthias Pfefferle, Dr. Wilfried Reichardt, Dr. Marco Reisert, Cris Lovell-Smith, Dr. Felix Staehle, Dr. Aurélien Stalder, Frederik Testud, Dr. Matthias Weigel, Ara Yeramian, Dr. Benjamin Zahneisen, and many others. You have made my PhD a great time. Especially I wish to mention Dr. Nico Splitthoff with whom I have shared offices for more than four years; I had never thought that late-night (or rather early-morning) ISMRM conference deadlines can be so much fun!

Commitment to the PatLoc project of many people from partners in industry and academia was also essential for this thesis. I highly acknowledge the work of Heinrich Lehr, Stéphanie Ohrel, Dr. Hans Post, Johannes Schneider and Dr. Peter Ullmann from Bruker BioSpin GmbH, and the on- and off-site assistance provided by Dr. Andrew Dewdney from Siemens Healthcare with support from Dr. Franz Schmitt. It has been very interesting to perform common PatLoc projects with Dr. Zhenyu Liu and Prof. Dr. Jan G. Korvink from the Department of Microsystems Engineering at the University of Freiburg, with Prof. Dr. Oliver Speck from the University of Magdeburg, with Fa-Hsuan Lin, PhD, from the Massachusetts General Hospital in Boston, USA, and with Dr. Florian Knoll and co-workers from the University of Graz, Austria. It has also been an honor to welcome guests who perform research on nonlinear encoding at the cutting edge, like Kelvin Layton from the University of Melbourne, Australia, and Jason Stockmann, PhD, from Yale University, USA.

Also the financial support of the *Wissenschaftliche Gesellschaft Freiburg* to cover publishing costs is greatly acknowledged.

Last but not least I thank my parents Uta and Wolfgang, my whole family, and especially my beloved wife Charlotte for all the patience and continuous encouragements. It's like Beppo Roadsweeper. One sweep after another. And in the end, it's finished.

It has been many hours that I have worked on this thesis. Each hour has been worthwhile. Thank you all!

Gerrit Schultz

Contents in Brief

Contents in Detail

Introduction

"ANY sufficiently advanced technology is indistinguishable from magic." The British writer Arthur C. Clarke, famous for his science-fiction novel *2001: A Space Odyssey*, formulated his "third law" in 1973 [23], the very same year Paul Lauterbur published the first image [92] acquired with a technology which later has come to be known as *magnetic resonance imaging* (MRI, Fig. 1a). This technology allows physicians to literally see what is going on inside the human body - and this in a completely non-invasive way.

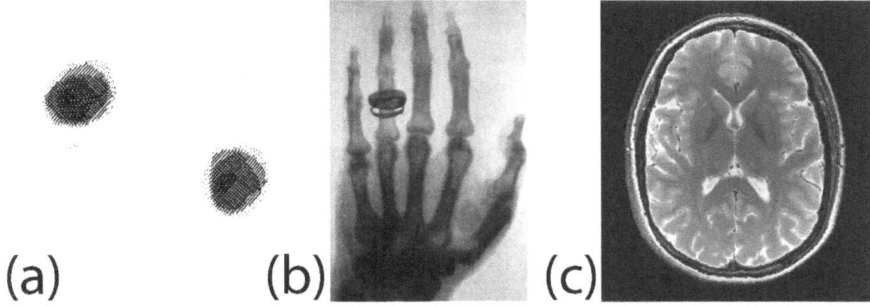

Figure 1: Medical imaging: a look inside. (a) The very first MR image. (b) X-ray of von Kölliker's hand, acquired 1896 by Wilhelm Conrad Röntgen. (c) Typical anatomical MR image acquired on a modern system.

MRI is not the first non-invasive medical imaging technology. Already in the late 19th century, X-rays were discovered and it definitely must have been a magical moment for the audience when Wilhelm Conrad Röntgen presented an X-ray image of Albert von Kölliker's hand on January 23rd, 1896, in a public lecture (Fig. 1b taken from [202]). Compared to plain X-rays and computed tomography, MRI does not involve high-energy radiation and it is much more versatile, offering a range of different contrasts and diagnostic applications that can hardly be catalogued nowadays. If anyone would have shown a typical state-of-the-art MR image with all its fine anatomical details (Fig. 1c) to Arthur C. Clarke, he (and probably also Paul Lauterbur) would have called this image to be *magical*. The author Clarke might have used this image right away in some of his novels. On the other hand, the scientist Lauterbur would have had to face yet another huge challenge. In fact, there is a decisive difference between science-fiction and objective science: The collective work of hundreds, even thousands of scientists and engineers was required to be able to routinely acquire images like the one shown in Fig. 1c. The novelist can describe a phenomenon and call it magic, the scientist, however has to explain this phenomenon. To the scientist, the third law therefore comes along rather prosaic: "A scientist should be able to understand any technology." Nevertheless, most MRI scientists will probably confirm that even though we (sometimes) understand nowadays how an image like the one shown in the above figure is formed, the effect still has not lost its magical aura.

What about the two first laws of Arthur C. Clarke? The author formulated them in this way:

1. When a distinguished but elderly scientist states that something is possible, he is almost certainly right. When he states that something is impossible, he is very probably wrong.
2. The only way of discovering the limits of the possible is to venture a little way past them into the impossible.

There is much truth in these laws also for non-fictitious science. It is undisputed that each researcher bases his insight on knowledge gained by, maybe not elderly, but often elder and more experienced scientists. As the history of science has shown even the brightest minds can be mistaken, and declare something that is in fact possible to be impossible; but to quote Albert Einstein: "Only the one who does not question is safe from making a mistake". Also, science and technology would not have evolved as they have if no one would have questioned established concepts, if no one would have ventured a little way past what had already been discovered before.

Milestones of Magnetic Resonance Imaging   MRI is based on a physical phenomenon which seemed impossible at first: the observation that an atomic nucleus has an intrinsic magnetic moment, caused by the nuclear spin. Gerlach and Stern observed in 1922 an unusual line spreading which could not be explained with the classical physical theory [45]. Several brilliant scientists, among them Wolfgang Pauli, dared to think the impossible and elaborated, starting in the 1920s, the quantum theory, which could consistently describe the observed effect. More than one decade later, in 1938, Isidor I. Rabi designed an experiment for the precise measurement of nuclear magnetic moments by applying a transverse radio frequency (RF) field at the Larmor frequency, thereby discovering the nuclear magnetic resonance (NMR) phenomenon [140]. In 1946, Edward Purcell [137] and Felix Bloch [11] independently detected an NMR signal from bulk matter. Only a few years later the first commercial NMR spectrometers were available and could be used with success to analyze chemical compositions of fluids and solids.

The birth of MRI finally came in 1973, when Paul Lauterbur [92] and Peter Mansfield [108] realized independently that additional gradient fields can encode information about the location of the signal sources. In the following years, significant improvements in hardware design were made and a prolific research activity started - which is still growing nowadays - in controlling the hardware components to enhance the efficiency and variety of methods for the extraction of diagnostic information. An excellent example is the fast RARE (turbo spin echo) sequence developed by Jürgen Hennig and co-workers in 1986 [60]. About the mid-1980s, MRI technology had advanced to a point where scanners became routinely available for medical diagnostics.

A further important technological improvement came with the realization of parallel imaging (PI) in the 1990s, especially by Peter B. Roemer [145], Dan Sodickson [173] and Klaas Prüssmann [135]. Originally, scanners had been equipped with only one RF coil for the reception of MR signals. It was later realized that MR signals from receiver coils with non-homogeneous sensitivity bear encoding information supplementary to the information obtained from gradient encoding. Instead of using only one volume coil, several smaller surface coils are placed close to the measured object in PI. The advantage of this technique is that the additional information provided by the several coils is recorded *in parallel* in contrast to the time-intensive *sequential* gradient encoding. Since the advent of PI, major research activity has been conducted - and is being conducted - in evaluating how this additional information can be exploited to improve image acquisitions. Important benefits are the increase of the signal-to-noise ratio (SNR) and especially the acceleration of image acquisitions by reducing the amount of gradient encoding steps while retaining full image resolution.

PatLoc[1]   At the time the PatLoc project started, PI had an influence on the gradient encoding schemes, but not on the gradient hardware itself.[2] Gradient coils are usually designed to produce linear *spatial encoding magnetic fields* (SEMs). Benefits of strongly curvilinear SEMs or even SEMs with locations of vanishing field gradients inside the imaging region had occasionally been discussed before [193, 110, 208, 131]; however, no general approach had been presented up to that point which had tackled the question if the advent of PI would allow gradient systems to be more effective under certain circumstances if designed to generate such *nonlinear and non-bijective SEMs* (NB-SEMs[3]) instead of linear SEMs.

The PatLoc project, part of the larger INUMAC[4] project, was intended to fill this gap. PI offered the possibility to compensate for encoding deficiencies introduced by ambiguous SEMs. Initial investigations suggested already interesting implications to MRI [62], [[61]][5]. The non-rectilinear geometry of the NB-SEMs seemed to be better adapted to the anatomical structures, for example, cortical imaging would profit from such geometries.

Another interesting property was hypothesized: NB-SEMs should reduce the problem of peripheral nerve stimulation (PNS). Typically, PNS manifests as an involuntary muscle twitching and is therefore displeasing for the patient. In extreme cases, stimulation with gradients can even be dangerous, when heart muscle fibers are stimulated. PNS is caused by the time-varying magnetic fields generated by the gradient coils. NB-SEMs offer the possibility to reduce the magnetic field variations while preserving high local gradients, thus reducing the problem of PNS. These hypotheses were very promising and it could be expected that research with NB-SEMs would open new perspectives to MRI which made PatLoc a very exciting project.

When I entered the PatLoc project in spring 2007, it had just been started a couple of months earlier with Prof. Dr. Jürgen Hennig as project initiator,

---

[1]Acronym for P̲arallel Imaging T̲echnique using L̲ocalized Gradients.

[2]There are only rare exceptions like the publication of Dennis L. Parker and J. Rock Hadley [126]. In this publication, applications for a novel type of gradient hardware are analyzed. The hardware generates non-bijective encoding fields; the field geometry is, however, very special: Modifications occur only along one spatial dimension with alternating, quasi-linear regions. A general investigation of MRI with non-bijective encoding fields is not presented.

[3]In this thesis, the acronym *NB-SEM* is used in opposition to the term *linear SEM*. In a broad sense, it denotes any magnetic gradient field which intentionally deviates from linearity in order to achieve a certain encoding effect.

[4]Acronym for I̲maging of N̲euro Disease U̲sing high field M̲R A̲nd C̲ontrastophores.

[5]Double brackets, [[·]], indicate own (co-)authorship throughout this thesis.

Dr. Maxim Zaitsev as project leader and one other PhD student, Anna Masako Welz working on the project. The timing was perfect because little had been explored up to that point, and much was to be discovered in this exciting research field of using strongly curvilinear SEMs in MRI.

Concerning the Research Carried Out During the Course of This Thesis
Retrospectively, Arthur Clarke's three laws might have served as a guideline for my PhD research. For the situation of a PhD student, it appears not unreasonable that the following three rules can be inferred from Clarke's laws:

1. A PhD student should learn from his colleagues, but, most importantly, learn to pave his own way.
2. A PhD thesis should cover unexplored material.
3. A PhD thesis should be written to be understandable by a scientist.[6]

At the beginning of the project, we had to solve the most urgent problems of designing a first PatLoc prototype coil and performing initial experiments. This first period was basically shared work, where I focused more on theoretical issues and Anna Masako Welz more on the technical problems. We decided on building a coil with two orthogonal quadrupolar SEMs, fields which are flat at the center and steep at the periphery. From my rather theoretical point-of-view, those fields seemed to be the natural generalization to the linear SEMs. But also from the technical point-of-view, those fields seemed useful because they provided more encoding efficiency at the periphery where the fields have steep gradients. Encoding with such quadrupolar fields is ambiguous, but Prof. Dr. Jürgen Hennig anticipated that the additional information obtained from several RF-receiver coils should be sufficient to resolve these ambiguities. And indeed, it turned out that a reconstruction algorithm could be developed which was capable of resolving these ambiguities under realistic imaging conditions. In 2008, we had finished a first prototype coil with support from Dr. Zhenyu Liu, Dr. Feng Jia and Prof. Dr. Jan G. Korvink from the Department of Microsystems Engineering at the University of Freiburg and in collaboration with Bruker BioSpin GmbH in Ettlingen, Germany, where Dr. Peter Ullmann, Heinrich Lehr, Stéphanie Ohrel and Dr. Hans Post were involved and in

---

[6]Follows from the third law in its form adapted here to the situation of real science: "A scientist should be able to understand any technology".

collaboration with Siemens Healthcare, Erlangen, Germany. We successfully performed the first experiments in the first half of 2008.

The initial experiments were promising; the next steps were even more ambitious. It would have been a long way for our small team to bring the project to the next level alone and therefore I am grateful that more people entered the project: Hans Weber, Dr. Daniel Gallichan, Chris Cocosco, Dr. Walter Witschey and recently also Sebastian Littin. The increased team size allowed us to divide the work more clearly between us without giving up close collaboration. One sub-group was concerned with the development of a powerful PatLoc coil for multi-channel in vivo brain imaging. Others aimed at developing innovative imaging sequences. Another long-term goal was the development of medical applications for PatLoc imaging. We decided that I should extend my initial, more theoretically-oriented, studies and focus primarily on the elaboration of adequate image reconstruction techniques. This focus allowed me not only to pave my own way in research and be in line with the above second rule that "a PhD thesis should cover unexplored material," but also to have a distinctive portion of purely individual work inside this collective project.

The initial image reconstruction seemed to work well; however, further insight had to be gained for the elaboration of a first ambitious high-quality publication. The reconstruction was very fast, but it was restricted to one specific imaging situation. It turned out that an iterative reconstruction method applicable to a broad range of imaging situations could be implemented. Such a method is, however, very slow and therefore we decided that algorithms should be developed tailored to other, more or less specific, imaging situations. The most important of those methods are discussed in this thesis. Especially when the PatLoc head insert, designed for human brain imaging, was available during the course of 2009 on, these methods could be tested on data generated with a powerful SEM system. An important date marked May 2010 when the Ethics Committee of the University of Freiburg approved measurements on human volunteers for Cartesian trajectories. With this approval, we could finally start to perform imaging in vivo. The data allowed us to evaluate the performance of the system and we could start developing new applications for medical imaging. A lot has been achieved so far, but there is much work to be done in the future to further explore the capabilities of NB-SEMs.

Concerning This Dissertation The third rule, stating that "a PhD thesis should be written to be understandable by a scientist," immediately concerns this text and I hope to have succeeded in adequately conveying the most relevant information of the performed work. At first, this seemed to be a difficult task because I had worked on a multitude of projects myself and contributed work to other projects. Apart from recent and/or less significant work, contributions from my part were published (or are to be published) in scientific journals [[61, 156, 158, 42, 207, 101, 43, 86, 189]], in conference proceedings, mainly at ISMRM, [[155, 159, 199, 105, 161, 162, 100, 213, 121, 160, 157, 44, 24, 190, 102, 154, 153, 191, 103, 25, 205, 206]] and in patent applications. Two patents have been granted already [[63, 192]]. Two more patent applications with co-inventorship contribution are currently under review at the European Patent Office. At second sight, I realized that not all, but most of these contributions could be considered in this thesis while maintaining unity of presentation without giving the impression of concatenating unrelated individual projects.

In this thesis, fundamental implications that the usage of NB-SEMs might have on MRI are presented with a special emphasis on adequate image reconstruction methods. While planning the present text, it was particularly important to me to present my own contributions not isolated from state-of-the-art MRI, but to link this work to what has been known before. It seemed obvious to me how the linking should be performed. PatLoc imaging uses PI hardware, but the restrictions of the conventional gradient hardware are relaxed to NB-SEMs. In this regard, PatLoc imaging generalizes conventional parallel imaging. Therefore, I tried to identify a theoretical formalism which was capable of explaining the most important state-of-the-art image reconstruction methods for conventional PI, while being abstract enough to be useful for PatLoc imaging.

Fortunately, a similar situation had occurred before because PI effectively generalizes standard single-coil imaging. Klaas Prüssmann presented in his seminal SENSE publication [135] a mathematically reliable image reconstruction framework abstract enough to be in principle applicable also to PatLoc imaging. In this thesis, this framework is extended to non-rectilinear reconstruction grids to be able to derive particular reconstructions for PatLoc. The relation of conventional imaging, PatLoc and the reconstruction framework is depicted in Fig. 2. The framework effectively describes image reconstruction as a simple matrix-vector multiplication and is therefore

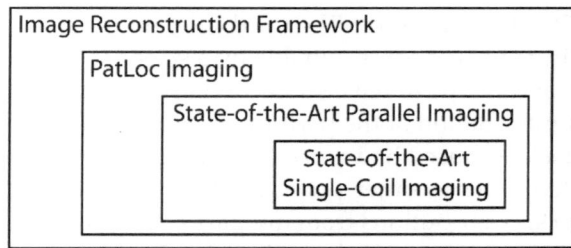

Figure 2: Hierarchy of imaging modalities and reconstruction framework. Whereas parallel imaging generalizes single-coil imaging, PatLoc imaging can be interpreted as a generalization of state-of-the-art parallel imaging because it also makes use of several receiver coils, but the encoding fields are not required to have linear spatial variations. The reconstruction theory used in this thesis is abstract enough to be applicable to all of these imaging modalities.

the basis for direct linear reconstruction methods. This matrix approach is closely linked to existing iterative reconstruction methods and it is also linked to methods which incorporate prior knowledge. I therefore believe that the matrix method concerns a fundamental approach to MR image reconstruction, and consequently this thesis is based on this framework as far as possible.

The presentation of this dissertation benefits from this abstract approach because, having a common background, the different reconstruction methods do not have to be presented independently from each other. There are basically only four fundamental equations in this thesis. These are the signal equation (Eq. 4.9) from which the encoding matrix is derived (Eq. 4.18). The reconstruction matrix is then found with the help of Eq. 4.20, basically by inverting the encoding matrix, and the image is reconstructed by evaluating the matrix-vector multiplication of the reconstruction matrix with the signal data (Eq. 4.16).

The main problem of image reconstruction is that the encoding matrix is very large and direct inversion is only feasible for very special situations. It is therefore important to analyze the structure of the encoding matrix in detail for each imaging situation. If inversion is not practical it can be beneficial to use iterative methods instead based on the insight gained from the performed matrix analysis. The same matrix approach was used to present reconstruction methods for PatLoc as well as for state-of-the-art methods. Strict adherence to this matrix approach might be unusual and it partly involves mathematical technicalities. I believe, however, that the attempt to link all presented methods to one common principle is worthwhile because it adds clarity to the overall presentation and it might help to better understand the implications that the generalization of linear SEMs to NB-SEMs has to MRI.

Brief Outline The thesis is conceptually divided into two main parts. The first part presents conventional state-of-the-art MRI where linear SEMs are employed (chapters 1 and 2). The second part from chapter 3 on deals with PatLoc imaging and the usage of NB-SEMs.

Chapter 1: Physical and Technical Background The purpose of the first chapter is to derive the fundamental signal equation in conventional imaging (Eq. 1.31) from the ground up. The derivation reveals basic physical and technical concepts relevant to this work.

Chapter 2: Basics of MR Image Reconstruction The basics of linear image reconstruction are presented using a matrix approach and the most common reconstruction methods are introduced from single-coil acquisitions as well as from multi-coil acquisitions.

Chapter 3: Overview of PatLoc Imaging and Presentation of Initial Hardware Designs The concept of PatLoc imaging is introduced, some of the expected benefits are discussed, and the hardware measurement environment is presented.

Chapter 4: Signal Models and Basics of Image Reconstruction in PatLoc Imaging The PatLoc signal model (Eq. 4.9) is derived, in parallel to chapter 1, and the basics of image reconstruction in PatLoc imaging are presented. This chapter provides principles that are common to the individual methods that are discussed in chapters 5, 6 and 7.

Chapter 5: Direct Reconstruction for Cartesian PatLoc Imaging Image space and k-space image reconstruction for a two-dimensional Cartesian PatLoc k-space trajectory is presented in this chapter. Conceptually, the image space reconstruction method is probably the most fundamental reconstruction in PatLoc imaging. Therefore, this method and its consequences are analyzed in thorough detail.

Chapter 6: Direct Reconstruction for Radial PatLoc Imaging The topic
in this chapter is a non-Cartesian radial PatLoc trajectory. Its properties are
analyzed and efficient direct image reconstruction methods are presented.

Chapter 7: Iterative Reconstruction in PatLoc Imaging In this chapter,
several iterative image reconstruction methods are developed and analyzed
with the Cartesian and the radial trajectories of the two previous chapters
as well as with a more complex multi-dimensional imaging trajectory.

Chapter 8: Summary and Outlook The final chapter summarizes the main
results of the thesis, some conclusions are drawn and open problems are
addressed that need to be solved in the future.

Appendix Besides remarks on notation and abbreviations, some supplementary material is given, in particular proofs whose results are of particular
interest to this thesis.

Common Knowledge, Team Contributions and Own Contributions Almost all contents of Chapter 1 are common knowledge. The image reconstruction methods that are introduced in Chapter 2 are also well-known; a
significant contribution of this thesis is the attempt to use a unified matrix
approach as a point of reference for all methods, thereby establishing interesting connections between them. The second part of the thesis (chapters 3
to 7), where PatLoc imaging and reconstruction is described, entirely forms
original scientific work, including the appendix (except for section A.2).
PatLoc is a team-oriented project and therefore it is impossible to completely
isolate individual contributions. Chapter 3 serves as introduction to PatLoc
imaging with work presented also performed by other group members.
This is different for the subsequent chapters, which only have little overlap
with others' work. The individual contributions are acknowledged in detail
at the location of occurrence.

Chapter 1

Physical and Technical Background

THE fundamental physical phenomenon of magnetic resonance is the existence of nuclear spin. With each spin a magnetic moment is associated making it sensitive to its magnetic environment. In MR(I) a very large ensemble of spins exists. Therefore quantum statistics describes well the behavior of the macroscopic quantities. Whereas the *local* magnetic interactions are responsible for the large amount of available diagnostic information, it is the *external* fields which allow one to retrieve this information and make it observable for the diagnosing physician in modern medical examinations.

This dissertation is based on the development of an external hardware component and therefore the focus of this thesis are interactions with the external magnetic fields and local interactions are ignored unless necessary to understand the discussed imaging behavior. To this end, the spin ensemble is mostly treated as non-interacting. Based on this assumption, the basic equation of motion for the magnetization vector in an external magnetic field is derived. This equation is purely classical and therefore the further physical treatment can be performed with classical electromagnetic theory. To produce image contrast, relaxation effects are exploited, which are the result of spins interacting with their magnetic neighborhood. At some places in this thesis, these effects are considered by extending the equation of motion for the magnetization to the famous Bloch equations.

MRI signals are created by first magnetizing the object under examination with a constant, strong magnetic field, then perturbing the equilibrium magnetization with a transverse RF field before encoding the object with magnetic gradient fields and finally receiving the signal with RF-receiver coils. The frequency and phase content of the received signals strongly depends on the geometric and temporal characteristics of the magnetic fields involved. This implies that a very high standard of coil design and electronic integration is required for high-quality spectra or images in MR(I), one reason among others, which make MR(I) an extremely powerful, but also challenging technology.

The basic physical principles of MR(I) are well understood. Far from being complete, only the most important results are reviewed here. For a detailed physical treatment of the magnetic resonance phenomenon consult [95]. Similarly, only the basic technical features of those hardware components are presented, which are used to generate the required external magnetic fields. A thorough description of the technical realization of an MR scanner is presented in chapter 15.1 of [123], page 540 - 598. Considering that within the PatLoc project a different kind of encoding hardware has been developed, special emphasis is placed on the gradient system and its main purpose: signal localization. In PatLoc, signal localization with a modified gradient hardware is not sufficient in general and should therefore be accompanied with parallel image acquisition; this topic is therefore also touched at the end of this chapter.

1.1   Nuclear Magnetic Resonance

In this section, the physical principles of MR are presented and the basic NMR experiment, fundamental to MR spectroscopy and MR imaging, is analyzed involving

- magnetization of the object under examination with the main magnet,
- excitation of the magnetization with an RF-transmit pulse and
- signal reception with the RF-receiver unit.

1.1.1   Physical Principles

The physics of MR is based on the physics of the nuclear spin. The spin is a non-classical property and therefore quantum mechanics is the correct framework for describing its dynamics. The basic observation is that a spin can be regarded as an intrinsic angular momentum of the nucleus. A nucleus consists of charged particles and therefore with the spin a magnetic moment $\hat{\mu}$[1] is associated, which points along the direction of the spin angular momentum $\hat{S}$:

$$\hat{\mu} = \gamma\hat{S}. \tag{1.1}$$

---

[1]The hat indicates quantum mechanical operators.

The proportionality constant γ is termed *gyromagnetic ratio*. This ratio is different for each nucleus. For the most important nucleus in MR, hydrogen, with spin 1/2, it has the value $\gamma = 267.52 \ 10^6 \ \mathrm{rad/Ts}$, also denoted as $\gamma = \gamma/(2\pi) = 42.58 \ \mathrm{MHz/T}$.

Having a magnetic moment, the spin interacts with the magnetic field $\vec{B}$ at its location. The interaction energy is described by the Hamiltonian:

$$\hat{H} = -\hat{\mu}\vec{B}. \tag{1.2}$$

In the NMR experiment, a macroscopic voltage is measured in the receiver chain. The voltage is induced by the magnetization of the measured object, which can itself be regarded as a macroscopic (spatially-dependent) property. Quantum statistics can be used to bridge the gap between microscopic quantum theory and macroscopic measurements. In NMR, quantum statistics gives very accurate results because the (local) sample sizes involve around 10^{22} spins.

These large spin ensembles exhibit a macroscopic magnetization under the influence of external magnetic fields. But what is the exact effect of those fields onto the magnetization?

To answer this question, a non-interacting spin ensemble is assumed, which is a very good assumption within the scope of this thesis. The relevant findings can be deduced based on the density operator formalism. The density operator is defined as $\hat{\sigma} := \overline{|\psi\rangle\langle\psi|}$, where the overbar indicates averaging over all independent sample quantum states.

The (macroscopic) magnetization density $\vec{M}$ at location $\vec{x}$ and time t is then found by calculating

$$\vec{M}(\vec{x}, t) = n(\vec{x}) \cdot < \hat{\mu} >= n(\vec{x}) \cdot Tr\left\{\hat{\sigma}(\vec{x}, t)\hat{\mu}\right\}, \tag{1.3}$$

where $n(\vec{x})$ is the spin density. The dynamics of the magnetization is therefore entirely defined by the dynamics of the density operator. The time evolution of this operator is described by the von Neumann equation:

$$\frac{d\hat{\sigma}}{dt} = -\frac{i}{\hbar}[\hat{H}, \hat{\sigma}]. \tag{1.4}$$

In this equation, $\hbar$ denotes the reduced Planck constant, which has a value of 1.05×10^{-34} Js. The time derivative of the individual components of the magnetization is found by combining Eqs. 1.2 - 1.4:

$$\frac{\dot{M}_i}{n} = \frac{\mathrm{d}}{\mathrm{d}t} Tr\left\{\hat{\sigma}\hat{\mu}_i\right\} = -\frac{\mathrm{i}}{\hbar} Tr\left\{[\hat{H},\hat{\sigma}]\hat{\mu}_i\right\} = +\frac{\mathrm{i}}{\hbar}\sum_j Tr\left\{\hat{\sigma}[\hat{\mu}_i,\hat{\mu}_j]B_j\right\}.$$

According to Eq. 1.1, the commutator relations of the magnetization operator follow the common relations of the spin angular momenta:

$$[\hat{\mu}_i,\hat{\mu}_j] = \gamma^2[\hat{S}_i,\hat{S}_j] = \mathrm{i}\hbar\gamma^2\sum_k \epsilon_{ijk}\hat{S}_k = \mathrm{i}\hbar\gamma\sum_k \epsilon_{ijk}\hat{\mu}_k,$$

where ϵ_{ijk} is the Levi-Civita symbol. The time derivative of M_i is therefore found to be:

$$\dot{M}_i = -n\sum_{j,k}\epsilon_{ijk}Tr\left\{\hat{\sigma}\hat{\mu}_k\right\}(\gamma B_j) = -\sum_{j,k}\epsilon_{ijk}M_k(\gamma B_j) = (\vec{M}\times(\gamma\vec{B}))_i,$$

and the dynamics of the magnetization vector is described with a simple equation:

$$\dot{\vec{M}} = \vec{M}\times(\gamma\vec{B}). \tag{1.5}$$

This equation is the macroscopic equation of motion of the magnetization vector. This equation is also known from classical physics. Most results in this thesis are based on this classical equation, and therefore mostly a quantum mechanical treatment can be omitted and established techniques from classical electrodynamics are employed instead.

1.1.2 Main Magnetic Field

Starting from an initial state, the equation of motion presented in Eq. 1.5 can be integrated for known magnetic fields. However, the initial state requires at least some magnetization. The most important purpose of the main magnetic field $B_0\vec{e}_z$ is to polarize the object under examination.

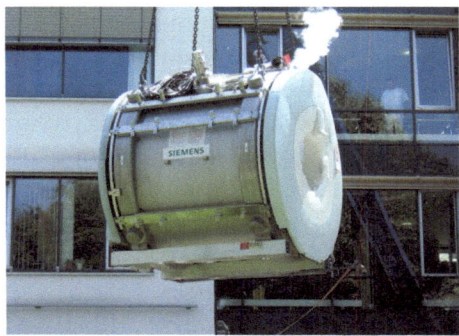

Figure 1.1: This MR scanner (MAGNETOM Trio, A Tim System 3T, Siemens Health-care, Erlangen, Germany) was equipped with a PatLoc insert coil while this thesis was conducted. The scanner is shown during delivery to the site of installation. Visible from outside is the vacuum chamber that contains the main magnet, the largest component of the scanner.

a) Main Magnet

The magnetic field is generated with the large main magnet (cf. Fig. 1.1). The field strength determines the precession frequencies of the magnetization. A major engineering criterion is spatio-temporal homogeneity of the precession frequencies. Therefore, the magnet design is based on a superconducting solenoid which generates very homogeneous fields with an accuracy of around $0.1 - 10ppm$ in the typical imaging region. Typical field strengths for imaging patients range from $0.2\,\mathrm{T} - 3\,\mathrm{T}$. An $11.75\,\mathrm{T}$ system (Iseult/INUMAC project) is planned to be delivered in April 2013 to the Neurospin site in Saclay, France [187]. It will be largest and strongest whole-body system ever built. Experimental or pre-clinical scanners often have even stronger fields of up to $20\,\mathrm{T}$. One advantage of such strong systems is an increase in SNR. Most clinical magnets are shielded with a second superconducting coil. The shield reduces efficiency in favor of enhanced patient safety and siting costs resulting from fast decaying magnetic fields outside of the examination area.

b) Polarization

With the main magnet, the measured object is polarized. But how does the generated constant magnetic field $B_0\vec{e}_z$ actually create the nuclear magnetization in the sample? In order to find a reliable value of the initial magnetization methods from quantum statistics should be used. The initial magnetization is established in the thermodynamic equilibrium. In this equilibrated state, the off-diagonal elements (coherences) of the density operator are zero. The diagonal elements (populations) are weighted according to their corresponding Boltzmann factors:

$$\sigma_{mm}^{eq} = \frac{1}{Z} exp(-E(m)/k_B T). \tag{1.6}$$

The value $Z = \sum_m exp(-E(m)/k_B T)$ represents the canonical partition function, k_B is the Boltzmann constant with value $k_B = 1.38 \times 10^{-23} J K^{-1}$, T is the temperature and $E(m)$ is the energy of the corresponding Zeeman quantum state. For a constant field $B_0 \vec{e}_z$ the energy levels $E(m)$ are, according to Eqs. 1.1, 1.2, given by:

$$E(m) = m\hbar\gamma B_0,$$

where m is the quantum number of the z-angular momentum $\hat{S}_z$. In NMR, the Boltzmann factor $B = \hbar\gamma B_0/k_B T$ is typically only about 10^{-5}. Therefore, the exponentials in Eq. 1.6 can be simplified using a Taylor series expansion and for a spin 1/2 system with only two Zeeman states ($m = \pm 1/2$) the equilibrium density operator reduces to:

$$\hat{\sigma}^{eq} = \begin{pmatrix} \frac{1}{2} + \frac{1}{4}B & 0 \\ 0 & \frac{1}{2} - \frac{1}{4}B \end{pmatrix}.$$

The initial magnetization $\vec{M}^{eq}$ is then found with the relations presented in Eqs. 1.1, 1.3:

$$M_x^{eq} = M_y^{eq} = 0,$$

$$M_z^{eq} = n \cdot \gamma \cdot Tr\left\{\hat{\sigma}^{eq}\hat{S}_z\right\} = \frac{1}{4}\frac{\hbar^2\gamma^2}{k_B T}nB_0 \overset{B_0=1.5\,\mathrm{T}}{\approx} 5 \times 10^{-3}\,\mathrm{J/Tm^3} \tag{1.7}$$

$$\approx 4 \times 10^{-9} B_0/\mu_0, \quad \mu_0 = 4\pi \cdot 10^{-7}\,\mathrm{Tm/A}.$$

The resulting nuclear paramagnetism of water has a susceptibility of only 4×10^{-9}. It is about 2000 times weaker than the actual diamagnetism of water. The contribution of the nuclear spins to the longitudinal magnetization is therefore negligible. Nevertheless, it is strong enough to be detected once being moved out of equilibrium as shown below.

c) Precession

In the thermodynamic equilibrium, $\vec{M}^{eq}$ does not change in magnitude and direction. If the thermodynamic equilibrium is disturbed, a magnetization vector $\vec{M}_0$ might result with non-zero transverse components. For a constant magnetic field $B_0 \vec{e}_z$ the equation of motion, given by Eq. 1.5, can be solved analytically. With an initial magnetization $\vec{M}_0$ the solution is simply:

$$\vec{M}(t) = \mathbf{R}(\vec{e}_z, \omega_L t)\vec{M}_0.$$

The matrix $\mathbf{R}$ is just a standard 3D rotation matrix that describes a rotation by the angle $\omega_L t$ around the z-axis (cf. definition of $\mathbf{R}(\cdot, \cdot)$ in Appendix A.1 on page 291). As the angle increases linearly with time, the motion of the magnetization is indeed a precessional motion around the z-axis (cf. Fig. 1.2) with the *Larmor frequency* ω_L:

$$\omega_L = -\gamma B_0. \tag{1.8}$$

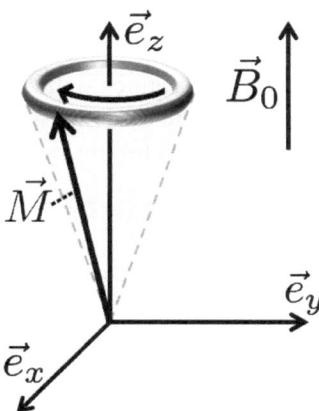

Figure 1.2: Precession of the magnetization vector around the direction of the static main magnetic field.

d)   Relaxation and the Bloch Equations

For the assumed non-interacting spin ensemble, the precessional motion goes on forever. In reality, however, the spins interact with each other and their charged neighborhoods. The magnetization therefore slowly relaxes toward its equilibrium value $\vec{M}^{eq}$. The longitudinal relaxation gives rise to the diagnostically very important T_1-contrast and the transverse relaxation to the T_2-contrast. This macroscopic relaxation effect is described by the Bloch equations [11], which modifies the basic equation of motion presented in Eq. 1.5:

$$\dot{\vec{M}} = \vec{M} \times (\gamma \vec{B}) - T_2^{-1}(M_x \vec{e}_x + M_y \vec{e}_y) - T_1^{-1}(M_z - M_z^{eq})\vec{e}_z. \qquad (1.9)$$

There are many other interaction effects, like for example chemical shift or diffusion, which can correctly be treated with an appropriate model. These effects give rise to a modification of the above Bloch equations [182]. Within the scope of this thesis, these effects are, however, irrelevant and therefore they are ignored.

e)   Rotating Frame Formalism

Consider a reference frame, which rotates with $\vec{\omega}$ compared to the laboratory frame. If ∂_t^{rot} describes the time derivative in the rotating frame, the equation of motion (Eq. 1.5) takes the following form:

$$\partial_t^{rot} \vec{M} = \vec{M} \times (\gamma \vec{B} + \vec{\omega}). \qquad (1.10)$$

For a reference frame which follows exactly the precessional motion of the magnetization, i.e., $\vec{\omega} = \omega_L \vec{e}_z = -\gamma B_0 \vec{e}_z$, the effect of the constant main magnetic field $\vec{B} = B_0 \vec{e}_z$ is formally eliminated: Equation 1.10 reduces to $\partial_t^{rot} \vec{M} = 0$; the magnetization vector in the rotating reference frame is therefore fixed in time.

1.1.3   RF Excitation

The RF-transmit system serves to "excite" the magnetization by moving it out of thermodynamic equilibrium. RF excitation is essential

- because the static longitudinal magnetization is very weak and cannot be measured effectively. It is the dynamic motion in the transverse plane, which induces measurable currents in the RF-receiver coils.
- because the return of the magnetization back to thermodynamic equilibrium is tissue-dependent and provides image contrasts with a high relevance for medical diagnostics.

a) RF-Transmit System

The object is excited by irradiating appropriate RF pulses into this object. Fig. 1.3 schematically shows the hardware typically involved in the signal transmission process and the caption explains the purpose of the individual components of the transmit chain.

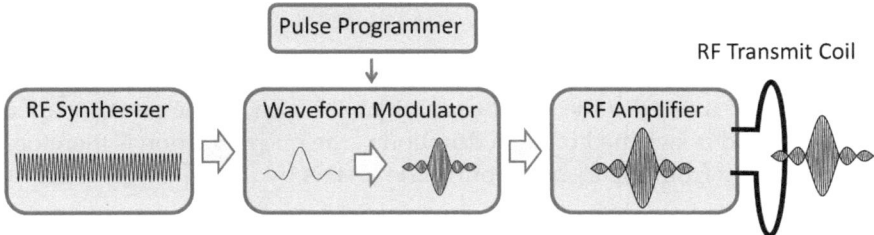

Figure 1.3: Typical RF-transmit chain. An RF synthesizer generates a continuous waveform typically oscillating at the Larmor frequency, from which pieces of the desired pulse duration are cut. A waveform modulator adjusts the pulse in amplitude and phase according to the digital instructions of the sequence programmer and sends it to the RF-power amplifier. Finally, the amplified pulse is coupled to the RF-transmit coil, which irradiates the RF field into the object under examination.

b) Excitation

Consider on-resonance excitation with a transmitting RF field $\vec{B}_1(t)$. On-resonance means that the field rotates with the Larmor frequency, given by Eq. 1.8, in the direction of the rotating reference frame. Even if the transmit field has a longitudinal component along the z-axis or an opposing rotational component, it is sufficient to only consider the rotation along the rotating Larmor frame as those other components have a negligible impact on the dynamics of the magnetization under normal imaging conditions (cf. note 7 of chapter 8 in [95]). The transmit field can therefore be assumed to be directed in the transverse plane. With an initial direction along the x-axis it is given by:

$$\vec{B}_1(t) = B_1(t)(\cos(\omega_L t)\vec{e}_x + \sin(\omega_L t)\vec{e}_y) = B_1(t)\mathbf{R}(\vec{e}_z, \omega_L t)\vec{e}_x = B_1(t)\vec{e}'_x.$$

The vector $\vec{e}'_x$ describes the fixed x'-axis in the rotating reference frame and the vector $\vec{e}_x$ describes the fixed x-axis in the laboratory frame. The latter equality holds because the two vectors $\vec{e}'_x$ and $\vec{e}_x$ are linked via $\vec{e}'_x = \mathbf{R}(\vec{e}_z, \omega_L t)\vec{e}_x$. In the rotating reference frame, the transmit field therefore points along the $\vec{e}'_x$-direction. The magnetic field envelope $B_1(t)$ might have a time-dependency, which is assumed to be slowly varying compared to the Larmor frequency. When the transmit field is added to the main magnetic field, the equation of motion (Eq. 1.10) reduces to:

$$\partial_t^{rot}\vec{M} = \gamma B_1(t)(\vec{M} \times \vec{e}'_x).$$

The dynamics described by this equation is just a precessional motion around the x'-axis with the *Rabi frequency* $|\omega_R| = \gamma B_1$. If the on-resonance transmit field is switched on for a duration τ, the magnetization is therefore flipped away from the z'-axis around the x'-axis by the flip angle α given by:

$$\alpha = \gamma \int_{t=0}^{\tau} B_1(t)\,\mathrm{d}t. \tag{1.11}$$

This flip affects the magnetization vector accordingly:

$$\begin{aligned} \vec{M}(\alpha, t) &= M_z^{eq}\left(\cos(\alpha)\vec{e}'_z + \sin(\alpha)\vec{e}'_y\right) \\ &= M_z^{eq}\left(\cos(\alpha)\vec{e}_z + \sin(\alpha)\mathbf{R}(\vec{e}_z, \omega_L t)\vec{e}_y\right). \end{aligned} \tag{1.12}$$

The same applies to any initial magnetization $\vec{M}_0$ other than the equilibrium magnetization. The resulting flip of the magnetization vector is the physical interpretation of what is normally referred to as "excitation". Off-resonance excitations, where the transmit field rotates with a slightly different frequency than the Larmor frequency, lead to more complicated motions of the magnetization vector. The dynamics are, however, fully described by the Bloch equations. Closed-form solutions to these equations exist only under special imaging conditions (an example is discussed in section 1.2.3, page 32ff). In general, the dynamics of the magnetization vector is found by numerical integration.[2]

1.1.4   NMR Signal Detection

The final step in acquiring an NMR signal is to detect the excited magnetization. This is done with receiver coils which are sensitive to the fast magnetic field variations caused by the precessing magnetization.

a)   RF-Detection System

A typical RF-detection system is schematically depicted in Fig. 1.4 and explained in detail in the caption. Consult the textbook [111] for a detailed presentation of RF coil and circuit design.

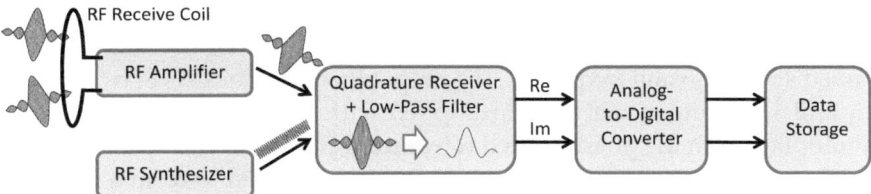

Figure 1.4: Typical RF-receiver chain. First, the signal is received with one or more receiver coil probeheads. The small signals are amplified before being sent to the quadrature receiver. In this hardware component, the signals are multiplied with sinusoidal waveforms from an RF synthesizer having a reference carrier frequency of the same frequency as used for signal transmission. There are two reference signals, shifted by $90°$. The outgoing signals form, after low-pass filtering and digitization in an analog-to-digital converter (ADC), real and imaginary part of the NMR signal, which is finally stored using appropriate hardware.

b)   Free Induction Decay

The influence of the individual components of the RF-detection system onto the NMR signal can also be quantified, which is the topic of this section.

First, consider that the precessing magnetization generates a magnetic field which is induced in an RF-receiver coil. Based on Faraday's law of induction

---

[2]Nice animations of spin dynamics can found at [150].

and a reciprocity law [68][3], it can be shown that the induced voltage U in the receiver coil is given by:

$$U(t) = -\dot{\Phi}(t) = -\frac{\mathrm{d}}{\mathrm{d}t} \int_V \vec{\mathfrak{B}}^{re}(\vec{x})\vec{M}(\vec{x},t)\,\mathrm{d}\vec{x}. \tag{1.13}$$

Here, Φ is the magnetic flux through the receiver coil, V is the excited volume and $\vec{\mathfrak{B}}^{re}$ is the magnetic field generated by the receiver coil per unit current.[4] The time derivative of M_z can be neglected because the precessional motion is restricted to the xy-plane. Therefore, introduction of Eq. 1.12 into the above equation leads to a voltage of:

$$U(t) = \omega_L \int_V M_z^{eq}(\vec{x})\sin(\alpha)\left(\mathfrak{B}_x^{re}(\vec{x})\cos(\omega_L t) - \mathfrak{B}_y^{re}(\vec{x})\cos(\omega_L t + \frac{\pi}{2})\right)\mathrm{d}\vec{x}. \tag{1.14}$$

The signal is amplified by a factor β_A, it is split in two and modulated in the quadrature receiver. The effect of the quadrature receiver can be explained with a multiplication of the signal, represented by Eq. 1.14, with a sinusoid tuned at the transmit frequency. The output therefore consists of two signals s_1 and s_2, where s_1 has been multiplied with $2\cos(\omega_L t)$ and s_2 has been multiplied with the phase-shifted reference signal $2\cos(\omega_L t + \pi/2)$. After a low pass filter, the two signals are formally combined to form a complex signal $s(t)$:

$$s(t) = s_1(t) + \mathrm{i}s_2(t) = \int_V m(\vec{x})c(\vec{x})\,\mathrm{d}\vec{x}, \tag{1.15}$$

$$\begin{aligned} m(\vec{x}) &:= \omega_L \beta_A M_z^{eq}(\vec{x})\sin(\alpha), \\ c(\vec{x}) &:= \mathfrak{B}_x^{re}(\vec{x}) - \mathrm{i}\mathfrak{B}_y^{re}(\vec{x}). \end{aligned} \tag{1.16}$$

The quantity $c(\cdot)$ is usually termed *RF-coil sensitivity*. *Spin density* is a common term to denote the quantity $m(\cdot)$. This definition is problematic,

---

[3]The used model is valid for field strengths of up to about $1.5\,\mathrm{T}$ on whole-body systems. The model assumes that the magnetic field generated by the excited magnetization has an immediate effect on the magnetic flux in the receiver coil (near-field). For higher field strengths however, time lags must be considered [67]. Consult for example [66] for a correct treatment beyond the near field or Appendix E in [163], where a formula for the induced voltage is presented.

[4]Here, too, the limited validity of Eq. 1.13 becomes apparent. The derivation of Eq. 1.13 models the receiver coil as a simple wire loop and not as a resonant structure, as it should correctly be done [163]. It is assumed that the coil's DC sensitivity equals its RF sensitivity. Interactions with the measured object are ignored. In practice the RF sensitivity depends on the electromagnetic properties of the object and the frequency (also cf. [201]), and therefore the RF sensitivity is typically determined for each scan separately (also cf. chapter 2.1.2b, page 48).

but might be justified because, according Eqs. 1.7, 1.16, m is actually proportional to the spin density. However, small deviations occur when the transmit field is not homogeneous because, in this case, the flip angle is not constant over the entire excitation volume (cf. Eq. 1.11). Though not exact as well, it is also common to denote $m(\cdot)$ as *magnetization*. In this thesis both terms, *spin density* and *magnetization*, are used to describe $m(\cdot)$. In the following, the dependency of m on the amplification β_A will be suppressed by assuming w. l. o. g. $\beta_A := 1$.

The signal presented in Eq. 1.15 is the measured signal of the NMR experiment. This signal is constant because relaxation effects have been ignored in these calculations. In reality the presence of transverse relaxation causes the signals to decay. This decaying signal is called the *free induction decay*, or in short, the *FID*.

c) Signal-to-Noise Ratio

Physical measurements are always of a statistical nature. The main sources of noise for MRI are thermal motions of charged particles. It is obvious that the electrons in the receiver electronics add to the resulting noise. However, in NMR, it is the charged ions of the objects under examination, which typically form the dominant part of the resulting noise. Whereas elaborate designs of the receiver electronics can lead to a significantly reduced noise contribution, thermal motion of the ions of the measured object cannot be influenced by the experimenter. Noise in the electronic devices might pose a problem with micro-architectures [55]. However, in this work, micro-coils were not used and therefore the discussion of noise is uniquely restricted to thermal noise originating from the object under examination.

How does it happen that the sample contributes noise to the measured signal? The principle can be understood in a fairly simple way: The human body mainly consists of water, in which different ions like for example Na^+, K^+ or Ca^{2+} are dissolved. These ions are thermally agitated and move. This motion is responsible for a fluctuating current density which is accompanied by an electromagnetic field. The resulting electric field generates a fluctuating voltage across the terminals of the receiver electronics, and is considered as noise.

This noise, in a basic situation, has been described quantitatively by Johnson in 1928 already [77]. Basic theoretical work considering AC-currents has elucidated the basic principle in the same year by Nyquist in [116]. More suitable for NMR reception is, for example, the theoretical description as presented in the section *A conducting sample* in Appendix A in a publication by Hoult [67]. The derivation is based on the Langevin equation and the law of equipartition of energy from statistical mechanics leading to the following result for the noise squared $< \eta^2 >$:

$$< \eta^2 >= 4k_B T B_W R, \tag{1.17}$$

where T is the temperature of the measured object, B_W the bandwidth of the receiver, and R is the resistance of the measured object seen from the terminals of the receiver electronics. This resistance expresses a principle of reciprocity: The effect of moving ions in the sample onto the noise in the received signal is analyzed by considering the resistance of the sample to a current flowing in the circuit of the receiver!

The macroscopic resistance of the measured object can be calculated with the help of Ohm's law: Because of Ohm's law, the resistance R is equivalent to the power P deposited in the body per unit current in the receiver coil ($U = RI \Rightarrow R = P/I^2$). The dissipated power can be calculated also on a local scale, where Ohm's law states that the current density $\vec{j}$ generated by an electric field $\vec{E}$ depends on the electric conductivity σ: $\vec{j} = \sigma \vec{E}$. The electric field caused by the current in the receiver has two effects: On the one hand, it is responsible for local currents flowing with the velocity $\vec{v} = \vec{j}/\rho = \sigma \vec{E}/\rho$, where ρ is the electric charge density. On the other hand, the field exerts a Lorentz force $\vec{f} = \rho \vec{E}$ onto the moving particles. This force acts on the local currents and performs the work $a = \vec{f} \cdot \vec{v} = \rho \vec{E} \cdot \vec{E} \sigma/\rho = \sigma \vec{E}^2$. By considering that this work is dissipated the resistance can be calculated by integrating over the volume V of the measured object:

$$\begin{aligned} R = \frac{P}{I^2} &= \int_V \sigma(\vec{x})|\vec{E}(\vec{x})|^2 \, \mathrm{d}\vec{x} \Big/ I^2 = \int_V \sigma(\vec{x})|E(\vec{x})/I|^2 \, \mathrm{d}\vec{x} \\ &= \int_V \sigma(\vec{x})|\vec{\mathcal{E}}(\vec{x})|^2 \, \mathrm{d}\vec{x}, \end{aligned} \tag{1.18}$$

where $\vec{\mathcal{E}}$ is the electric field $\vec{E}$ per unit current, denoted as *electric sensitivity* of the receiver coil in this thesis. Note that in the derivation of the latter equation, it has been disregarded that, in MRI, the electromagnetic quantities are high-frequency RF signals. Nevertheless, the latter equation is still valid (see e.g. Eq. 3 in [200]) with the electric sensitivity $\vec{\mathcal{E}}$ being a complex-valued quantity (just as the magnetic sensitivity $\vec{\mathcal{B}}$).

The signal-to-noise ratio of the acquired signal can then, within the limits of the used model, be expressed with the electromagnetic properties of the receiver coil and the measured object by combining Eqs. 1.7, 1.15, 1.16, 1.17, 1.18:

$$SNR = \frac{|s|}{\sqrt{(<\eta^2>)}} = C \cdot \frac{|\int_V n(\vec{x})(\mathcal{B}_x^{re}(\vec{x}) - i\mathcal{B}_y^{re}(\vec{x}))\,d\vec{x}|}{\sqrt{\int_V \sigma(\vec{x})|\vec{\mathcal{E}}(\vec{x})|^2\,d\vec{x}}},$$

$$\text{with} \quad C = \frac{1}{8}\frac{\hbar^2\gamma^3|\sin(\alpha)|}{(k_B T)^{3/2}}\frac{B_0^2}{B_W^{1/2}}. \tag{1.19}$$

1.2 Magnetic Resonance Imaging

With the main magnet and the RF-transmit/receive system, a signal is obtained which has information about the whole object. However, according to Eq. 1.15, all locations are encoded nearly equivalently. Therefore signal localization is not achieved with these hardware components; it cannot be differentiated whether the signal originates from one location or another. In MR imaging, the bulk part of spatial encoding is obtained by an additional hardware component: the gradients.

1.2.1 The Gradients

The purpose of the three gradients is to encode information about the locations of the individual signal sources. This task is traditionally solved by generating three spatial magnetic encoding fields (SEMs), whose B_z-components vary linearly along the three different axes of the magnet. An important result of this section is that it is possible to apply these linear SEMs such that the signal data and the spatial distribution of the excited magnetization form a simple Fourier pair. Such a strategy is often used by imaging sequences like the gradient echo or the spin echo, which differ from each other in the way how signal relaxation is exploited to produce a different image contrast (also cf. section 1.2.4, page 33f).

The involved electronics is schematically depicted in Fig. 1.5. The wire windings of gradient coils are typically supported by a cylindrical structure. This geometry is advantageous for hardware integration and especially useful in handling patient scans. The basic gradient coil design, along with one more realistic fingerprint design of an x-gradient coil, is depicted in Fig. 1.6. For practical designs, the wire windings are optimized to compromise between gradient linearity, efficiency, minimal B_x and B_y field strength (=concomitant fields), inductivity, power dissipation and other important coil characteristics.

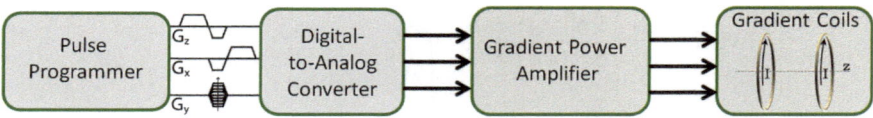

Figure 1.5: Typical gradient driving electronics. The sequence programmer defines the trapezoidal pulse shapes for each gradient channel. The digital instructions are converted to an analog voltage level using a digital-to-analog converter. This voltage is amplified with gradient power amplifiers and finally sent to the gradient coils. The coils generate the linear encoding fields with magnetic field time-courses according to the programmed pulse shapes.

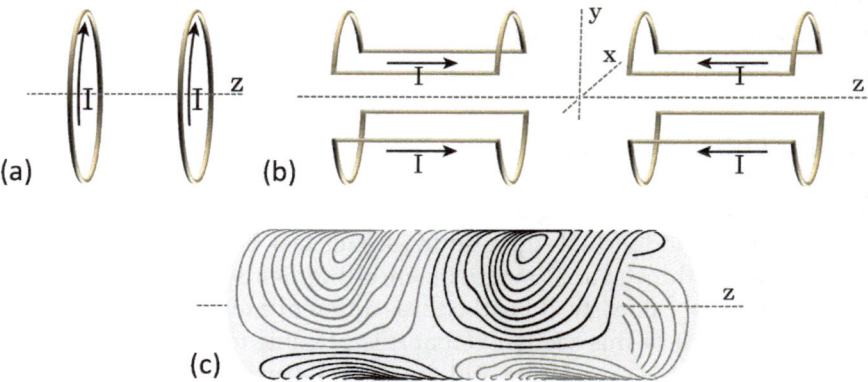

Figure 1.6: Simple and more practical gradient coil wire designs. (a) The basic z-gradient is a Maxwell pair. (b) The basic x- and y-gradients are double-saddle coils (= Golay coils). (c) Fingerprint design of a linear x-gradient coil. The pattern has been optimized using a stream function method with high order smoothness (see chapter 4 in [76]). The image shown is courtesy of Dr. Feng Jia and corresponds to Fig. 4.15a in [76].

1.2.2 Gradient Encoding: Signal Equation for a Single Receiver Coil

The physical principle, which eventually makes localization possible, is simple: The additional linear gradient field changes the precession frequency of the spins along the direction of the field gradient. The received signal therefore has a broadened frequency distribution with a one-to-one correspondence between frequency and location along the direction of the field gradient. With three orthogonal gradients, it is therefore possible to extract the spin density at each location in a unique way. The physical relation between gradient encoding and localization is sketched in Fig. 1.7.

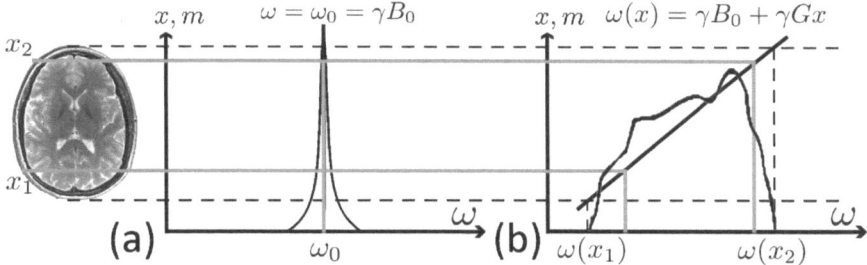

Figure 1.7: The principle of gradient encoding. (a) Without a gradient the magnetic field is constant over the entire object. Therefore the magnetization precesses at the same frequency in the whole object and the frequency content of the signal is represented by a very narrow peak. There is a finite line width in reality because of chemical shift, susceptibility effects and T_2^*-relaxation, among others (the line width shown is vastly exaggerated for reasons of illustration). (b) With a linear gradient field applied along one axis, magnetization vectors perpendicular to that axis still precess with the same frequency. However, along the gradient axis the Larmor frequency is different for each location. This results in a broadened frequency distribution with a one-to-one-correspondence to the spatial coordinate of the signal source.

A rigorous derivation of this result may begin with the dynamics of the magnetization in the fixed frame system, mathematically described by Eq. 1.5. The effective encoding field $\vec{B}_{enc}$, resulting from the superposition of the applied gradient fields, disturbs the main magnetic field. The fields vary slowly in comparison to the precessional motion. The gradient field dynamics can therefore be treated as being static in the equation of motion, given by Eq. 1.5. The resulting motion is a precessional motion with a

frequency corresponding to the magnitude of the overall external magnetic
field:

$$\omega = -\gamma \left| B_0 \vec{e}z + \vec{B}_{enc} \right| = \omega_L + (-\gamma B_{enc}^z) + (-\gamma B_\perp)\mathcal{O}\left(\frac{B_\perp}{B_0}\right) \quad (1.20)$$

$$\approx \omega_L + (-\gamma B_{enc}^z).$$

For a scanner with a B_0 on the order of $1 - 3\,\mathrm{T}$, the gradient field B_{enc}^z
is typically below $10\,\mathrm{mT}$. The magnitude of the concomitant fields $B_\perp =$
$[(B_{enc}^x)^2 + (B_{enc}^y)^2]^{1/2}$ is of the same order as B_{enc}^z; in the region of interest
(ROI), it is most often even below B_{enc}^z. As a consequence of the large difference between gradient field strengths and main magnetic field strength, the
approximation of Eq. 1.20 is very good. Therefore, only the z-components
of the gradient fields have a significant impact on the precession frequency
of the magnetization vector and the direction of the precessional motion is
almost not affected by the gradient fields.

With gradient encoding, the precession frequency of the magnetization (cf.
Eq. 1.12) gets a spatial dependency that deviates from the Larmor frequency
ω_L in most parts of the object. After the quadrature receiver the complex
signal is then modulated with a time and space dependent phase factor
$\phi(\vec{x}, t)$:

$$s(t) = \int_V m(\vec{x})c(\vec{x})e^{-i\phi(\vec{x},t)}\,\mathrm{d}\vec{x}. \quad (1.21)$$

This phase factor can be manipulated by the gradient fields in two different
ways: application of a gradient field *during* signal readout or *before*. Reconsider Fig. 1.7b. There, it is shown that the application of a SEM *during* signal
readout alters the frequency content of the signal. Therefore, this strategy is
denoted as *frequency encoding*. The frequency content is different only for
spins experiencing a different field strength - therefore localization with
pure frequency encoding is only feasible along one spatial direction. Several
signal readouts, each encoded with a different gradient direction, could be
used to complete signal localization. However, it is also possible to combine
frequency encoding with a strategy, where SEMs are applied *before* signal
readout. These SEMs do not affect the frequency content of the received
signals directly, but spins at different locations acquire a different phase
during the application of the SEMs and this phase information modulates
the signal when being read out. In this thesis, the term *phase encoding* is
used to describe such an encoding strategy.[5]

---

[5]Note that this definition is broader than often encountered in the MR literature.

Based on Eq. 1.13, it can be shown that, when both strategies are combined, the phase factor in Eq. 1.21 consists of an initial phase from phase encoding and a time-dependent part resulting from frequency encoding:

$$\phi(\vec{x}, t; r) = \phi(\vec{x}, 0; r) + \gamma \int_{\tilde{t}=0}^{t} B_{enc}^{z}(\vec{x}, \tilde{t}; r) \, d\tilde{t}. \tag{1.22}$$

The index r has been added because typically (apart from single-shot imaging) a number of signal readouts ($r = 1, \dots, N_{pe}$) are acquired. The magnetic gradient encoding field $B_{enc}^{z}(\vec{x})$ is a superposition of the three linear gradient fields $B_{j}^{z}(\vec{x})$:

$$B_{enc}^{z}(\vec{x}, \tilde{t}; r) = \sum_{j=1}^{3} B_{j}^{z}(\vec{x}, \tilde{t}; r) = \sum_{j=1}^{3} G_{j}(\tilde{t}; r) x_{j} = \vec{G}(\tilde{t}; r) \vec{x}. \tag{1.23}$$

The introduced parameters $G_{j}, j = 1, 2, 3$, are the *gradient strengths* of the corresponding gradient field.

The latter equation shows that the effective encoding field decomposes into a spatial and a temporal component. The spatial component is predefined by the geometries of the gradient fields.[6] However, the temporal component can be influenced freely by defining the time-courses of the gradient pulse shapes. These temporal degrees of freedom are captured by the introduction of k-space. With the k-space notation the phase distribution of Eq. 1.22 reads:

$$\phi(\vec{x}, t; r) = \left(\vec{k}_r + \vec{k}(t; r) \right) \vec{x}, \tag{1.24}$$

where the initial k-space position $\vec{k}_r$ and the k-space traversal during readout $\vec{k}(t; r)$ are defined as:[7]

$$\vec{k}_r := \gamma \int_{\tilde{t}=0}^{\tau} \vec{G}(\tilde{t}; r) \, d\tilde{t} \quad \text{and} \quad \vec{k}(t; r) := \gamma \int_{\tilde{t}=0}^{t} \vec{G}(\tilde{t}; r) \, d\tilde{t}. \tag{1.25}$$

---

[6]This is where PatLoc imaging becomes interesting: The generalization to arbitrary field geometries introduces new spatial degrees of freedom for MRI signal encoding (cf. chapter 4, page 135ff).

[7]In the literature, it is also not uncommon to define k-space slightly differently with γ replaced by $(\gamma/2\pi)$, see for example [7, 12, 125]. Depending on which definition is used, the factor 2π may, or may not, occur in other equations related to k-space.

In this definition, it was assumed w. l. o. g. that the duration of phase encoding τ is the same for each readout r. Introducing the k-space notation (Eqs. 1.24, 1.25) into the signal equation (Eq. 1.21) leads to:

$$s(t; r) = \int_V m(\vec{x}) c(\vec{x}) e^{-i(\vec{k}_r + \vec{k}(t;r))\vec{x}} \, d\vec{x}. \tag{1.26}$$

In the general case, the temporal dimension of the sampling trajectory is important. For example, image contrast, caused by relaxation, is determined by the timing of data sampling. However, in the latter equation explicit time-dependent effects like relaxation have been ignored to focus on spatial encoding rather than temporal effects. Under these assumptions, the signal does not change if the k-space trajectory is traversed differently as long as the set $\mathcal{K} = \{\vec{k}_r + \vec{k}(t;r); t \in [0;T], r = 1, \ldots, N_{pe}\}$ of acquired k-space locations remains the same. Thus, it is possible to eliminate the temporal dependency from the signal equation and Eq. 1.26 adopts a simpler form by only considering the signal values at the sampled k-space location $\vec{k} \in \mathcal{K}$:

$$s(\vec{k}) = \int_V m(\vec{x}) c(\vec{x}) e^{-i\vec{k}\vec{x}} \, d\vec{x}. \tag{1.27}$$

This equation is one of the most important equations in the field of MRI. It shows that signal and spin density, modulated by the RF-coil sensitivity have a Fourier relation. There is only one caveat: The set of sampled k-space locations $\mathcal{K}$ is only a one-dimensional trajectory of finite length within the d-dimensional full k-space $K = \mathbb{R}^d$ required for a true Fourier relation. In chapter 2.2.1c it is shown on page 61 that the finite length of the trajectory is closely linked to image resolution. More subtle is the problem that a true d-dimensional ($d = 2, 3$) image is to be reconstructed from a *one*-dimensional trajectory. It turns out that for sufficiently dense sampling, it is possible to treat the one-dimensional trajectory $\mathcal{K}$ as a d-dimensional subset K of $\mathbb{R}^d$. The reason for this surprising result is described in the paragraph "Completeness of k-Space Encoding" on page 64 in the following chapter. In this thesis, the extended subset $K \supset \mathcal{K}$, $K \subset \mathbb{R}^d$ is called *effective k-space coverage*, or simply *effective k-space*, whereas $\mathcal{K}$ is called *sampled k-space (coverage)*. The concepts of k-space trajectory, sampled k-space coverage and effective k-space coverage are illustrated in Fig. 1.8.

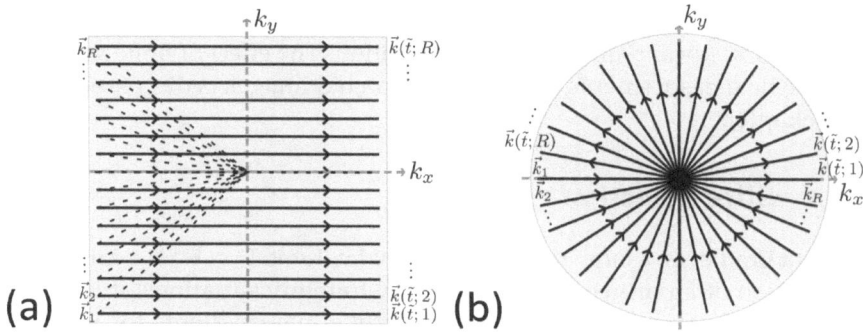

(a) **(b)**

Figure 1.8: k-space trajectory and k-space coverage. (a) Cartesian trajectory. Shown are 16 phase-encodes. The effect of phase encoding, according to how this term is defined in this thesis, is to define the initial k-space position before readout. With the x-gradient, the initial k-space location is shifted along the k_x-axis (often denoted as a *prewinder*) and with the y-gradient along the k_y-axis (phase encoding in the narrow sense). During acquisition, the x-gradient is switched, and k-space is traversed along the corresponding direction. The direction of k-space traversal is indicated by the arrows accompanying the trajectory. When time-dependent effects like signal relaxation are ignored, the direction of k-space traversal can be ignored. The *sampled k-space* is given by the black lines. However, the *effective k-space* extends around the black lines and is indicated by the gray area. In chapter 2.2.1c it is shown under which conditions this extension occurs. (b) Radial trajectory. By combining x-and y-gradients, the initial k-space positions define locations on a circle in k-space. During readout, the same combination of the gradients, with opposite flow of the coil currents, is used. The trajectory leads to a higher sampling density at the center. A sufficient number of readouts ensures a gap-free effective circular k-space coverage.

For simplicity, consider here complete k-space coverage $K = \mathbb{R}^d$, and a homogeneous RF-coil profile $c(\vec{x}) = 1$ for all $\vec{x} \in V$. Under these special conditions, signal $s(\vec{k})$ and spin density $m(\vec{x})$ form a Fourier transform pair:

$$s(\vec{k}) = \int_V m(\vec{x}) e^{-\mathrm{i}\vec{k}\vec{x}} \, \mathrm{d}\vec{x} = \mathcal{FT}\{m\}(\vec{k}),$$

$$m(\vec{x}) = \int_K s(\vec{k}) e^{\mathrm{i}\vec{k}\vec{x}} \, \mathrm{d}\vec{k} = \mathcal{FT}^{-1}\{s\}(\vec{x}). \tag{1.28}$$

The latter equation mathematically expresses the effect of gradient encoding as the capability to uniquely localize an MRI signal: Under the assumption of infinitely long sampling, the spin density of the measured object can be retrieved exactly and uniquely at each location. The effect of finite sampling in realistic measurements on the reconstructed images is discussed in the next chapter.

1.2.3 Slice Selection

Without gradients, a large three-dimensional volume $V \subset \mathbb{R}^3$ is excited after application of an on-resonance RF pulse. In many situations, it is useful to excite only thin slices and use two orthogonal gradients for in-plane encoding. This process is called *slice selection* and is achieved by applying a gradient field during transmission of the RF pulse.

Consider a gradient field $B_{enc}^z(\vec{x}) = G_z z$ along the z-axis (= z'-axis) switched during an RF pulse $\vec{B}_1(t) = B_1(t)\vec{e}_x'$. According to Eq. 1.10, the motion of the magnetization in the rotating reference frame is given by:

$$\partial_t^{rot} \vec{M} = \vec{M} \times \gamma(B_1(t)\vec{e}_x' + G_z z \vec{e}_z'). \tag{1.29}$$

In general, a closed-form solution to this equation does not exist and must be found numerically [26, 129]. Under the *small-tip-angle assumption*[8] $M_z(t) = M_z(0) = const$ a closed-form solution exists, revealing insight into the relationship between excited magnetization and pulse shape. With the initial condition $\vec{M}(0) = M_z^0 \vec{e}_z'$, in Eq. 1.29 only the transverse components of the magnetization need to be considered further. For symmetric pulse envelopes $B_1(t)$ of duration τ_p, the complex-valued solution $M_\perp = M_x + iM_y$ to Eq. 1.29 right after the pulse is found to be:

$$M_\perp(\tau_p, \vec{x}) = i\gamma M_z^0(\vec{x}) e^{-i\gamma G_z z \tau_p/2} \mathcal{FT}^{-1}\{B_1\}(\gamma G_z z). \tag{1.30}$$

The main result from this equation is that slice profile and pulse envelope form a Fourier transform pair - under the small-tip-angle assumption. In theory, this assumption seems to be good only for flip angles below $20°$; notwithstanding, the above Fourier relation is in practice often acceptable for flip angles up to $90°$ [96]. An approximately rectangular-shaped slice of thickness Δz is therefore excited with an apodized pulse envelope mimicking a sinc-function of frequency $f = \gamma/2 G_z \Delta z$. This result is depicted in Fig.

---

[8]described for example in chapter 5.1.3.2 of [96].

1.9. When slice selection is performed, it is useful to reduce the signal equation (Eq. 1.28) to a two-dimensional (2D) problem with $\vec{x} \in V \subset \mathbb{R}^2, \vec{k} \in \mathbb{R}^2$ and $\bar{m}(x, y) = \int_z m(x, y, z)\mathrm{d}z$. When the bar over $\bar{m}$ is ignored 2D and 3D imaging problems can be handled with the same notation.

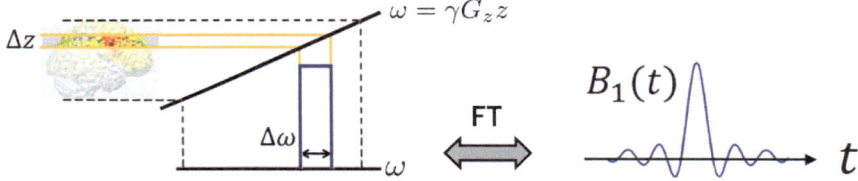

Figure 1.9: Relationship of slice profile and pulse shape. Under the small-tip-angle assumption and linear gradient fields employed, slice profile and pulse envelope form a Fourier transform pair. Note that the Fourier relation is not valid for high flip angles. In this case, no analytic solution to the Bloch equations exists and therefore numerical methods must be used to establish the exact relationship between pulse shape and slice profile.

1.2.4 Basic Imaging Sequences

An important part of MRI research is devoted to the development of various imaging sequences; i.e., the definition of RF and gradient pulse shapes and the timing of signal reception. In the context of this thesis, only two of the most basic imaging sequences are considered: the *gradient echo* [53] and the *spin echo* [56, 59]. Extensive information regarding sequence design is found in the textbook of Bernstein et al. [10].

a)   Gradient Echo

The (two-dimensional) gradient echo is a very simple imaging sequence. With Cartesian sampling, k-space is traversed as depicted in Fig. 1.8a. The corresponding pulse sequence is presented in Fig. 1.10a: After slice selection, a phase encoding step brings the k-space vector to the desired position. From this position a line in k-space is read out with a gradient of a fixed amplitude. In contrast to single-shot imaging, an RF-transmit pulse is played out for each acquired k-space line with the repetition time T_R. This ensures reduced signal dephasing, which is due to magnetic field inhomogeneities, mainly caused by susceptibility differences, which have been ignored in the signal equation (cf. Eq. 1.27). For long echo times T_E (i.e., the time between RF pulse and center of signal readout) and long T_R, the resulting contrast is often referred to as the T_2^*-*contrast*.

b)   Spin Echo

An important advantage of a spin echo is that the effect of static magnetic field inhomogeneities is eliminated. Whenever magnetic field inhomogeneities would deteriorate the image quality, a spin echo will produce superior image quality. The imaging sequence is depicted in Fig. 1.10b. In contrast to a gradient echo, two RF pulses are played out prior to data acquisition. The effect of the second pulse is to reverse the signal dephasing taken place since the application of the first pulse. Repetition time T_R and echo time T_E (i.e., the time between the first RF pulse and the center of signal readout) are chosen according to the desired imaging contrast. For long T_E and long T_R the contrast is often referred to as the T_2-*contrast*.

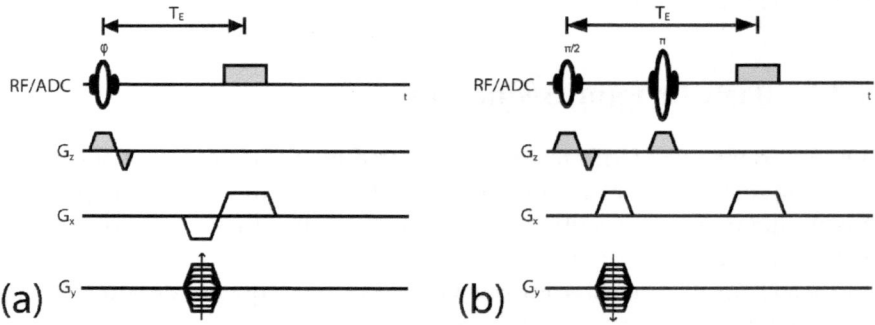

Figure 1.10: Two basic imaging sequences. (a) Gradient echo. (b) Spin echo.

1.3 Parallel Imaging[9]

In the early years, only a single RF coil was used for MRI measurements. From about 1990 on, initial experiments were performed with multi-coil receiver arrays. Initially, such arrays were used to improve SNR [145]. The potential of multi-coil arrays to accelerate MR image sequences [173, 135] was recognized only in the late 1990s and since then research in the field of parallel imaging has exploded. In this section, imaging with an RF array is introduced, some of the most important implications of parallel imaging to MRI are briefly discussed and the signal equation for multi-coil acquisitions is presented.

1.3.1 RF-Receiver Array

Before the advent of multi-coil RF arrays, MRI scanners were typically equipped with one large RF-volume coil. Such a volume coil is typically designed to have a homogeneous sensitivity. This is beneficial because then the coil is equally sensitive to all parts of a measured object. In contrast to such homogeneous large volume coils, small RF coils, placed near the surface of the object under examination, are not sensitive to the whole object. Nevertheless, Roemer et al. realized in 1990 that such surface coils can be useful in MRI when several of those surface coils are combined to an array of coils surrounding the measured object (cf. Fig. 1.11a). Even though the individual elements are only sensitive to a limited region of the imaging volume (cf. Fig. 1.11b), the combination of all coils is sensitive to the whole volume with a tendency of a higher sensitivity near the surface of the object, and for field strengths above about 1 T for human systems a high sensitivity can also be observed at the center; this phenomenon is sometimes termed *dielectric resonance* (see for example the root-sum-of-squares[10] sensitivity image in Fig. 1.11c). Fortunately, the sensitivity variations have proven to be rather unproblematic in practice.

---

[9]In this thesis, the term *parallel imaging (PI)* is used in a broad sense. Sometimes, PI is used in a narrower sense comparable to the term *partially parallel imaging (PPI)*, typically used to denote accelerated imaging with the help of an RF array. Here, however, PI refers to all imaging experiments where data are acquired with several RF coils. PI is therefore defined here as *multi-coil imaging* opposed to *single-coil imaging*.

[10]The root-sum-of-squares involves: (a) multiplication of each voxel value with its complex-conjugate and (b) formation of a single image from the several coil images by summing up the (squared) voxel values and (c) taking the square root of the formed single image.

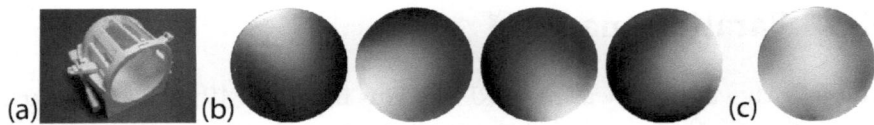

Figure 1.11: RF-receiver coil array with sensitivity maps. (a) Twelve-channel head receiver coil array for a MAGNETOM Trio, A Tim System 3T, Siemens Healthcare, Erlangen, Germany. (b) Four RF-coil sensitivity maps at $3\,\text{T}$ of the coil shown in (a), where each map has been combined from three others. The maps were determined by dividing images of each receiver channel, acquired with a homogeneous phantom, by the corresponding RF-transmit field maps, which were measured similar to the method described in [34]. (c) Root-sum-of-squares image of the RF-sensitivity profiles.

It is an important feature of a receiver array that it consists of several coils, each of which generating a separate signal - in parallel. Each signal channel should provide as much independent information as possible. Thus, it is important that the individual coils are not strongly coupled to each other. RF-coil decoupling strategies (see e.g. chapter 3.4.2 in [90]) are therefore of great interest to the RF engineer with important consequences for the optimal coil geometries. At the same time, the coils should be placed as near as possible to the measured object in order to enhance the SNR. These and other concerns explain why modern whole-body MR scanners are often equipped with a multitude of different RF-receiver arrays, where each array is optimized for a different medical application. For example, there are cardiac, spine or knee arrays. Another example is Fig. 1.11a, where a head coil array is shown.

1.3.2   Implications of Parallel Imaging

Signal reception with several coils has the advantage over single-coil measurements that each RF coil is sensitive in different object regions; thus, an RF-receiver array provides spatial information in addition to gradient encoding. And this additional information is not generated sequentially as done with gradients, but in parallel; i.e., at the same time. Therefore, the information gained with an array almost comes "for free". The additional information can be used in various ways. Some of the most important implications to MRI are presented here.

a) Increased SNR

In 1990, Roemer et. al presented in their seminal publication [145] that parallel acquisition can significantly enhance the SNR of the reconstructed images. The basic idea relies on an optimal combination of the different coil images. An adequate optimization can be formulated as a reconstruction problem and is therefore discussed in more detail in the next chapter, see in particular the *Remark* on page 78.

b) Acceleration of MR Measurements

Even more important is that PI can be used to significantly accelerate MRI scans. The duration of patient examination is not only a question of sufficient resources or patient comfort. Among others, shorter measurements significantly reduce motion artifacts. For single-shot techniques, such as EPI [109] (also cf. chapter 3.4.2 in [212]), it is advantageous to shorten measurements in order to reduce susceptibility artifacts. Also functional MRI [113] profits from a higher temporal resolution such that even 3D single-shot acquisitions become feasible.[11] The usage of PI in this context has already been suggested in the late 1980s and early 1990s [18, 70, 82, 88, 139]. Further technological and theoretical developments in the late 1990s [173, 135] leveraged the original ideas to the wide-spread acceptance of PI in research and clinical environments. The role of PI for the acceleration of MR measurements is best understood in the context of image reconstruction and is therefore discussed in chapter 2.3, page 72ff.

c) Further Applications

Further applications of PI are reviewed in [90] including artifact removal caused by coherent k-space inconsistencies and the reduction of motion artifacts. Another interesting application of PI is the fast determination of B_0-inhomogeneities [175, 174]. In the context of parallel imaging, the presented PatLoc imaging concept can also be regarded as a further interesting application of PI.

---

[11] A modern example of an ultra-fast 3D trajectory is found in [211].

1.3.3   Signal Equation for Several Receiver Coils

When several receiver coils are considered in an RF array, cross-talk between
the coils can occur. With modern decoupling techniques, this cross-talk is
often reduced to a negligible level in high-quality receiver arrays and the
received signals behave nearly independently from each other. Therefore,
the signal equation derived for the single-channel case in Eq. 1.27 is valid
also in multi-coil arrangements. An array with N_c signal channels then
generates separate signals $s_\alpha(\vec{k})$:

$$s_\alpha(\vec{k}_\kappa) = \int_V m(\vec{x})c_\alpha(\vec{x})e^{-i\vec{k}_\kappa\vec{x}}\,\mathrm{d}\vec{x} \quad \text{for all} \quad \alpha = 1,\ldots,N_c. \tag{1.31}$$

The index κ has been introduced to indicate that only a finite number of
data points at $\vec{k} = \vec{k}_\kappa$ are stored for post-processing. The difference between
the individual signals results from the different spatial distributions $c_\alpha(\vec{x})$
of the RF-coil sensitivities. Note that, even when the individual channels
cannot be regarded as being completely decoupled, the above equation is
still valid. If needed, the RF-coil sensitivities are measured in a separate
scan using the same hardware configuration. Therefore the cross-talk is
implicitly accounted for when the sensitivities are extracted from the data.
A detailed analysis of the effects that coupled RF coils have on MRI signals
and reconstructed images is found in [118], chapter 3, page 73ff.

Chapter 2

Image Reconstruction in MRI

WHEREAS the first chapter has described the basics of MRI signal formation, the present chapter deals with the reverse process: the problem of recovering the object information from the acquired signals. This is a difficult task because MRI measurements only indirectly represent the object, and there is only a finite amount of measurement data available for the vast amount of object information.

This inherently inverse problem has been solved for standard multi-coil acquisitions with a rigorous mathematical framework for linear image reconstruction [135]. In the preface, it has already been mentioned that conventional multi-coil imaging has more stringent imaging requirements than PatLoc because, conventionally, field linearity is required for gradient encoding; notwithstanding, the rigorous mathematical framework can easily be extended to be applicable also to PatLoc imaging (see chapter 4.2, page 140ff). Therefore this linear reconstruction framework is important for this thesis and it is reviewed at the beginning of the present chapter. The most important image reconstruction methods for single-coil imaging as well as multi-coil imaging are derived in this chapter using the same abstract framework.

Though this approach is more technical than standard descriptions of the different algorithms, it has the advantage of a unified portrayal of some of the most important reconstruction methods currently used in MRI. As a consequence, relations between individual methods can be elaborated (such as between SENSE and GRAPPA or between gridding reconstruction and the general matrix inversion approaches). The presentation tries to use a mathematical language which is as precise as possible. One consequence is for example the description of the SENSE reconstruction matrix with the help of the Kronecker product. New is also the explanation of the superresolution effect for certain PI reconstructions.

This chapter focuses on the essentials of MR image reconstruction. Not covered are dynamic imaging modalities like for example cardiac imaging, where several frames are recorded within the cardiac cycle (see e.g. [176]). A good description of spatio-temporal reconstruction methods is found in [5]. Also not covered are nonlinear reconstruction methods. Such methods have proven advantageous in special situations like for example reconstruction from sparse data [28, 106] or reconstruction from subsampled radial imaging data [13, 83]. A problem with such nonlinear algorithms is that image properties are not easy to predict. This is different for linear reconstruction methods, where concrete results can be derived. Image properties like image resolution, aliasing and SNR can be calculated explicitly, and this is done in the present chapter for the general case and some of the discussed image reconstruction methods.

2.1 Basics of Linear Image Reconstruction

Linear image reconstruction is particularly beneficial because reconstruction can be described as a simple matrix-vector operation. Image reconstruction involves the inversion of the *encoding matrix*, which comprises the relevant information of the imaging process. With known gradient encoding scheme and RF-coil sensitivity data, the encoding matrix can easily be calculated. After presentation of the image reconstruction framework, a short section is devoted to the problem of obtaining reliable data from gradient and RF sensitivity encoding. After that, it is shown how basic image properties like image resolution, aliasing artifact and SNR can be calculated if reconstructed with the presented matrix approach.

2.1.1 Fundamental Reconstruction Algorithms

The basic principles of linear reconstruction theory for standard PI [135] are reviewed below before special imaging situations are discussed in later sections. The reconstruction theory is based on the signal equation presented in Eq. 1.31, which describes the general imaging process of PI. It is repeated here:

$$s_\alpha(\vec{k}_\kappa) = \int_V m(\vec{x}) c_\alpha(\vec{x}) e^{-i\vec{k}_\kappa \vec{x}} \, d\vec{x} \quad \text{for all} \quad \alpha = 1, \ldots, N_c. \quad (2.1)$$

The encoding basis for parallel imaging at measured k-space positions $\vec{k}_\kappa$ ($\kappa = 1, \ldots, N_\kappa$) is defined as:

$$\text{enc}_{\alpha,\kappa}(\vec{x}) = c_\alpha(\vec{x})e^{-i\vec{k}_\kappa\vec{x}}. \tag{2.2}$$

With this definition signal formation can be interpreted as the projection of the magnetization onto the encoding functions:

$$s_{\alpha,\kappa} := s_\alpha(\vec{k}_\kappa) = \int_V m(\vec{x})\text{enc}_{\alpha,\kappa}(\vec{x})\,\mathrm{d}\vec{x}. \tag{2.3}$$

The linear relationship between signal and magnetization favors linear reconstruction methods, where the magnetization, collected in a vector **m** of length N_ρ,[1] is reconstructed by adequately weighting the signal measurements $s_{\alpha,\kappa}$. The reconstruction is therefore described by a matrix **F**, often termed *reconstruction matrix*:

$$\mathbf{m} = \mathbf{F}\mathbf{s}. \tag{2.4}$$

The reconstruction problem can then be formulated as finding a reconstruction **F**, which produces a magnetization vector **m** with elements m_ρ that approximate the magnetization at the corresponding position as closely as possible:

$$m_\rho = \sum_{\alpha,\kappa} F_{\rho,(\alpha,\kappa)} s_{\alpha,\kappa} \approx \int_V m(\vec{x})i_\rho(\vec{x})\,\mathrm{d}\vec{x}. \tag{2.5}$$

The reconstructed values m_ρ might represent the total magnetization within the voxel of interest or the average density of the magnetization within the voxel. In the following, it is assumed that the goal of the reconstruction is the latter. The right hand side of Eq. 2.5 is the desired value for m_ρ. It depends on the chosen ideal voxel shape i_ρ. Often Dirac delta functions are chosen as ideal voxel shapes. This choice simplifies the involved calculations. Even though box functions are a better representation of image voxels it is usually acceptable to use delta functions because, typically, reconstruction grids are

---

[1]The one-to-one procedure of mapping a matrix to a vector is often denoted as *vectorization*. The inverse mapping from the vector back to the matrix is termed in this thesis *de-vectorization*.

chosen not coarser than the encoded image resolution. Inserting Eq. 2.3 into the latter equation yields:

$$m_\rho = \int_V m(\vec{x}) f_\rho(\vec{x}) \, d\vec{x}. \tag{2.6}$$

where the voxel function f_ρ is given by:

$$f_\rho(\vec{x}) = \sum_{\alpha,\kappa} F_{\rho,(\alpha,\kappa)} \mathrm{enc}_{\alpha,\kappa}(\vec{x}). \tag{2.7}$$

The voxel function f_ρ can also be interpreted as the *spatial response function*. The spatial response function and its relationship to the point spread function is explained in section 2.1.3, page 50ff. The reconstruction problem is thus reduced to finding good approximations of the voxel functions to the ideal voxel shapes:

$$f_\rho(\vec{x}) \approx i_\rho(\vec{x}).$$

Two different approaches are considered here. These approaches have been termed *weak* and *strong* reconstructions in [135].

a)   Weak Matrix Approach

The weak approach only requires that ideal voxel shapes and voxel functions satisfy the orthogonality relation:[2]

$$\int_V i_\rho^*(\vec{x}) f_{\rho'}(\vec{x}) \, d\vec{x} = (\Delta V)^{-1} \delta_{\rho,\rho'}. \tag{2.8}$$

In chapter 4.2.2b, page 148ff, it is shown that the quantity ΔV represents the nominal voxel volume.[3] For 2D imaging, it is given by $(\Delta x)^2$, where

---

[2]If the goal of the reconstruction is to find the total magnetization within the reconstructed voxels, $(\Delta V)^{-1}$ must be replaced by its inverse ΔV.

[3]This dependency on the voxel volume has not been observed in [135]. For standard rectilinear reconstruction grids, this dependency on the voxel volume can usually be ignored because the diagnostic value of MR images lies in *relative* intensity differences. Note however, that, without the introduction of the voxel volume in the latter equation, the physical units of that equation are no longer consistent. Under certain circumstances, the dependency on the voxel volume becomes important in PatLoc imaging, for example in chapter 5.1, page 155ff.

Δx is the discretization distance of the reconstruction grid.[4] The entries of the encoding matrix are defined as:

$$E_{(\alpha,\kappa),\rho} := \int_V i_\rho^*(\vec{x}) \mathrm{enc}_{\alpha,\kappa}(\vec{x}) \, d\vec{x} = \mathrm{enc}_{\alpha,\kappa}(\vec{x}_\rho) = c_\alpha(\vec{x}_\rho) e^{-i\vec{k}_\kappa \vec{x}_\rho}. \qquad (2.9)$$

In the latter equation the ideal voxel shapes were assumed to be delta functions $(i_\rho^*(\vec{x}) := \delta(\vec{x} - \vec{x}_\rho))$. With the definitions of voxel functions and encoding matrix the orthogonality relation of Eq. 2.8 reduces to a matrix equation:

$$\mathbf{F}\mathbf{E} = (\Delta V)^{-1} \mathbb{1}. \qquad (2.10)$$

Solving this matrix equation for the reconstruction matrix $\mathbf{F}$ solves the reconstruction problem. Typically, the Moore-Penrose pseudo-inverse (MPPI) is taken as the solution:

$$\mathbf{F} = (\Delta V)^{-1} \mathbf{E}^+. \qquad (2.11)$$

Note that the MPPI has different interpretations under different circumstances. Three different situations may occur:

1. Equation 2.10 has infinitely many solutions. This is generally the case when $N_c N_\kappa \geq N_\rho$, i.e., when a reconstruction grid is chosen which is not much finer than the corresponding grid of acquired data points.[5] The MPPI then takes the solution with the smallest Euclidian norm. Problems like for example an underestimation of the spin density may therefore occur when the reconstruction grid is chosen too coarsely. The explicit solution then reads:

$$\mathbf{F} = (\Delta V)^{-1} (\mathbf{E}^H \mathbf{E})^{-1} \mathbf{E}^H. \qquad (2.12)$$

---

[4]For 2D imaging it would be more precise to talk about *pixels* rather than *voxels*. In this thesis this imprecise terminology is accepted in favor of a unified presentation suited for 2D as well as 3D imaging. Also consider that, in reality, a 2D slice has a finite thickness. The discrepancy of calling quantities like $(\Delta x)^2$ "volumes" is therefore also resolved by simply multiplying such areas with the slice thickness.

[5]For $N_c N_\kappa \geq N_\rho$, the condition $\mathbf{F}\mathbf{E} = (\Delta V)^{-1}\mathbb{1}$ represents an *underdetermined* system of equations. Notwithstanding, this situation is usually considered as an *overdetermined* acquisition in the MRI literature because the amount of signal data exceeds the number of image voxels to be solved for. This terminology is also justified because the corresponding discretized signal equation $\mathbf{s} = \mathbf{E}\mathbf{m}$ represents an *overdetermined* system of equations, used for example for iterative CG reconstructions, cf. section 2.3.1f, page 89ff. In order to avoid confusion in this regard, only rare use of the terms *overdetermined/underdetermined* is made in this thesis.

2. No solution exists. This is the case when a very fine reconstruction grid is chosen. The MPPI is then the minimizer of a least-squares problem $\|[\Delta V \cdot \mathbf{FE} - \mathbb{1}]\mathbf{W}\|_F^2$, where the diagonal matrix $\mathbf{W}$ is a weighting function and the subscript F denotes the Frobenius matrix norm. Equal weighting for all image voxels is ensured if $\mathbf{W}$ is chosen to be the unity matrix. Then the explicit solution is given by:

$$\mathbf{F} = (\Delta V)^{-1}\mathbf{E}^H(\mathbf{EE}^H)^{-1}.$$

3. There is exactly one solution. This is a very special case. In this case, the two explicit solutions stated above are equivalent: $\mathbf{F} = (\Delta V)^{-1}(\mathbf{E}^H\mathbf{E})^{-1}\mathbf{E}^H = (\Delta V)^{-1}\mathbf{E}^H(\mathbf{EE}^H)^{-1}$.

The solutions to the three cases rely on the property that either the matrix $\mathbf{E}^H\mathbf{E}$ or $\mathbf{EE}^H$ is invertible. Invertibility is ensured only if $\mathbf{E}$ has full rank. This can, however, not always be guaranteed. One example would be an image acquisition, where some k-space locations are sampled several times and subsequent reconstruction is performed onto a dense grid. It is therefore necessary to use a reconstruction, which can cope with this potential problem. And the MPPI can! To show this, consider the singular value decomposition (SVD) of a matrix $\mathbf{A}$: $\mathbf{A} = \mathbf{P}\boldsymbol{\Sigma}\mathbf{Q}^H$, where $\mathbf{P}$ and $\mathbf{Q}$ are unitary and $\boldsymbol{\Sigma}$ is a potentially non-square matrix with entries only along the main diagonal. These entries form the singular values of $\mathbf{A}$. Then, the MPPI of $\mathbf{A}$ is given by: $\mathbf{A}^+ = \mathbf{Q}\boldsymbol{\Sigma}^+\mathbf{P}^H$. The MPPI solution $\boldsymbol{\Sigma}^+$ is simply defined as the transpose of $\boldsymbol{\Sigma}$ with inverted singular values. In [170] it is recalled that the MPPI of a matrix $\mathbf{A}$ has two different kinds of expansions, which are mathematically equivalent to the MPPI[6]:

$$\mathbf{A}^+ = (\mathbf{A}^H\mathbf{A})^+\mathbf{A}^H = \mathbf{A}^H(\mathbf{AA}^H)^+.$$

The first expansion reduces to the first case above if $\mathbf{E}^H\mathbf{E}$ is invertible and the second expansion reduces to the second case above if $\mathbf{EE}^H$ is invertible. These equivalences show that all discussed cases are covered by the MPPI.

Remark: In the MRI literature, one often encounters reconstructions based on the discretization of the forward model using a Riemann sum approximation. The resulting equation $\mathbf{s} = \mathbf{Em}$ is then solved using the MPPI with solution $\mathbf{m} = \mathbf{E}^+\mathbf{s}$. Such a "forward" approach is problematic because

---

[6]That result can be proved easily with the help of the SVD of $\mathbf{A}$.

reconstruction solves an inverse problem; however, the discussion above shows that the forward discretization is justified because the more sophisticated inverse approach has the same solution under the conditions of (a) weak reconstruction (b) delta functions as ideal voxel shapes (c) Cartesian reconstruction grids.[7]

b)   Strong Matrix Approach

In the strong reconstruction approach voxel shapes are chosen to represent the least-squares approximation to the ideal voxel shapes. In Appendix B in [135] it is shown that this approach results, with $\Delta V := 1$, in the solution:

$$\mathbf{F} = \mathbf{E}^{H}\mathbf{B}^{+}, \tag{2.13}$$

where $\mathbf{B}$ is the correlation matrix of the encoding functions:

$$B_{(\alpha,\kappa),(\alpha',\kappa')} = \int_{V} \mathrm{enc}_{\alpha,\kappa}(\vec{x})\mathrm{enc}^{*}_{\alpha',\kappa'}(\vec{x})\,\mathrm{d}\vec{x}. \tag{2.14}$$

and V is the volume over which the least-squares approximation of the voxel function to the ideal voxel shape is calculated. For comparison, the concepts of weak and strong reconstruction are illustrated in Fig. 2.1.

Remark: If additional factors are added to the encoding functions, defined in Eq. 2.2, this formalism can incorporate effects such as relaxation, field inhomogeneities due to non-uniform B_0-field, susceptibility differences, or, in a slightly modified form, chemical shift imaging. Interesting in the context of this thesis is also that RF pulses can be designed to influence the phase of the magnetization. This effect can also be considered with an additional factor in the encoding functions. In chapter 4 it is shown that this formalism can also be used in PatLoc imaging with a modified encoding matrix.

c)   Relationship Between Weak and Strong Reconstruction

Both reconstruction methods have in common that the solution is determined from a comparison with an ideal reconstruction. The strong reconstruction aims at approximating the ideal voxel shapes in a least-squares

---

[7]This approach of discretizing the forward model prior to inversion is also justified for non-Cartesian reconstruction grids. The discretization (see Eq. 4.25) results in Eq. 4.20.

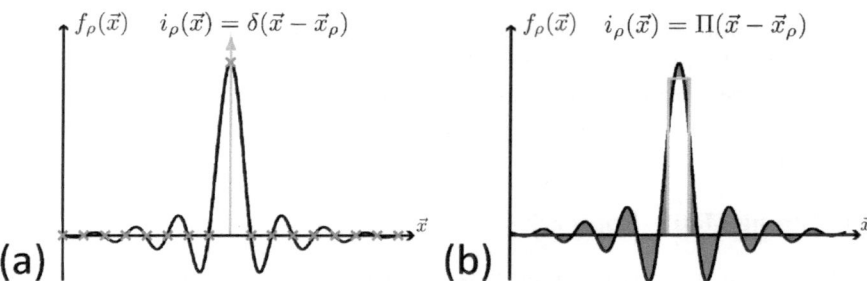

Figure 2.1: The concepts of weak and strong reconstruction. Illustrated are voxel functions (black) and ideal voxel shapes (gray); in the shown example, a delta function ($\delta(\cdot)$) has been chosen as ideal voxel shape for the weak approach, and, a box function ($\Pi(\cdot)$) for the strong approach. With both approaches a voxel function is sought that resembles the ideal voxel shape as closely as possible. (a) The weak reconstruction requires that, for a delta function as ideal voxel shape, the voxel function is unity at the voxel center and zero at the centers of the neighboring voxels. No conditions are imposed on the behavior in-between. (b) The strong reconstruction aims at minimizing the least-squares deviation from the ideal voxel shape; thus, a reconstruction is chosen which minimizes the (square of the) gray-shaped area. Close inspection shows that, in the depicted example, both approaches lead to voxel functions which differ only very slightly from one another.

sense, whereas the weak reconstruction only requires that the voxel function is defined at a finite number of grid points.[8] For the weak reconstruction, no condition is stated for what happens in between the grid points. The strong approach is therefore more convincing and should in general provide higher reliability than the weak approach.

But also the weak approach normally leads to reliable reconstructions: The reconstruction grid is typically chosen dense enough to avoid loss of acquired image information. Correspondingly, the encoding functions vary smoothly on a voxel scale and high amplitude variations of the voxel function are unlikely between the undefined grid points. This is particularly true when $\mathbf{FE} = \mathbb{1}$ can be fulfilled. If not (i.e., for dense reconstruction grids) the minimum-norm solution serves a similar purpose.

Both approaches are in fact closely related to each other. In the limit of infinitely dense reconstruction grids both methods are equivalent because in this case $\mathbf{B} = \mathbf{EE}^H$ and therefore the strong approach has the recon-

---

[8]At least when delta functions are chosen as ideal voxel shapes.

struction $\mathbf{F} = \mathbf{E}^H (\mathbf{E}\mathbf{E}^H)^+$, which corresponds to the MPPI solution of the weak reconstruction. This perfect congruence of the weak and the strong approach is technically broken, once realistic reconstruction grids of finite density are considered. However, note that in most cases the correlation matrix $\mathbf{B}$ cannot be calculated analytically, but has to be determined by means of numerical integration. If a Riemann-sum is chosen with a step-size corresponding to the voxel size of the (sufficiently dense) reconstruction grid, the correlation matrix is again given by $\mathbf{B} = \mathbf{E}\mathbf{E}^H$, and both, weak and strong reconstruction, yield exactly the same results once again. Closely related to this discussion is the minimum-norm reconstruction presented in [170].

d) Conclusion

With sufficiently dense reconstruction grids, it is appropriate to consider only delta functions as ideal voxel shapes in favor of minimizing reconstruction time. Owing to the fact that in this case, weak and strong approach have similar solutions, the following presentation is oriented toward the solution of the weak approach, unless stated otherwise:

$$\mathbf{F} = \mathbf{E}^+, \quad \text{with} \quad E_{(\alpha,\kappa),\rho} = \mathrm{enc}_{\alpha,\kappa}(\vec{x}_\rho) = c_\alpha(\vec{x}_\rho)e^{-i\vec{k}_\kappa \vec{x}_\rho}, \qquad (2.15)$$

where the $\mathbf{E}$ must be replaced by $\Delta V \cdot \mathbf{E}$ if the volume information is of interest. This reconstruction is denoted in this thesis as the *MPPI reconstruction* or *MPPI solution*.

In theory, the MPPI approach is straightforward. Once the encoding matrix is determined, images can be reconstructed by simply inverting this matrix. In practice, however, two issues must be addressed: The first has already been mentioned above and concerns the problem that the large dimensions of the encoding matrix complicate direct inversion. One focus of this chapter is to tackle this inversion problem for different situations. Depending on the structure of the encoding matrix, direct inversion can be an option. If not, iterative methods often lead to acceptable results. The second issue relates to the fact that image reconstruction is based on accurate knowledge of the encoding matrix. This issue is the topic of the following section.

2.1.2 Determination of the Encoding Matrix

The correct determination of the encoding matrix is crucial for image reconstruction. According to Eq. 2.15, this matrix consists of two factors: the gradient encoding factor $e^{-i\vec{k}_\kappa \vec{x}_\rho}$ and the RF-sensitivity encoding factor $c_\alpha(\vec{x}_\rho)$. The determination of these two factors is treated separately here.

a) Gradient Encoding

The gradient encoding part $e^{-i\vec{k}_\kappa \vec{x}_\rho}$ of the encoding matrix is based on two assumptions: First, it is assumed that the trajectory $\vec{k}_\kappa$ matches the true trajectory. Second, it is assumed that the gradients generate exactly linear encoding fields (cf. Eq. 1.23).

The hardware of state-of-the-art MRI systems is particularly well optimized for accurate control of the k-space trajectories. For many standard imaging sequences and applications it can therefore be assumed that the desired k-space trajectory is accurate. If a certain application requires a higher accuracy, established calibration methods (see e.g. chapter 2.2.4 of [211]) or promising new methods like for example magnetic field monitoring [4] could be considered to improve the reliability of gradient encoding.

Typically less demanding are the requirements on gradient linearity. Linearity is very accurate only at the isocenter of the MRI bore. Outside of the center, non-linearities occur. The non-linearities are often accepted in order to permit improvements in other performance measures such as power consumption or especially switching speed of the gradients. Typical artifacts resulting from gradient non-linearities are image distortions. The distortions can be corrected if the spatial distributions of the magnetic gradient fields are known. The spatial distributions can be measured indirectly with the help of calibration phantoms [149] or directly by acquiring field maps of the gradient fields (cf. chapter 5.1.2c, page 178ff, and 6.2.1b, page 220f; further references may be found in [29]). These methods are particularly important in the context of PatLoc imaging, where strong deviations from gradient linearity are generated intentionally.

b) Sensitivity Encoding

Reconstruction also requires the determination of the complex-valued (cf. Eq. 1.16) spatial distributions $\mathbf{c}(\cdot) := (c_1(\cdot), \ldots, c_{N_c}(\cdot))^T$ of the RF-coil sensitivities. These can be estimated by acquiring a gradient echo image. Typically, a 64×64-acquisition is sufficient to capture the spatial variations of the sensitivities. If the RF-coil sensitivities are estimated directly from the gradient echo images, they will be corrupted by the magnetization $m = |m|e^{i\Phi}$ of the object: $\mathbf{c}^{(est)} = m\mathbf{c}$. One therefore has to adopt a method to suppress the influence of the object in the estimated sensitivity maps.

One possibility is to acquire an additional image with a homogeneous volume coil and divide the individual components by this image [135]. This, however, requires one additional scan. Another disadvantage is the noise amplification of the resulting estimate. A different method is to calculate the sum-of-squares of the acquired images $(\mathbf{c}^{(est)})^H \mathbf{c}^{(est)} = c^2 m^2$ and divide the individual coil images by the square-root of those. The resulting sensitivity estimate is then: $\mathbf{c}^{(est)} = f \cdot \mathbf{c}$, where $f = e^{i\Phi}/c$. The coil estimates are weighted with the root-sum-of-squares of all coil sensitivities and a phase factor. All coil sensitivities are affected by the same variation f. The only consequence of using these coil estimates instead of the unknown true coil sensitivities is that the reconstructed image will be weighted by $1/f$. For typical industrial coil geometries, the root-sum-of-squares of the coil sensitivities is fairly homogeneous (cf. e.g. Fig. 1.11c). Therefore, these coil estimates are generally good enough for adequate image reconstruction.

The coil estimates can be improved by averaging over neighboring voxels, which is often possible because the coil sensitivities contain only low spatial frequencies. A similar result with improved SNR is achieved with a method based on the stochastic matched filter presented in [188]. This method has been used to generate the RF-coil sensitivity maps in this thesis. With the technological progress in the computer industry more computation-intensive methods become feasible such as the nonlinear iterative reconstruction method proposed in [184].

Note that there is a fundamental difference to the gradient fields: For higher field strengths (> 1.5 T for human systems), wave effects cannot be neglected any more and the RF-coil sensitivities depend on the object under investigation - in contrast to the gradient fields. Therefore, it is not sufficient to measure the profiles only once, but the sensitivity maps should be reacquired for separate examinations.

2.1.3   Image Resolution and Aliasing Artifacts

Image resolution and aliasing artifacts can be analyzed with the spatial response function (SRF). The SRF has already been introduced above in a different context, where it was interpreted as a voxel function (cf. section 2.1.1, page 40ff); the SRF is calculated from Eq. 2.7, which is repeated here:

$$f_\rho(\vec{x}) = \sum_{\alpha,\kappa} F_{\rho,(\alpha,\kappa)} \mathrm{enc}_{\alpha,\kappa}(\vec{x}). \tag{2.16}$$

Following Eq. 2.6, the SRF describes the (continuous) spatial distribution of the magnetization that contributes signal to the voxel of interest. As a consequence, image resolution and aliasing artifacts are fully described with the SRF. Apart from very fundamental situations such as standard Fourier imaging, the SRF varies from voxel to voxel. Therefore, the SRF should be calculated for several voxels whenever possible. This is not always an easy task and it is often more convenient to analyze image resolution and aliasing alternatively with the point spread function (PSF), which can be determined straightforwardly by data simulation.

The PSF is in some respect the opposite of the SRF: The PSF $p_{\vec{x}_0}(\rho)$ describes the effect of a single source point $\delta(\vec{x} - \vec{x}_0)$ at a certain location $\vec{x}_0$ onto the intensities of each voxel in the reconstructed image. However, it is closely related to the SRF:

$$p_{\vec{x}_0}(\rho) \stackrel{(2.6)}{=} \int_V \delta(\vec{x} - \vec{x}_0) f_\rho(\vec{x})\, \mathrm{d}\vec{x} = f_\rho(\vec{x}_0) = [\mathbf{F}\mathbf{s}(\delta(\vec{x} - \vec{x}_0))]_\rho. \tag{2.17}$$

The vector $\mathbf{s}(\delta(\vec{x} - \vec{x}_0))$ is the signal generated by a point source located at $\vec{x}_0$. The concepts of SRF and PSF may be explained with the help of Fig. 2.2.

The PSF approach can be useful for sufficiently high-resolved image reconstructions.[9] An interesting relationship between SRF and PSF is established with the following lemma: *Consider evaluation of the SRF only on the reconstruction grid $\mathcal{G}$ and evaluation of the PSF only for source locations on $\mathcal{G}$. Then, the SRF is given by the rows of the matrix product $\mathbf{FE}$, whereas the PSF is described by the columns of that product.* This lemma follows directly from the above definitions of SRF and PSF. Crucial is the observation that $\mathbf{FE}$ is Hermitian

---

[9]The condition of sufficient resolution should generally be fulfilled when $\mathbf{FE} = \mathbb{1}$ cannot be satisfied exactly.

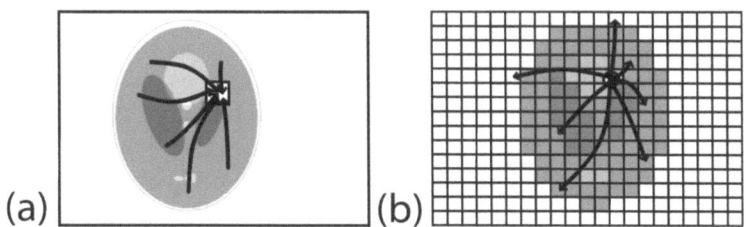

Figure 2.2: Concepts of SRF and PSF. (a) The SRF describes the signal contributions of the object to a certain reconstructed image voxel. (b) The PSF describes the contribution of a single source point to the different reconstructed image voxels. SRF and PSF therefore describe - in some way - opposite processes. In practice, however, they are often very similar.

for both the weak and the strong reconstruction approach.[10] The SRF of a voxel ρ evaluated at the grid points is therefore equivalent to the Hermitian of the PSF evaluated for a source located at $\vec{x}_\rho$ and it is sufficient to analyze either of them.

Most measures of image resolution focus on the width of the main peak of the absolute value of the SRF or, alternatively, of the PSF [53]. The width of the main peak may be estimated in various ways. In this thesis, the width is defined as the full width at half maximum (FWHM) of the SRF. If numerical simulations are performed the FWHM of the PSF is determined instead. This definition is useful whenever image resolution is not the focus of an analysis because it allows an estimation of image resolution with only one single number. The effect of a finite width of the main peak is image blurring.

A secondary criterion for image resolution is signal contamination from neighboring voxels. Neighboring voxels contribute when the main peak of the SRF is broader than one voxel. Also, the sidelobe behavior of the SRF leads to signal contamination. The sidelobe contribution is normally classified as an artifact (truncation artifact, Gibbs ringing artifact) rather than a feature of image resolution. Note, however, that it is possible to

---

[10]Such a Hermitian relation between PSF and SRF has been observed in [170] for a similar reconstruction method. A corresponding relation also exists for the weak and the strong reconstruction: For the weak reconstruction, this statement follows from the fact that $\mathbf{FE} = \mathbf{E}^+\mathbf{E}$, which is Hermitian. For the strong reconstruction, $\mathbf{FE} = \mathbf{E}^H\mathbf{B}^+\mathbf{E}$, which is also Hermitian.

reduce the height of sidelobes at the expense of the width of the main lobe by filtering the data. On the other hand, it is also possible to reduce the width of the main lobe at the expense of the sidelobes. To some degree, it is even possible to design reconstructions with heavily asymmetric SRFs. The sidelobe behavior and width of the main peak can therefore be traded against each other, giving flexibility in designing adequate reconstructions depending on the application. In order to inspect image resolution in detail, it is therefore necessary to explore not only the width of the main peak, but the complete shape of the SRF (or alternatively of the PSF), for example by analyzing function plots of the SRF of several voxels.

Especially when undersampling is driven to its limit, the well defined main peaks are deteriorated with high sidelobes in the SRF, which might even evolve into secondary aliasing peaks. The effect is often denoted as the *aliasing artifact*. Depending on the trajectory, the aliasing artifact can be very prominent with a perfectly coherent structure (for example for Cartesian trajectories), with a less pronounced coherency (for example for radial trajectories), or even rather noise-like with an incoherent structure (for example for random undersampling).

An academic example of an SRF and the corresponding reconstructed image is shown in Fig. 2.3. In this figure, also the relation of characteristic features of the SRF like width of main peak, sidelobe behavior and secondary aliasing peaks with artifacts consisting of blurring, Gibbs ringing and aliasing are depicted. In particular, it is shown that Gibbs ringing and aliasing artifacts are not always clearly differentiable by analyzing a single SRF of one image location.

2.1.4   Signal-to-Noise Ratio

Image reconstruction may enhance noise in the reconstructed image voxels. Two important methods for the analysis of noise propagation are discussed here.

Condition Number   The condition number describes the worst case effect of a small change in the signal to the image after reconstruction. More specifically, the relative condition number κ_{rel} of a general reconstruction algorithm $\mathbf{f}(\cdot)$ for a measured signal $\mathbf{s}$ is the maximum ratio of the frac-

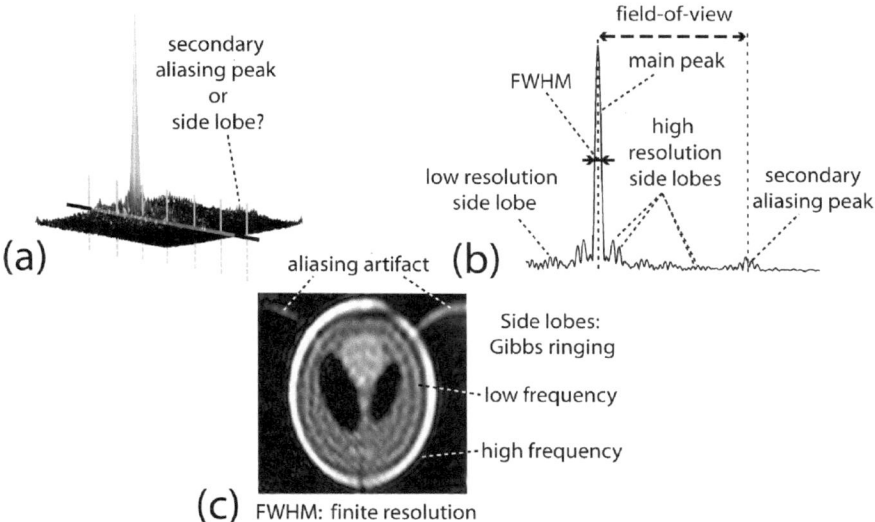

Figure 2.3: Analysis of image artifacts with the help of the SRF. (a) 2D plot of the SRF for a certain image location. (b) A 1D cross section through the main peak as indicated by the grid in subplot (a). (c) Image reconstruction of an example numerical phantom. The finite width of the main peak leads to a finite image resolution. The example shown represents an unusual reconstruction: Two types of sidelobes with different frequencies occur. The resulting Gibbs ringing also exhibits two different frequencies. In the SRF, a very small aliasing peak is visible. In conformity to this fact, the reconstructed image shows no visible aliasing in most parts of the image. However, at the top part of the image, substantial aliasing results. In the 2D function plot of the SRF several small peaks occur, which cannot be classified exactly as pronounced Gibbs ringing sidelobes or secondary aliasing peaks.

tional change in the image $\mathbf{f}(\mathbf{s})$ to any fractional change in the signal s (cf. definition 2.4.6 on page 131 in [27]):

$$
\begin{aligned}
\kappa_{rel}(\mathbf{s}) &= \lim_{\epsilon \to 0^+} \sup_{\|\delta\mathbf{s}\| < \epsilon} \left[\frac{\|\mathbf{f}(\mathbf{s}+\delta\mathbf{s}) - \mathbf{f}(\mathbf{s})\|}{\|\mathbf{f}(\mathbf{s})\|} \Big/ \frac{\|\delta\mathbf{s}\|}{\|\mathbf{s}\|} \right] \\
&= \frac{\|\partial\mathbf{f}/\partial\mathbf{s}\|\|\mathbf{s}\|}{\|\mathbf{f}(\mathbf{s})\|} \overset{\mathbf{f}(\mathbf{s})=\mathbf{Fs}}{=} \frac{\|\mathbf{F}\|\|\mathbf{s}\|}{\|\mathbf{Fs}\|} = \frac{\sigma_{max}(\mathbf{F})}{\|\mathbf{Fs}\|/\|\mathbf{s}\|}.
\end{aligned}
$$

The result on the right hand side has been derived based on the assumption that the reconstruction is linear; i.e., $\mathbf{f}(\mathbf{s}) = \mathbf{Fs}$. The value $\sigma_{max}(\mathbf{F})$ is the maximum singular value of the reconstruction matrix $\mathbf{F}$. Depending on the signal, the condition number of the reconstruction is therefore limited by:

$$1 \leq \kappa_{rel}(\mathbf{s}) \leq \frac{\sigma_{max}(\mathbf{F})}{\sigma_{min}(\mathbf{F})}. \tag{2.18}$$

The worst case signal with a condition number equaling the eigenvalue spread of the reconstruction is often simply denoted as the condition number $\kappa(\mathbf{F})$ of the reconstruction matrix $\mathbf{F}$.

(Co-)Variance Analysis   Often, it is useful to have information about the noise propagation on a voxel-by-voxel basis. As MRI measurements are statistical processes, the resulting image voxel values can be regarded as random variables, whose variances and correlations with respect to other image voxels are in general adequately described with a covariance matrix, occasionally denoted as the *image noise matrix* $\mathbf{X}$ [135]. Assuming zero-mean noise in the individual receiver channels (which is generally the case) and a linear reconstruction $\mathbf{F}$ it is straightforward to show that

$$\mathbf{X} = \mathbf{F}\tilde{\boldsymbol{\Psi}}\mathbf{F}^{H}, \quad \text{with} \quad \tilde{\boldsymbol{\Psi}} = \overline{\boldsymbol{\eta}\boldsymbol{\eta}^{H}}. \tag{2.19}$$

The vector $\boldsymbol{\eta}$ represents the noise contribution of the acquired signal data. The *sample noise matrix* $\tilde{\boldsymbol{\Psi}}$ has a very sparse structure: Note that the temporal correlations of the signal data have the time scale of collisions between the charged particles in the object, thus they are very short, such that there are no correlations between different signal acquisitions κ. Moreover, each signal acquisition of the same receiver coil has the same statistical properties. Therefore, the signal noise matrix can be decomposed into the product $\tilde{\boldsymbol{\Psi}} = \mathbb{1}_{N_\kappa} \otimes \boldsymbol{\Psi}$. The matrix $\boldsymbol{\Psi} = \overline{\boldsymbol{\eta}_r\boldsymbol{\eta}_r^{H}}$ is of size $N_c \times N_c$ only. It is often referred to as the *receiver noise matrix*. The subscript r indicates that in contrast to the much larger matrix $\tilde{\boldsymbol{\Psi}}$, there is only one entry in the noise vector $\boldsymbol{\eta}_r$ for each receiver channel. The receiver noise matrix $\boldsymbol{\Psi}$ is determined by simply acquiring noise on each coil channel and then averaging over the outer product. This might be done, for example, by playing out a gradient echo sequence without exciting the sample.

The matrix $\tilde{\boldsymbol{\Psi}}$ describes the noise covariances of the individual signal channels $\mathbf{s}_\alpha$. But what is the theoretical relation of the noise to the physical properties of the sample and the receiver coil? In chapter 1.1.4c, page 23ff, such a relation (Eq. 1.18) is established for a single channel based on the principle of reciprocity. The principle also holds for several receiver channels and Roemer presents in [145] how the noise is related to sample and coil properties. This relation can be explained with a concept similar to the elegant "net" coil combination presented by Wiesinger et al. [200]. Consider a linear signal combination $s = \sum_\alpha w_\alpha s_\alpha = \mathbf{w}^T \mathbf{s}$. As discussed in the previous paragraph, the variance of the combined signal is $\overline{s^2} = \mathbf{w}\Psi\mathbf{w}^H$. Consider now a single virtual coil, which would generate exactly the same signal. Because of the linearity of the Maxwell equations the electric sensitivity $\vec{\mathcal{E}}$ would simply be $\vec{\mathcal{E}}(\vec{x}) = \sum_\alpha w_\alpha \vec{\mathcal{E}}_\alpha(\vec{x})$. According to Eq. 1.18, the resistance R of the sample seen by this virtual coil would then equal to:

$$R = \int_V \sigma(\vec{x})|\vec{\mathcal{E}}(\vec{x})|^2 \,\mathrm{d}\vec{x} = \int_V \sigma(\vec{x})|\sum_\alpha w_\alpha \vec{\mathcal{E}}_\alpha(\vec{x})|^2 \,\mathrm{d}\vec{x} = \mathbf{w}\mathbf{R}\mathbf{w}^H,$$

$$\mathbf{R}_{jk} = \int_V \sigma(\vec{x})\vec{\mathcal{E}}_j(\vec{x})\vec{\mathcal{E}}_k^*(\vec{x}) \,\mathrm{d}\vec{x}. \tag{2.20}$$

Combining this result with Eq. 1.17, it can be concluded directly that the noise covariance matrix is related to the physical properties of sample and receiver in the following way:

$$\Psi = 4k_B T B_W \mathbf{R}. \tag{2.21}$$

Signal-to-Noise Ratio   The signal-to-noise (SNR) ratio measures how strongly the reconstructed magnetization is affected by noise. It is calculated by dividing the absolute value of the signal m_ρ in a voxel ρ by the standard deviation $\sqrt{X_{\rho,\rho}}$ of the noise in that voxel. Recall that the reconstructed signal m_ρ represents the "average" magnetization m_ρ^{avg} in the corresponding voxel (where "average" is defined by Eq. 2.6). It can therefore often be considered as being independent of the reconstruction. The SNR is then given by:

$$SNR = \frac{|m_\rho|}{\sqrt{X_{\rho,\rho}}} \overset{(2.19)}{=} \frac{|m_\rho^{avg}|}{\sqrt{(\mathbf{F}\tilde{\Psi}\mathbf{F}^H)_{\rho,\rho}}} \overset{(2.6,2.21)}{=} \frac{|\int_V m(\vec{x})f_\rho(\vec{x})\,\mathrm{d}\vec{x}|}{\sqrt{4k_B T B_W (\mathbf{F}(\mathbb{1}\otimes\mathbf{R})\mathbf{F}^H)_{\rho,\rho}}}. \tag{2.22}$$

2.1.5   SNR-Optimized Reconstructions

The MPPI reconstruction $\mathbf{F} = \mathbf{E}^+$, presented in Eq. 2.15, is only one out of several possibilities to solve the weak reconstruction condition $\mathbf{FE} = \mathbb{1}$ if the number of reconstruction points is less than the number of signal data, which is often the case when several receiver coils provide separate data. This ambiguity leaves room to improve the SNR in the reconstructed image while still fulfilling the condition of weak reconstruction. Keep in mind that the reconstructed image values should represent the magnetization density of the object independent of the type of reconstruction. Therefore, instead of maximizing SNR, it is also possible to simply minimize the noise propagated to the reconstructed image voxels. The reconstruction weights $F_{\rho,(\alpha,\kappa)}$ are determined independently for each voxel and therefore the optimization can be performed for all voxels at the same time by minimizing the trace of the image noise matrix:

$$\min_{\mathbf{F}} \mathrm{Tr}\{\mathbf{F}\tilde{\mathbf{\Psi}}\mathbf{F}^H\} \quad \text{subject to} \quad \mathbf{FE} = \mathbb{1}.$$

The optimization problem represents a complex-valued quadratic program with very good properties: There are no inequality constraints and the image noise matrix $\mathbf{X} = \mathbf{F}\tilde{\mathbf{\Psi}}\mathbf{F}^H$ is a positive-definite, Hermitian matrix (cf. Eqs. 2.20, 2.21), for which an inverse always exists. The above problem can be solved with the help of the corresponding Lagrange function. This function is formed by multiplying the left hand side of the constraint $\mathbf{FE} - \mathbb{1} = \mathbb{0}$ with Lagrange multipliers $\mathbf{\Lambda}$ and adding this term to the cost function. Then, the derivative of the Lagrange function is set to zero. Together with the constraint $\mathbf{FE} = \mathbb{1}$, a set of two equations have to be fulfilled at the same time:

$$2\mathbf{F}\tilde{\mathbf{\Psi}} + \mathbf{\Lambda}\mathbf{E}^H = \mathbb{0} \quad \text{and} \quad \mathbf{FE} = \mathbb{1}.$$

Solving the first equation for $\mathbf{F}$, inserting the result in the second equation, the Lagrange multipliers can be determined and inserted back in the first equation resulting in the solution:[11]

$$\mathbf{F} = (\mathbf{E}^H \tilde{\mathbf{\Psi}}^{-1} \mathbf{E})^{-1} \mathbf{E}^H \tilde{\mathbf{\Psi}}^{-1}. \tag{2.23}$$

---

[11]For the real-valued problem of this kind, compare chapter 10.4.2 in [15]. A different, but elegant proof that makes use of the Cholesky factorization of the image noise matrix is found in Appendix A of [200].

The inverse of $\mathbf{E}^H\tilde{\boldsymbol{\Psi}}^{-1}\mathbf{E}$ should usually exist whenever the amount of signal data exceeds the number of image voxels. In [134] Prüssmann et al. point out that the reconstruction formally reduces again to the simpler standard form as presented in Eq. 2.15 by virtue of the Cholesky factorization $\tilde{\boldsymbol{\Psi}} = \mathbf{LL}^H$ and by redefinition of the encoding matrix and the signal data: $\mathbf{E} \rightarrow \mathbf{L}^{-1}\mathbf{E}$ and $s \rightarrow \mathbf{L}^{-1}s$. The advantage of this redefinition is that uncorrelated signals result. This process is therefore sometimes denoted as *decorrelation* [134]. This discussion also shows that SNR optimization is only useful when significant signal correlations between different channels exist. Many state-of-the-art RF coils show only minor correlations and therefore SNR optimization does often not improve image quality significantly and can often be neglected.

2.2 Image Reconstruction from a Single Receiver Coil

The development of image reconstruction methods for PatLoc imaging benefits a lot from an understanding of the basic methods that are used to reconstruct imaging data acquired with a single RF-receiver coil. When spatial encoding is done exclusively with linear gradient fields, the term *Fourier imaging* is often used.[12] Some of the most commonly used reconstruction methods are presented and analyzed for Cartesian imaging, radial imaging and arbitrary sampling trajectories. The presentation follows an unconventional approach. The properties of Cartesian image reconstruction are typically described by analyzing the properties of the discrete Fourier transform (DFT) [53, 96]. Despite the undisputed effectiveness of such an approach, the context of this thesis requires taking on a more abstract point of view. Therefore the most important image properties from Cartesian sampling are derived directly from the general matrix approaches presented in the previous section. Then, it is demonstrated for radial trajectories that direct matrix inversion results in feasible reconstructions also for other sorts of trajectories as well. However, for non-Cartesian trajectories such an approach is not efficient, and the section concludes with the presentation

---

[12]In this thesis, the term *Fourier imaging* is used in a broad sense. The term shall not only encompass Cartesian trajectories, but any trajectory like for example a radial acquisition scheme.

of two useful algorithms that are often encountered in practice: filtered back-projection and gridding reconstruction.

2.2.1   Standard Cartesian Method

a)   Image Reconstruction

The most basic and also most wide-spread imaging modality is Fourier imaging with Cartesian k-space traversal (see Fig. 1.8a). Assume an acquisition with N phase-encoding lines and constant k-space increment $2\pi\Delta k$ from one phase-encode to the next. For quadratic images the same parameters, N samples at distance $2\pi\Delta k$, are typically chosen along the frequency encoding direction.[13] Image reconstruction in Cartesian Fourier imaging is straightforward: The desired images are found by simply applying an inverse 2D discrete Fourier transform (DFT) to the signal data, implemented as a fast Fourier transform (FFT). In order to conform to later notation, the reconstruction is written as a matrix equation. To this end, the 2D signal data as well as the reconstructed images are represented as vectors $\mathbf{s} \in \mathbb{R}^{N^2}$ and $\mathbf{m} \in \mathbb{R}^{N^2}$ respectively, and the inverse 2D-DFT operation is described with the matrix $\mathbf{iDFT}$. The reconstructed image is then found according to:

$$\mathbf{m} = \mathbf{iDFT} \cdot \mathbf{s}. \tag{2.24}$$

The entries of the matrix[14] $\mathbf{iDFT}$ describe a shifted and scaled version of the standard inverse 2D-DFT:

$$(\mathrm{iDFT})_{(p,p'),(q,q')} = (\Delta k)^2 \cdot e^{\frac{2\pi i}{N}(pq + p'q')}. \tag{2.25}$$

b)   Conformity with Linear Reconstruction Theory

It is shown here under which circumstances the same reconstruction is found with the general matrix approaches presented in section 2.1. Explicit calculations are shown only for the weak approach. It is left to the interested reader to show that the strong approach gives exactly the same results in the case of Cartesian Fourier imaging.

---

[13]On some MRI scanners the frequency direction is oversampled by a factor of two in order to avoid wrapping artifacts in this direction.

[14]The indices p, p', q, q' are defined to run from $-N/2$ to $N/2 - 1$.

From Eq. 2.11 it is known that the reconstruction matrix $\mathbf{F}$ for the weak approach is related to the encoding matrix via $\mathbf{F} = (\Delta V)^{-1}\mathbf{E}^+$. On the other hand, the reconstruction matrix should conform to $\mathbf{F} = \mathbf{iDFT}$, according to Eq. 2.24. Comparison of the two expressions immediately shows that the imaging process must be designed to generate an encoding matrix $\mathbf{E} = (\Delta V)^{-1} \cdot \mathbf{DFT}$. The matrix $\mathbf{DFT}$ is the inverse of $\mathbf{iDFT}$ and can be described as its Hermitian scaled with $N^{-2}(\Delta k)^{-4}$. Also consider that all voxels have the same size $\Delta V = (\Delta x)^2$. The (reference) encoding matrix therefore has the following entries:

$$E_{(p,p'),(q,q')} = b \cdot e^{-\frac{2\pi i}{N}(pq+p'q')}, \quad \text{where} \quad b = (N\Delta x\Delta k)^{-2}. \quad (2.26)$$

The encoding matrix is linked to the physical conditions of the acquisition process via Eq. 2.9. This equation is repeated here:

$$E_{(\alpha,\kappa),\rho} = \int_V i_\rho^*(\vec{x})\text{enc}_{\alpha,\kappa}(\vec{x})\,d\vec{x}, \quad \text{with} \quad \text{enc}_{\alpha,\kappa}(\vec{x}) = c_\alpha(\vec{x})e^{-\mathrm{i}\vec{k}_\kappa\vec{x}}. \quad (2.27)$$

In Fourier imaging, only one receiver coil with homogeneous sensitivity is used. Therefore, the index α can be skipped. Ignoring correct physical units it is assumed w. l. o. g. that $c(\vec{x}) = 1$. The k-space trajectory $\vec{k}_\kappa$ forms the Cartesian sampling grid $\mathcal{K}$:

$$\mathcal{K} = 2\pi\Delta k \cdot (\mathcal{I}_N \times \mathcal{I}_N), \quad \text{where} \quad \mathcal{I}_N := [-N/2, N/2 - 1]. \quad (2.28)$$

Under these conditions, it is helpful to identify the index κ with the ordered pair $(p, p') \in \mathcal{I}_N \times \mathcal{I}_N$ and the encoding functions of Cartesian Fourier imaging (cf. Eq. 2.27) are given by:

$$\text{enc}_{p,p'}(\vec{x}) = e^{-2\pi\mathrm{i}\Delta k(px+p'y)}. \quad (2.29)$$

The calculation of the corresponding encoding matrix involves an integration over the support of the ideal voxel shape. As mentioned above, a realistic voxel would have a square-shaped support. Comparison with the reference encoding matrix (2.26) shows, however, that the ideal voxel shapes of standard Fourier reconstruction are delta functions $i_\rho(\vec{x}) = \delta(\vec{x} - \vec{x}_\rho)$. As a consequence the integration is just an evaluation of the encoding function at the voxel centers of the reconstruction grid $\mathcal{G}$. Take into account that the image is reconstructed on a Cartesian grid $\mathcal{G} = \Delta x \cdot (\mathcal{I}_N \times \mathcal{I}_N)$ with the same number of grid points as $\mathcal{K}$. The voxel centers are therefore described by $\vec{x}_\rho = \Delta x \cdot (q, q')^T$ when the voxel position ρ is identified with the pair $(q, q') \in \mathcal{I}_N \times \mathcal{I}_N$. Then, the entries of the encoding matrix $E_{(\alpha,\kappa),\rho} \rightarrow E_{(p,p'),(q,q')}$ read:

$$E_{(p,p'),(q,q')} = \int_V \delta(\vec{x} - \vec{x}_\rho)\text{enc}_{p,p'}(\vec{x})\,\mathrm{d}\vec{x} = e^{-2\pi\mathrm{i}\Delta k\Delta x(pq+p'q')}.$$

Finally, the comparison with Eq. 2.26 reveals that the weak reconstruction (under the discussed assumptions) is equivalent to standard Cartesian Fourier reconstruction if the following relation between k-space distance Δk and voxel size Δx holds:

$$\Delta x \Delta k = 1/N. \tag{2.30}$$

This relation discloses what k-space sampling distance Δk should be chosen for the object under investigation: First, it often makes sense to choose a reconstruction grid, which covers the whole object. Assume that the object lies inside the square-shaped region $V = [-a/2, a/2] \times [-a/2, a/2]$. Then, the object is covered by the reconstruction if and only if $N\Delta x > a$. Correspondingly, according to Eq. 2.30, the k-space sampling distance should be chosen smaller than

$$\Delta k < 1/a. \tag{2.31}$$

Summary   With the assumption of delta functions as ideal voxel shapes, both strong (not explicitly shown here) and weak reconstruction approaches are equivalent to the standard reconstruction of Cartesian Fourier imaging. The reconstruction is a scaled and shifted version of the standard inverse DFT. This result is found by choosing a k-space sampling distance Δk, which equals the inverse of the desired extent $N\Delta x$ of the image.

c)   Image Properties

The most important image properties - resolution, field-of-view (FOV) and image noise - are the topic of this section. They are analyzed in detail with the general theoretical considerations presented above, sections 2.1.3 and 2.1.4, page 50ff. It is shown that, for Cartesian Fourier reconstruction, the investigated image properties are characterized by simple analytical expressions.

Spatial Response Function and Point Spread Function   Image resolution and the concept of FOV can be analyzed with the SRF or, alternatively, with the PSF. First, a definition is made in order to simplify the calculations:

$$g_N(x) := \frac{1}{N} \sum_{p=-N/2}^{N/2-1} e^{\frac{2\pi i}{N}px} = \frac{1}{N} \cdot e^{-\frac{\pi i}{N}x} \frac{\sin(\pi x)}{\sin(\pi x/N)}. \tag{2.32}$$

The definition involves a geometric sum and can thus be transformed according to the equality on the right hand side. Note that the factor $1/N$ has been chosen to ensure that $g_N(0) = 1$.

The SRF of Cartesian Fourier reconstruction can be derived by combining the definition above with Eqs. 2.7, 2.24, 2.25, 2.29, 2.30:

$$f_{q,q'}(\vec{x}) = \frac{1}{(\Delta x)^2} \cdot g_N\left(q - \frac{x}{\Delta x}\right) g_N\left(q' - \frac{y}{\Delta x}\right). \tag{2.33}$$

According to Eq. 2.17, the PSF of a source located at $\vec{x}_0$ reads correspondingly:

$$p_{\vec{x}_0}(q,q') = \frac{1}{(\Delta x)^2} \cdot g_N\left(q - \frac{x_0}{\Delta x}\right) g_N\left(q' - \frac{y_0}{\Delta x}\right). \tag{2.34}$$

SRF and PSF of Cartesian Fourier reconstruction are illustrated in Fig. 2.4 for the parameters $\Delta k = 1$ and $N = 32$. Whereas the SRF is shift-invariant, the PSF changes depending on where the source location lies within a particular voxel. This is considered in the figure, where PSFs are shown for two different source locations, whereas only a single SRF plot is depicted. The figure confirms the statement that the SRF should be preferred over the PSF for image analysis whenever possible. An explanation is found in the figure caption.

Resolution   For Cartesian Fourier imaging, the FWHM of the main peak of the SRF, a primary measure for image resolution (cf. page 51 in section 2.1.3), can be calculated from Eq. 2.33. High-resolution applications have a FWHM of ≈ 1.21 voxels. In low-resolution applications the FWHM is only negligibly larger. The actual image resolution (as defined here) is therefore slightly lower than suggested by the voxel dimensions of the reconstructed image. The reason for this fact is that the voxels share object information resulting from convolution with the SRF. The fundamental relation between voxel size and k-space sampling distance, as presented in Eq. 2.30, casts

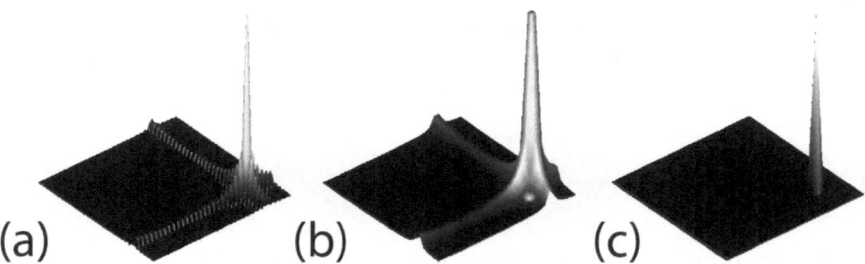

(a)   (b)   (c)

Figure 2.4: SRF and PSF of Fourier imaging. (a) SRF. (b) PSF with source location between two voxel centers. (c) PSF with source location exactly at a voxel center. The comparison of SRF and PSFs shows that only the SRF exhibits the correct Gibbs ringing oscillations. In the shown magnitude images, the PSFs only show smoothly decaying envelope functions. On-center source locations even give the wrong impression that no voxel contamination from neighboring voxels occurs. From these examples it can be concluded that the SRF should be analyzed and not the PSF if possible, unless justified otherwise.

image resolution into the realm of signal acquisition: Image resolution is defined by the extent $N\Delta k$ of the acquired k-space.

What about the sidelobe behavior? The SRF oscillates with zero-crossings at intervals of exactly one voxel. It is anisotropic; near the peak, the envelope of the SRF decreases as $1/r$ along the main coordinate axes and as $1/r^2$ along the diagonal direction. Along the main axes, the minimum value is $N/2$ voxels away from the main peak with value N^{-1}. Along the diagonal, the minimum value is $N/2$ voxels away from the center of the peak in each direction with a minimum value of N^{-2}. The envelope increases again for locations farther away than $N/2$ voxels from the central peak.

Field-of-View Whereas image resolution is a consequence of the finiteness of signal acquisition, a finite FOV is a direct consequence of the discrete nature of signal sampling. It has been argued above that the sampling interval Δk should be chosen smaller than the inverse of the extent of the measured object (cf. Eq. 2.31). Otherwise, the image reconstruction grid would be too small to cover the whole object. This is true, but it only describes part of what actually happens: Those image areas which fall outside of the reconstruction window are not merely cut out, but they wrap back into the image. Therefore, the size of the reconstruction grid is often referred to as the *field-of-view* and the wrapping behavior is denoted as the *fold-over artifact*. This artifact is illustrated in Fig. 2.5.

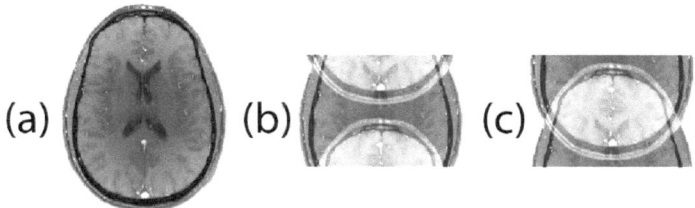

Figure 2.5: Fold-over artifact. (a) Sufficiently dense sampling results in non-aliased images. (b, c) If the sampling distance is chosen larger, the FOV becomes smaller and the image folds over. The aliased image is typically centered as in (b). The circularly shifted representation (c) is equivalent. It clearly shows that top half of the image and bottom half are aliased.

The argumentation above shows that the FOV equals the inverse of the k-space sampling distance. This is confirmed by a further analysis of the SRF and is a direct consequence of the fact that $g_N(\cdot)$ (cf. Eq. 2.32) is periodic:

$$g_N(x + N) = \text{sign}(N)g_N(x) = \pm g_N(x).$$

W. l. o. g. N is assumed to be even. Therefore, g_N is periodic with period N. According to Eqs. 2.33, 2.34, SRF and PSF are periodic with periodicity of exactly N voxels or equivalently with a periodicity of $FOV := N\Delta x$ in image space. Therefore, the SRF has a minimum at half distance between the periodic main peaks and increases again after half a FOV. The SRF indicates that magnetization vectors, located at positions with a distance FOV are superimposed, i.e., folded on top of each other. Therefore, it can be concluded that aliasing is avoided as long as the region W covered by the object lies within a square $\square_{FOV}$ having an edge length FOV in both directions:

$$W \subset \square_{FOV}. \tag{2.35}$$

This equation is the mathematical formulation of the famous Nyquist limit in the context of MR imaging. It conforms to Eq. 2.31, which establishes a relationship between image fold-over and signal acquisition. Whereas image resolution depends on the *extent* of the k-space sampling grid, fold-over occurs when the k-space sampling *distance* is chosen larger than the inverse

of the width of the object under investigation. In practice, fold-over artifacts occur only along the phase encoding direction because oversampling
the frequency encoding direction mainly just enlarges the amount of data
handling; it does not, however, prolong the acquisition time.

Completeness of k-Space Encoding   In MRI, only a one-dimensional path
$\vec{k}(t)$, $t \in \mathbb{R}$ through a higher-dimensional k-space $\vec{k} \in \mathbb{R}^d$ can be acquired.
In the first chapter it has already been mentioned that it is nevertheless
possible to treat the acquisition as though a finite higher-dimensional subset
$K \subset \mathbb{R}^d$ of the higher-dimensional k-space had been acquired (effective
k-space). This astonishing result can be understood with the concept of
FOV: The discrete nature of sampling leads to a finite FOV. Denser sampling
would only increase the size of the FOV with an infinitely large FOV if
d-dimensional continuous sampling was possible. However, as measured
objects are always of finite size, it is sufficient to acquire one-dimensional
k-space trajectories without losing image quality by leaving out data points
in-between. Of course, the same applies for the sampling along the path,
such that only a finite number of data points need to be stored. In case
of Fourier sampling, the Whittaker-Shannon interpolation formula [168]
goes one step further in that the formula gives an exact mathematical rule
of how the discrete signal data can be combined to "fill" the omitted k-
space between the data samples. With supplementary RF-encoding, the
density of k-space sampling can be reduced even further (cf. section 2.3,
page 72ff). The k-space sampling density is of uttermost importance in
MRI because gradient encoding is done in a time-consuming sequential
manner. Therefore a large amount of literature deals with the problem
of undersampling k-space as much as possible without losing significant
image information, among others [173, 135, 3, 200, 52, 112, 99, 69, 210].

Image Noise   The noise in the reconstructed images is analyzed here with
the two methods presented in section 2.1.4, page 52ff: Condition number
and (co-)variance analysis.

First, consider the condition number of the reconstruction matrix $\mathbf{F} = \text{iDFT}$.
This matrix is a scaled version of the normalized DFT. The normalized DFT
is unitary and therefore its singular values all equal unity. The singular
values of $\mathbf{F}$ are therefore also all equal and, according to Eq. 2.18, the
condition number of $\mathbf{F}$ is unity. The condition number cannot be below

unity, thus Cartesian Fourier reconstruction is *the* optimal reconstruction in terms of noise propagation.

Second, consider the statistical analysis using the image noise matrix. From Eq. 2.19 it can be concluded that the image noise matrix is proportional to the identity matrix:

$$\mathbf{X} = \mathbf{F}\tilde{\mathbf{\Psi}}\mathbf{F}^{H} = \psi \mathbf{F}\mathbf{F}^{H} = \psi(\Delta k)^{4}N^{2}\mathbb{1}_{N^{2}}.$$

The value ψ is the signal noise. It can be calculated from Eqs. 2.20, 2.21, and is a scalar because only one receiver coil is used for signal acquisition. The parameter N is the number of voxels in each dimension and Δk is the k-space sampling distance. The intensities of the image voxels are therefore not correlated and the variance is the same for all image voxels. The reconstructed image can therefore be regarded as being optimal in terms of statistical image properties.

With Eq. 2.22, the SNR of an image voxel ρ is given by:

$$SNR_{\rho} = \frac{|m_{\rho}^{avg}|}{\sqrt{\psi}}(\Delta x)^{2}N. \tag{2.36}$$

The SNR is therefore proportional to the voxel size. The linear dependency on the number of acquisition points refers to incoherent signal averaging via the FFT.

d) Conclusion

The general matrix approach can be used to derive the most important results for Fourier reconstruction. Strong and weak approach lead to the same reconstruction. The analysis of image properties like resolution and image noise shows that Cartesian Fourier imaging has remarkable properties. The image properties are the same for each voxel. Fourier reconstruction leads to uncorrelated voxels with optimal noise variance. The main reason for the beneficial properties of Fourier reconstruction is that it is basically the discrete Fourier transform. There is also a practical advantage: Even though the discrete Fourier transform matrix is dense, very fast reconstruction algorithms exist which solve the reconstruction with a complexity of $\mathcal{O}(N^{2}\ln(2N))$ for 2D imaging - much faster compared to direct computation of the Fourier transform, requiring $\mathcal{O}(N^{4})$ elementary operations.

2.2.2 Reconstruction Methods for Radial Imaging

The first MRI images were acquired with a radial acquisition trajectory [92]. Such a trajectory is sketched in Fig. 1.8b, page 31; a typical sequence diagram is shown in Fig. 2.6. Nowadays, radial imaging plays an important role in MRI, especially in clinical research settings. It offers unique and fast encoding options [151, 10, 141] and there are ongoing efforts to develop advanced imaging techniques [3, 47, 112] and investigate interesting applications [143, 214, 39]. One drawback of radial MRI is its susceptibility to gradient timing errors. However, effective techniques exist to bring these errors under control [130]. Other recent developments in improving acquisition and reconstruction methods add to the importance of radial imaging for MRI [148, 13]. If the k-space is traversed as in Fig. 1.8b, an initial k-space location has to be reached prior to frequency encoding similar to Cartesian imaging. In contrast to Cartesian imaging, however, the center of k-space (=echo) is acquired each readout. This results in oversampling of the center, which can be exploited in various advantageous ways (cf. e.g. chapter 2.3.4 in [210]).

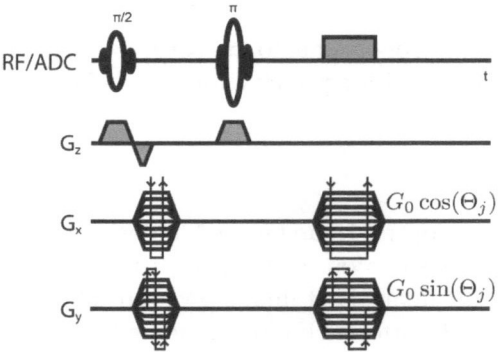

Figure 2.6: Basic sequence diagram for spin echo radial imaging. The mathematical formulas represent the gradient strengths of the x-gradient and the y-gradient for the different projection angles Θ_j. For reference, compare the diagram with the Cartesian analogue in Fig. 1.10b, page 34.

Radial measurements may be reconstructed in several ways. It is shown below that MPPI reconstruction is feasible, but computationally demanding. Faster alternatives are filtered back-projection and especially gridding reconstruction. Gridding reconstruction is also used for arbitrary sampling trajectories and discussed separately in section 2.2.3, page 69ff.

a) Direct Matrix Inversion

With the general matrix approach a matrix $\mathbf{F}$ can be derived that solves the reconstruction problem. The encoding functions are given by:

$$\text{enc}_{(p,j)}(\vec{x}) = e^{-2\pi i \Delta k p B_j(\vec{x})}, \quad \text{where} \quad B_j(\vec{x}) = \cos(\Theta_j)x + \sin(\Theta_j)y.$$

$B_j(\vec{x})$ is proportional to the magnetic field sensitivity during the jth signal readout ($j = 1, \ldots, N_p$), taken at the projection angle Θ_j, where the angles are typically distributed equidistantly on a semicircle. The index p denotes the pth sampling point along the corresponding readout of length N_r. The encoding matrix then has the following entries:

$$E_{(p,j),(q,q')} = e^{-\frac{2\pi i}{N} p B_j(q,q')}.$$

In the derivation, it has been assumed that $\vec{q} = (q, q') = \vec{x}/\Delta x$ by making use of the fact that with linear SEMs $B_j(\vec{x}) = B_j(\Delta x \cdot \vec{q}) = \Delta x \cdot B_j(q, q')$. It is useful to describe the reconstructions in the projection space, by taking the inverse *one-dimensional* DFT along the temporal dimension of the individual readouts: $\hat{s} = \text{iDFT}_t \cdot s$. With the definition $\hat{\mathbf{F}}_t = N^{-1} \cdot \mathbf{F} \cdot \mathbf{DFT}_t$ one finds $\mathbf{m} = \mathbf{Fs} = \hat{\mathbf{F}}_t \hat{s}$. Then, w. l. o. g. setting $\Delta V := 1$, the equation $\mathbf{F} = \mathbf{E}^+$ transforms accordingly:

$$\hat{\mathbf{F}}_t = N^{-1} \cdot \mathbf{F} \cdot \mathbf{DFT}_t = N^{-1} \mathbf{E}^+ \mathbf{DFT}_t = (\text{iDFT}_t \cdot \mathbf{E})^+ = \hat{\mathbf{E}}_t^+.$$

According to Eq. 2.32, the entries of $\hat{\mathbf{E}}_t = \text{iDFT}_t \cdot \mathbf{E}$ are given by:

$$(\hat{E}_t)_{(\omega,j),(q,q')} = g_N(\omega - B_j(q, q')).$$

In the limit $N \to \infty$ and for sufficiently dense sampling, the encoding matrix $\hat{\mathbf{E}}_t$, having been transformed to frequency space, becomes very sparse; it approaches a delta function. In this case, the signal acquisitions $\hat{s} \propto \hat{\mathbf{E}}_t \mathbf{m}$ represent projections along the isocontour lines of the projecting field (Fig. 2.7), and calculation of the forward operation $\hat{\mathbf{E}}\mathbf{m}$ can be accelerated by a factor of N_r. However, this does not immediately imply also fast calculation of the inverse operation. Another problem is that, in reality, the

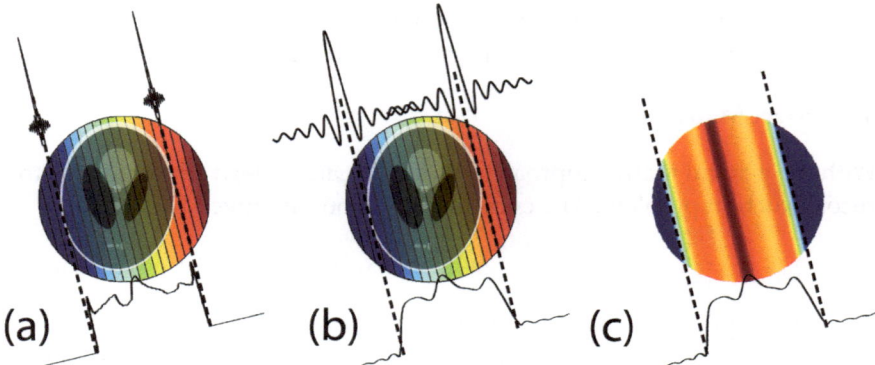

Figure 2.7: Radial projection imaging: an example of a projection and an example of back-projection. (a) For high-resolution readouts, the encoding matrix nearly represents exact projections along the field contour lines of the encoding field. The encoding matrix is therefore very sparse. (b) For low-resolution readouts, it is visible that the projections are in reality convolved with a sinc-function. Thus, the encoding matrix is not sparse for low-resolution imaging applications. (c) The back-projection operator projects the one-dimensional projections onto a two-dimensional plane.

number of samples N is finite and therefore $g_N(\cdot)$ cannot be approximated through a delta function. The encoding matrix is not sparse, thus direct inversion is impractical requiring $\mathcal{O}(N_r^3 N_p^3)$ elementary operations.[15] Explicit calculation of the correlation matrix $\mathbf{B}$ (cf. Eq. 2.14) shows that $\mathbf{B}$ is also dense and therefore the strong reconstruction has the same high numerical complexity as the weak reconstruction for radial imaging.

b) Filtered Back-Projection

Faster reconstructions are achieved with filtered back-projection (FBP). FBP is a well-established reconstruction technique in medical imaging [96, 32, 74], whose theory and discretization effects are well known. Because of the abundant literature on this topic, FBP is here given only a cursory discussion. There are several different possibilities for implementing filtered back-projection [32, 74]. A common implementation for MRI consists of

---

[15]For a more general case, that also includes standard radial imaging, it is shown in chapter 7.1.2, page 240ff, that it is possible to sparsify the encoding matrix with an appropriate filter, thereby significantly speeding up the forward operation. This can be exploited to accelerate iterative image reconstruction based on the CG method.

three steps. First, the N_p signal projections $s(k, \Theta_j)$ are multiplied by a filter function $H(k)$, which can be chosen as $H(k) = |k|$. Other filters and their properties are presented in [74], chapter 10. After filtering, an inverse 1D-FFT is performed on each filtered signal projection resulting in filtered projections $\bar{P}$:

$$\bar{P}(p, \Theta_j) = \sum_{l=-N_r/2}^{N_r/2-1} s(k_l, \Theta_j) H(k_l) e^{2\pi i l p / N_r},$$

where N_r is the number of readout points per projection. Finally, the reconstructed image $m(x, y)$ is found by back-projecting the filtered projections $\bar{P}(\cdot, \Theta_j)$ onto a Cartesian grid $(x, y) \in \Sigma_{cart}$:

$$m(x, y) = \sum_{j=1}^{N_p} B(\bar{P}(\cdot, \Theta_j))(x, y) \Delta\Theta,$$

where $\Delta\Theta$ is the angle increment between each projection and the back-projection operator $B(\cdot)$ is defined as:

$$B(\bar{P}(\cdot, \Theta_j))(x, y) = \bar{P}(x \cos(\Theta_j) + y \sin(\Theta_j), \Theta_j).$$

The operator $B(\cdot)$ thus back-projects a one-dimensional ray onto a two-dimensional plane. The discrete nature of the data has two effects. First, it is necessary to interpolate the projection data onto the positions $p = x \cos(\Theta_j) + y \sin(\Theta_j)$ [96, 74]. Typically, linear interpolation is used. This is, however, not compulsory and other methods like cubic spline interpolation may be employed. The second effect is that the target set of B must be a discrete subset $\Sigma \in \mathbb{R}^2$. Typically, a Cartesian grid Σ_{cart} is chosen large enough to cover the whole object. The FBP approach is illustrated in Fig. 2.8. The numerical complexity of the FBP approach is governed by the back-projection step, which has a complexity of $\mathcal{O}(N_p^3)$. Lookup tables may be used to speed up the reconstruction [146].

2.2.3 Further Non-Cartesian Methods

Not only radial imaging, but any non-Cartesian sampling strategy can be combined with the general matrix approaches of section 2.1. Similar to the special radial case, numerically much faster algorithms exist also

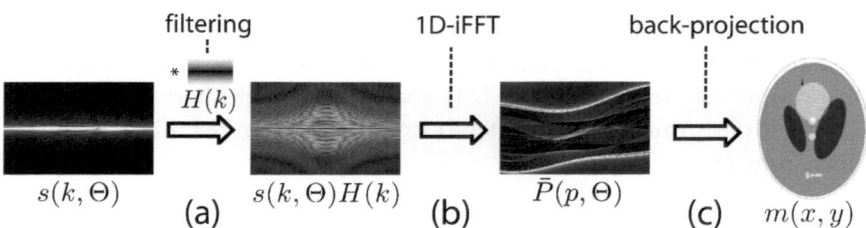

Figure 2.8: Typical filtered back-projection algorithm. (a) The signal projections are first multiplied with a filter along the readout direction. (b) The filtered signal projections are then Fourier transformed along the dimension of readout. (c) Finally, the image is reconstructed by back-projecting each filtered projection along the direction of the corresponding projection angle. The formulas correspond to the notation used in the main text.

for this more general situation of arbitrary sampling trajectories, among them implementations of the non-uniform FFT (nuFFT) such as gridding reconstruction or the min-max interpolation method of Fessler et al. [36]. An overview of nuFFT reconstruction is found in [69]; also cf. paragraph *Non-Uniform FFT* in chapter 7.1.3, page 248f. Here, only gridding reconstruction is roughly presented because of its fundamental relevance, simplicity and frequent use in MR image reconstruction. Consult [73, 132, 142, 8] for a deeper discussion of this method.

The idea of the gridding approach is simple: The signal data are interpolated (gridded) onto a grid with regular spacing in order to allow for an FFT. Crucial to this approach is a convolution with a gridding kernel. Associated with the convolution are two issues: First, the discrete implementation of the convolution operation requires that the non-uniform sampling density must be corrected in advance ("density compensation"). Second, as stated by the convolution theorem, the signal after the FFT-operation is weighted with the Fourier transform of the gridding kernel and this "roll-off" has to be corrected. After presentation of a typical gridding algorithm, the relationship of gridding to the MPPI solution is demonstrated here.

Gridding Algorithm   A typical gridding algorithm consists of 4 steps

1. Density compensation. Several methods exist to measure the local sampling density. Commonly used 2D and 3D methods include

Voronoi diagrams [2] or weight determination with the help of a convolution operation [78].

2. Convolution with gridding kernel and resampling onto a regular grid. In theory, the sinc-function would be an optimal kernel [124]. It is, however, impractical because of its infinite extent. Therefore, kernels with finite support are used in practice. One consequence is that it should be resampled onto an oversampled grid to avoid artifacts resulting from data fold-over [124, 73, 8]. A very common kernel is the Kaiser-Bessel kernel $f_{kb}(x; \alpha)$ whose effectiveness depends on the filter parameter α (also cf. [57]); with J_0 being the zero-order modified Bessel function of the first kind $f_{kb}(\cdot)$ is defined as:

$$f_{kb}(x; \alpha) = J_0\left(\alpha\pi \cdot \sqrt{1 - x^2}\right) \Big/ J_0(\alpha\pi), \quad \text{where } x \in [-1, 1]. \quad (2.37)$$

3. Performing an inverse FFT to the convolved and regularly resampled signal data.

4. "Roll-off" correction: division with the apodization function. The apodization function is the Fourier transform of the convolution kernel.

The individual steps are illustrated in Fig. 2.9. Gridding is very fast because the convolution can be performed with kernels of finite support. The complexity of the convolution is just $\mathcal{O}(N_{ker}N)$ and for the FFT an additional $\mathcal{O}(N \ln(N))$ operations are required, where N_{ker} is the size of the kernel and N the number of sampling points. For radial datasets, assuming $N_r \propto N_p$, gridding therefore has an improved complexity of $\mathcal{O}(N_p^2 \ln(N_p))$ compared to $\mathcal{O}(N_p^3)$ for standard FBP, which is not optimized via lookup tables [146].

Relationship to Direct Matrix Inversion It is useful to analyze the relationship of gridding reconstruction to an optimal solution via matrix inversion (cf. the above section 2.2.2a, page 67f). Such a relation can be established for the optimal sinc gridding kernel [164]. Consider that gridding reconstruction is a linear operation and can thus be represented by a reconstruction matrix $\mathbf{F}_{grid} = \mathbf{iDFT} \cdot \mathbf{T}^H \mathbf{D}$. In this equation, $\mathbf{iDFT}$ represents the usual inverse DFT, $\mathbf{T}$ the sinc-kernel and the diagonal matrix $\mathbf{D}$ the density compensation weights. The strong matrix approach, on the other hand, has the solution $\mathbf{F}_{ls} = \mathbf{E}^H \mathbf{B}^+$ (cf. Eq. 2.13). Optimally, reconstruction is performed on an infinitely dense grid. In this case, it can easily be shown that $\mathbf{E}^H = \mathbf{iDFT} \cdot \mathbf{T}^H$ and gridding reconstruction becomes

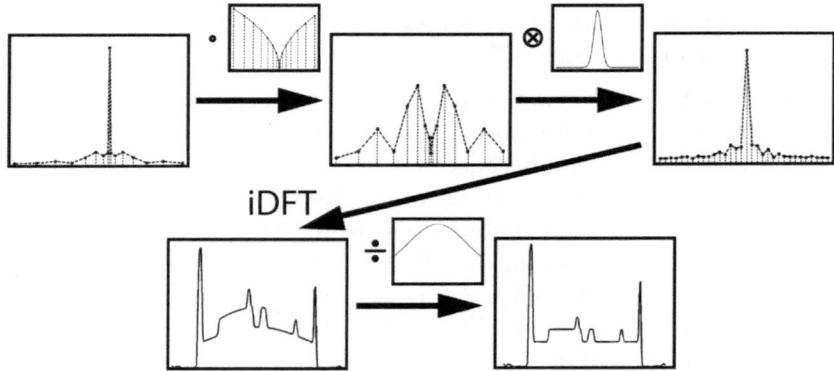

Figure 2.9: Typical gridding reconstruction algorithm. Starting at the top left of the image, the signal is multiplied with the density compensation weights. Then, the irregularly spaced signal values are convolved with the gridding kernel and resampled on a regular grid. The convolved signal is Fourier transformed and finally, the "roll-off" artifact is corrected by division with the apodization function. This illustration generalizes naturally to 2D and 3D gridding reconstructions.

$\mathbf{F}_{grid} = \mathbf{E}^H \mathbf{D}$ as opposed to the "least-squares" solution $\mathbf{F} = \mathbf{E}^H \mathbf{B}^+$. It follows immediately, that optimal gridding reconstruction approximates the "least-squares" solution by approximating the correlation matrix $\mathbf{B}$ with a diagonal matrix $\mathbf{D}$. From this matrix perspective, it is astonishing that this approximation does often not lead to image deterioration. However, situations have occurred in which gridding reconstruction fails and more accurate reconstruction methods must be used [107].

2.3 Image Reconstruction from Several Receiver Coils

Abundant literature is available on the topic of image reconstruction from several RF-receiver coils (cf. review article [90]). The most important reason for this major interest is certainly the significance attributed to PI: Many modern MRI systems are equipped with hardware for parallel reception. But also from a purely algorithmic perspective, the high level of ongoing research activity is not a surprise. Parallel image reconstructions are non-unitary. As a consequence, noise enhancement and artifacts introduced by the reconstruction become even more problematic than before.

Another key problem in PI image reconstruction is the amount of extra data to be handled from multiple receiver coils, thus making the inversion of the encoding matrix even more demanding than for single-coil acquisitions.

In Fourier imaging this problem could be solved with the application of the FFT. The simplest way of proceeding with several coil images is to perform an FFT separately for each coil. Then, the only problem that remains is how to combine the different coil images. Roemer et al. [145] have found a combination with optimal SNR of the resulting image; similar results were found by Walsh [188] based on statistical arguments. Also undersampled datasets are resolved on a coil-by-coil basis with Cartesian SENSE, a method developed by Prüssmann et al. [135].

Coil-by-coil approaches are very fast, however, the application of the DFT for each data channel bounds the image resolution according to the Nyquist criterion. In order to achieve "superresolution", simultaneous treatment of the coil images is required. In this section it is briefly explained that for low-resolution applications the general matrix approach can lead to higher-resolved image reconstruction.

PI image reconstruction methods are often divided into two large classes: image space algorithms, such as the optimal coil combination of Roemer et al. [145], PILS [50] or SENSE [135, 134], and k-space algorithms, such as SMASH [173], (Cartesian) GRAPPA [49] or pseudo-Cartesian GRAPPA [165]. In this section only the most common methods are presented. Special attention is given to Cartesian SENSE. The algorithm is derived from linear reconstruction theory and, as a by-product, the optimal coil combination of Roemer et al. [145] is found. Also, the most important image properties like image resolution, aliasing artifacts and image noise are analyzed in detail. Apart from Cartesian SENSE, iterative SENSE [134], often used to process non-Cartesian data, is presented and discussed. As representative for the k-space based reconstructions GRAPPA is described. It is shown that SENSE and GRAPPA are closely related to each other, thereby demonstrating that image space and k-space based reconstructions share a common background.

The analysis of the algorithms often reveals block-diagonal and block-circulant matrix structures. Such structures can be described with the

Kronecker product. The reader not used to this mathematical concept is encouraged to consult Appendix A.2, page 293f. A more detailed presentation can be found in chapter 13 of the textbook [91].

2.3.1   Image Space Reconstruction

Even though, historically, reconstruction in k-space was developed first in the context of PI, the presentation begins here with image space methods. Introduced in 1999, Cartesian SENSE (<u>SENS</u>itivity <u>E</u>ncoding) [135] has since then gained supreme importance for image reconstruction in PI besides the k-space based GRAPPA [49] algorithm (see section 2.3.2a, page 97ff). SENSE is very well suited to introduce into image reconstruction in PI because of its clarity and direct relationship to the general matrix approach presented above in section 2.1, page 40ff. The presentation begins with the basic Cartesian SENSE algorithm and an analysis of fundamental image properties like image resolution and aliasing as well as image noise. Then, capabilities of the general matrix approach to further improve image resolution are discussed. The presentation of image space reconstructions closes with a common adaptation of SENSE to non-Cartesian sampling trajectories.

a)   Cartesian SENSE (<u>SENS</u>itivity <u>E</u>ncoding)

Similar to Cartesian Fourier reconstruction, Cartesian SENSE is used to reconstruct images that are encoded with regular sampling trajectories. Therefore, the derivation of the encoding matrix follows arguments that are similar to those used in section 2.2.1, page 58ff, where standard Cartesian Fourier imaging is presented. The derivation is different because signal acquisition is accelerated along the phase encoding direction by skipping some of the encoding steps. Also, in contrast to Fourier reconstruction, SENSE is designed to cope with signals from several receiver coils $\alpha = 1, \ldots, N_c$. This methodological extension is reflected by labeling the encoding functions with the additional index α: $\mathrm{enc}_{p,p'}(\cdot) \to \mathrm{enc}_{\alpha,p,p'}(\cdot)$:

$$\mathrm{enc}_{\alpha,p,p'}(\vec{x}) = c_\alpha(\vec{x})e^{-2\pi \mathrm{i}(\Delta k_f p x + \Delta k_{ph} p' y)}. \tag{2.38}$$

In the previous section, it has been shown that without acceleration a quadratic FOV and isotropic resolution results when the same amount of data points are collected in the phase encoding direction as well as the frequency encoding direction with equal k-space sampling distances Δk_{ph} and Δk_f (cf. Eqs. 2.28, 2.29). Crucial with SENSE is that less encoding steps are acquired. Correspondingly, the k-space distance is increased along the phase encoding direction: $\Delta k_{ph} = R \cdot \Delta k_f$, with $R > 1$ (typically, integer acceleration factors $R = 2, 3, 4$ are used). Setting $\Delta k := \Delta k_f$, a reduced set of sampled k-space locations results: $\mathcal{K} = 2\pi\Delta k \cdot (\mathcal{I}_N \times R \cdot \mathcal{I}_{N/R})$, where the discrete intervals $\mathcal{I}_N, \mathcal{I}_{N/R}$ are defined as in Appendix A.1, on page 291. Similar to Cartesian Fourier reconstruction, the entries $E_{(\alpha,p,p'),(q,q')}$ of the encoding matrix are given by the encoding functions evaluated at the voxel centers of the (quadratic) Cartesian reconstruction grid $\mathcal{G} = \{\Delta x \cdot (q, q')^T | (q, q') \in \mathcal{I}_N \times \mathcal{I}_N\}$. Making use of the fact that $\Delta k \Delta x = 1/N$, the encoding matrix becomes:

$$E_{(\alpha,p,p'),(q,q')} = c_\alpha(q\Delta x, q'\Delta x)e^{-\frac{2\pi i}{N}(pq + Rp'q')}.$$

The weak approach requires the (pseudo-)inversion of the encoding matrix. However, the acceleration in the phase encoding direction makes the Fourier-terms non-bijective. They are periodic in q' as can be seen from the fact that $e^{-\frac{2\pi i}{N}(Rp'q')} = e^{-\frac{2\pi i}{N}(Rp'(q'+N/R))}$. Fourier-inversion of the undersampled data therefore leads to aliasing: R voxels with distance N/R are equally encoded (cf. Fig. 2.10). It is therefore useful to divide the reconstruction grid $\mathcal{G} = \Delta x \cdot (\mathcal{I}_N \times \mathcal{I}_N)$ into R equidistant non-overlapping sub-grids $\mathcal{G}_l = \Delta x \cdot (\mathcal{I}_N \times (\mathcal{I}_{N/R} + (l-1) \cdot N/R))$, $l = 1, \ldots, R$. The image space variable q' is then replaced by $q' \to (q', l)$ (see Fig. 2.10). The Fourier-terms are then independent of l and the encoding matrix decomposes into two matrices:

$$\mathbf{E} = \widehat{\mathbf{DFT}} \cdot \widetilde{\mathbf{C}}, \quad \text{where} \tag{2.39}$$

$$\begin{aligned}
\widehat{\mathrm{DFT}}_{(\alpha,p,p'),(\alpha',q'',q''')} &= \delta_{\alpha,\alpha'}e^{-\frac{2\pi i}{N}pq''}e^{-\frac{2\pi i}{N/R}p'q'''}, \\
\widetilde{C}_{(\alpha,q'',q'''),(q,q',l)} &= \delta_{q'',q}\delta_{q''',q'}c_\alpha(q\Delta x, (q' + (l-1)N/R\Delta x),
\end{aligned}$$

or, equivalently, where (with $\mathbf{I}_{q,q'}$ being zero except for one position, where the row and the column index is (q, q'), cf. the definition on page 293 in Appendix A.2):

$$\widehat{\mathbf{DFT}} = \mathbf{DFT} \otimes \mathbb{1} \quad \text{and} \quad \widetilde{\mathbf{C}} = \sum_{q,q'} \mathbf{I}_{q,q'} \otimes \mathbf{C}^{(q,q')}. \tag{2.40}$$

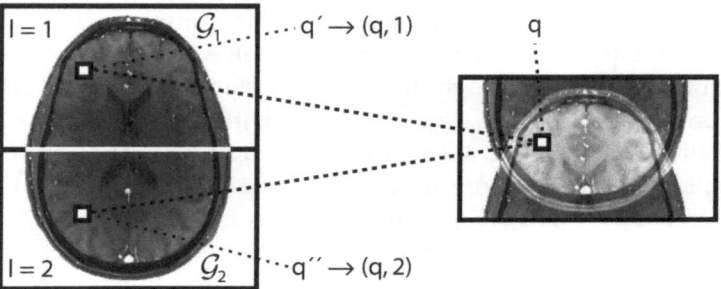

Figure 2.10: Aliasing in SENSE imaging. Shown is a situation with acceleration factor $R = 2$. The image illustrates that magnetizations at two different locations q' and q'' are equally encoded and cannot be differentiated. These positions are aliased to a common location q. The two locations are therefore denoted as $(q, 1)$ and $(q, 2)$ depending on if the location belongs to the top region $\mathcal{G}_1$ or to the bottom region $\mathcal{G}_2$.

The matrix $\widetilde{\mathbf{C}}$ is block-diagonal (cf. Eq. A.2, page 293) with very small blocks $\mathbf{C}^{(q,q')}$ of size $N_c \times R$. These blocks have the elements $C_{\alpha,l}^{(q,q')} = c_\alpha(q\Delta x, (q' + (l-1)N/R\Delta x)$. From these equations it can be seen that $\widetilde{\mathbf{C}}$ represents different sensitivity weighting on each sub-region $\mathcal{G}_l$. Consider the matrix $\widetilde{\mathbf{DFT}}$. With the commutation rule presented in appendix A.2, page 293f, one finds $\widetilde{\mathbf{DFT}} = \boldsymbol{DFT} \otimes \mathbb{1} = \mathbf{P}^H(\mathbb{1} \otimes \boldsymbol{DFT})\mathbf{P}$. The permutation $\mathbf{P}$ swaps the coil dimension and k-space dimension. According to Eq. A.3, $\mathbb{1} \otimes \boldsymbol{DFT}$ is block-diagonal and it follows that $\widetilde{\mathbf{DFT}}$ simply represents a coil-wise 2D-DFT.

For Cartesian SENSE $N_c N_\kappa \geq N_\rho$ and therefore, with Eq. 2.23 and with $\mathbf{E} \to (\Delta x)^2 \cdot \mathbf{E}$, the SNR-optimized weak reconstruction approach yields:[16]

$$\mathbf{F} = (\Delta x)^{-2} \cdot \widetilde{\mathbf{C}}^+ \widetilde{\mathbf{iDFT}} = (\Delta x)^{-2} \cdot (\widetilde{\mathbf{C}}^H \widetilde{\mathbf{\Psi}}^{-1} \widetilde{\mathbf{C}})^{-1} \widetilde{\mathbf{C}}^H \widetilde{\mathbf{\Psi}}^{-1} \widetilde{\mathbf{iDFT}}. \quad (2.41)$$

This result is found because $\widetilde{\mathbf{\Psi}}$ and $\widetilde{\mathbf{iDFT}}$ commute with each other. The block-diagonal structure (and thus sparsity) of the involved matrices is not

---

[16] For simplicity the symbol $\widetilde{\mathbf{C}}^+$ not only denotes the standard MPPI, but also the decorrelated MPPI for SNR-optimized reconstructions, described in this section (cf. section 2.1.5, page 56f).

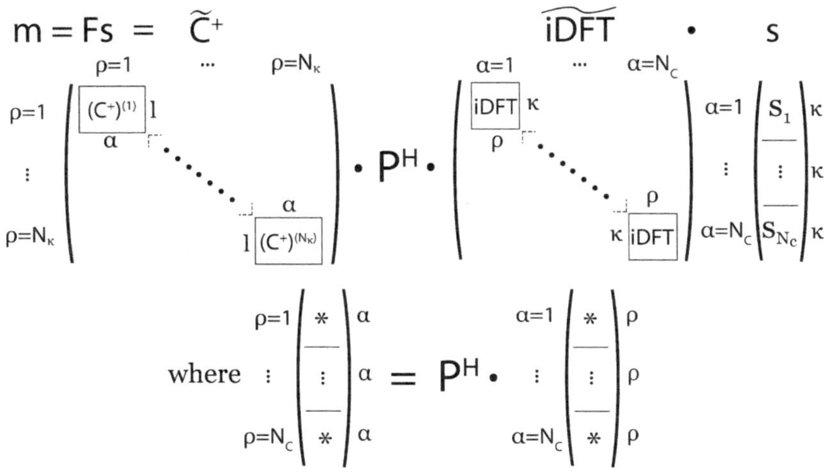

Figure 2.11: Structure of the SENSE reconstruction matrix. The reconstruction matrix is decomposable into two block-diagonal matrices and a permutation matrix. One block-diagonal matrix represents coil-wise inverse DFTs. The second block-diagonal matrix is formed by inverting a matrix, which contains the sensitivity profiles of the receiver coils. It is very sparse and can be structured voxel-group-wise. The block-diagonal structures of the matrices occur along different dimensions. Therefore, it is necessary to permute coil dimension and spatial dimension in between.

affected by the inversion: The matrix $\widetilde{\text{iDFT}} = \text{iDFT} \otimes \mathbb{1}$ represents a coil-wise inverse 2D-DFT and the MPPI of the sensitivity matrix separates to:

$$(\widetilde{\mathbf{C}}^H \widetilde{\boldsymbol{\Psi}}^{-1} \widetilde{\mathbf{C}})^{-1} \widetilde{\mathbf{C}}^H \widetilde{\boldsymbol{\Psi}}^{-1} = \sum_{q,q'} \mathbf{I}_{q,q'} \otimes \left[((\mathbf{C}^{(q,q')})^H \boldsymbol{\Psi}^{-1} \mathbf{C}^{(q,q')})^{-1} (\mathbf{C}^{(q,q')})^H \boldsymbol{\Psi}^{-1} \right].$$

The matrix $\mathbf{C}^{(q,q')})^H \boldsymbol{\Psi}^{-1} \mathbf{C}^{(q,q')}$ is only of size $R \times R$. The inversion of the sensitivity matrix is therefore very fast: Instead of having to invert one large matrix of size $N_\rho \times N_\rho$, it is sufficient to invert only very small matrices of size $R \times R$ for each voxel $(q, q') \in \mathcal{I}_N \times \mathcal{I}_{N/R}$ independently. The structure of the reconstruction matrix, particularly of $\widetilde{\text{iDFT}}$ and $\widetilde{\mathbf{C}}^+$, is illustrated in Fig. 2.11 (cf. the PatLoc analogue, Fig. 5.2, page 161).

The reconstruction algorithm is therefore very simple: First a coil-wise discrete 2D Fourier transform is performed. Then, for each voxel, the aliased signals are collected in a vector of length N_c and multiplied with the inverse of the sensitivity matrix consisting of the sensitivity values at the corresponding aliased locations. The algorithm is depicted in Fig. 2.12 in a form that shows the similarity to Cartesian PatLoc reconstruction as good as possible (cf. Fig. 5.3, page 163).

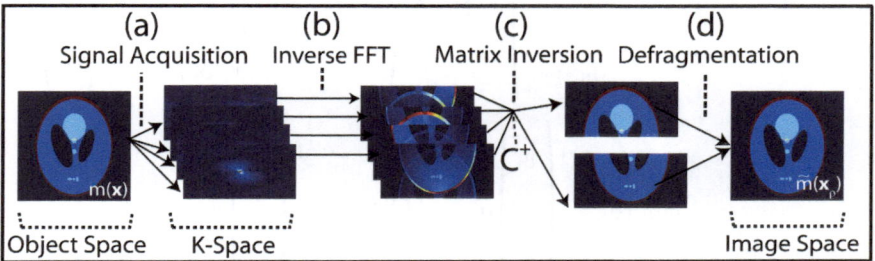

Figure 2.12: SENSE reconstruction algorithm. (a) Signals are acquired with several receiver channels. (b) A coil-wise inverse 2D-FFT is performed. (c) For each aliased voxel group a small matrix (pseudo-)inversion is performed in encoding space. (d) Finally, the unaliased image parts are pieced together. Typically, steps (c) and (d) are implemented as one single step. The reconstruction steps depicted are based on data simulated for four channels of a real-world RF-surface coil array and an acceleration factor of 2.

The reconstruction algorithm is very fast. The discussion of the latter paragraph has shown that the inversion of the sensitivity matrix has a numerical complexity of only $\mathcal{O}(N^2)$, which is less than the coil-wise Fourier inversion, that requires $\mathcal{O}(N^2 \ln(2N))$ operations.

Remark: For $R = 1$ the SNR-optimized reconstruction, presented in Eq. 2.41, reduces to the optimal complex-valued coil combination found by Roemer et al. in [145], Eq. 27, denoted as a *single uniform sensitivity image with optimized SNR at all points*:

$$m_\rho = \frac{\mathbf{c}_\rho^H \Psi^{-1}}{\mathbf{c}_\rho^H \Psi^{-1} \mathbf{c}_\rho} \mathbf{a}_\rho. \tag{2.42}$$

This equivalence is established by considering that the $N_c \times R$ matrix $\mathbf{C}^{(q,q')}$ is for $R = 1$ actually a $N_c \times 1$ vector $\mathbf{c}_\rho$, whose elements are the sensitivity values of the individual coil channels at a certain image location ρ. The vector $\mathbf{a}_\rho$ is also of length N_c; it consists of the image intensities in the ρ-th voxel from the different RF channels after Fourier transformation.

b) Image Resolution and Aliasing Artifacts

With Eqs. 2.7, 2.38, 2.41 and $\Delta k_{pe} = R \cdot \Delta k_f = R \cdot \Delta k$, the SRF of SENSE reconstruction is given by:

$$
\begin{aligned}
f_{(q,q',l)}(\vec{x}) &= \sum_{\alpha,p,p'} F_{(q,q',l),(\alpha,p,p')} \text{enc}_{(\alpha,p,p')}(\vec{x}) \\
&= \sum_{\alpha,\alpha',q'',q'''} \widetilde{C}^{+}_{(q,q',l),(\alpha',q'',q''')} c_\alpha(\vec{x}) \times \dots \\
&\dots \times (\Delta x)^{-2} \cdot \sum_{p,p'} \widehat{\text{iDFT}}_{(\alpha',q'',q'''),(\alpha,p,p')} e^{-2\pi i \Delta k (px + Rp'y)} \quad (2.43) \\
&= \left[\sum_{\alpha} \widetilde{C}^{+}_{(q,q',l),(\alpha,q,q')} c_\alpha(\vec{x}) \right] f^{Fourier}_{q,q',l}(\vec{x}) \\
&= c^{virt}_{q,q',l}(\vec{x}) \cdot f^{Fourier}_{q,q',l}(\vec{x}).
\end{aligned}
$$

The SRF is therefore a combination of the aliased Fourier SRF and a weighting function due to sensitivity encoding. The individual terms are given by:

$$
f^{Fourier}_{q,q',l}(\vec{x}) = \frac{1}{(\Delta x)^2} \cdot g_N\left(q - \frac{x}{\Delta x}\right) g_{N/R}\left(q' - \frac{y}{\Delta x}\right), \quad (2.44)
$$

$$
c^{virt}_{q,q',l}(\vec{x}) = \sum_{\alpha} \widetilde{C}^{+}_{(q,q',l),(\alpha,q,q')} c_\alpha(\vec{x}) \quad (2.45)
$$

$$
\text{with } \widetilde{C}_{(\alpha,q,q'),(q,q',l)} = c_\alpha(q\Delta x, (q' + (l-1)N/R\Delta x). \quad (2.46)
$$

The Fourier SRF has a reduced FOV and leads to aliasing in the phase encoding direction. According to the condition of weak reconstruction (Eq. 2.10), the sensitivity weighting[17] has the important property that

$$
c^{virt}_{q,q',l}(q\Delta x, (q' + (l'-1)N/R\Delta x) = \delta_{l,l'}. \quad (2.47)
$$

This relation expresses the fact that the sensitivity weighting suppresses the unwanted aliasing peaks in the Fourier SRF. In other words: The lack of gradient encoding in PI is compensated by sensitivity encoding. However, the SRF in SENSE is just an amplitude-modulated Fourier SRF. The frequency

---

[17]The notation as virtual coil sensitivity c^{virt} becomes comprehensible in section 2.3.1d, page 82ff, where ultimate SNR of SENSE images is discussed.

of the SRF, and therefore the primary measure for image resolution, is not affected by the reconstruction.

The latter equation states that the sensitivity weighting is defined exactly only at a small number of discrete positions. Complete suppression of the Fourier sidelobes between those positions is not demanded and also not possible, leading to residual aliasing. However, a beneficial property of the sensitivity weighting function ensures that residual aliasing does not pose a problem under normal imaging conditions and when acceleration is not driven to its limit: The MPPI solution $\widetilde{\mathbf{C}}^+$ is the solution to an underdetermined system and it therefore represents a feasible solution with minimum norm. This property ensures that the weighting is as small as possible in between the exactly defined values and excessive sidelobe amplification is avoided. Only under low-resolution conditions, as in spectroscopic imaging [17], residual aliasing might pose a problem in Cartesian SENSE reconstruction. Numerical examples of the Fourier SRF, the effective sensitivity weighting function and the resulting SENSE SRF are shown in Fig. 2.13. The examples show the SRF of a random voxel position for two different acceleration factors $R = 2$ and $R = 4$ and $32/R$ phase encodes.

c)   Image Noise

Image noise is analyzed here with the covariance analysis, presented on page 54f in section 2.1.4. For the SNR-optimized reconstruction of Eq. 2.41, the image noise matrix is calculated as:

$$\mathbf{X} = \mathbf{F}\widetilde{\boldsymbol{\Psi}}\mathbf{F}^H = R \cdot (\Delta k)^4 N^2 \cdot (\widetilde{\mathbf{C}}^H \widetilde{\boldsymbol{\Psi}}^{-1} \widetilde{\mathbf{C}})^{-1}$$

$$= R \cdot (\Delta k)^4 N^2 \cdot \sum_{q,q'} \mathbf{I}_{q,q'} \otimes \left[(\mathbf{C}^{(q,q')})^H \boldsymbol{\Psi}^{-1} \mathbf{C}^{(q,q')} \right]^{-1} .$$

It is block-diagonal with blocks of size $R \times R$. The spatial sensitivity variations of the RF-receiver coils introduce spatial variations of SNR in the image. Following Eq. 2.22, the SNR of voxel $\rho = (q, q', l)$ located at $\Delta x \cdot (q, (q' + (l-1)N/R)$ is then given by:

$$SNR_\rho^{red} = \frac{1}{\sqrt{R}} \frac{|m_\rho^{avg}|}{\sqrt{\left[(\mathbf{C}^{(q,q')})^H \boldsymbol{\Psi}^{-1} \mathbf{C}^{(q,q')} \right]_{l,l}^{-1}}} (\Delta x)^2 N.$$

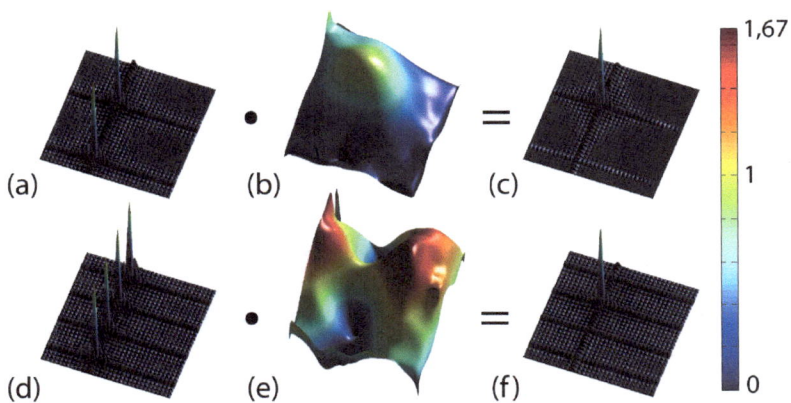

Figure 2.13: SRF of SENSE reconstruction. Top row: Acceleration factor $R = 2$. Bottom row: Acceleration factor $R = 4$. (a,d) Undersampling results in a reduced FOV with R aliasing peaks along the phase encoding direction for pure Fourier encoding. (b,e) "Virtual" sensitivity weighting (from 8 RF coils) ensures zero weighting at the aliased image positions and unity weighting at the location of interest. Outside of these discrete locations, the sensitivity weighting is as small as possible. For $R = 2$ and the chosen coil geometry, the weighting is almost everywhere below unity. This is not the case for the higher acceleration factor $R = 4$. (c,f) The SRF of SENSE reconstruction is formed by the multiplication of the Fourier SRF and the sensitivity weighting. All aliasing peaks are effectively suppressed. The beneficial behavior of the sensitivity weighting for $R = 2$ also improves the sidelobe behavior of the Fourier SRF. This is not everywhere the case for $R = 4$. However, the adverse effect is negligible.

It is useful to compare the SNR in the image voxels resulting from undersampling with the optimal SNR achievable without undersampling (i.e., for $R = 1$, where $\mathbf{C}^{(q,q')} \to \mathbf{c}_\rho$):

$$SNR_\rho^{full} = \frac{|m_\rho^{avg}|}{\sqrt{(\mathbf{c}_\rho^H \boldsymbol{\Psi}^{-1} \mathbf{c}_\rho)^{-1}}} (\Delta x)^2 N = |m_\rho^{avg}| \sqrt{\mathbf{c}_\rho^H \boldsymbol{\Psi}^{-1} \mathbf{c}_\rho} (\Delta x)^2 N$$

$$= |m_\rho^{avg}| \sqrt{\left[(\mathbf{C}^{(q,q')})^H \boldsymbol{\Psi}^{-1} \mathbf{C}^{(q,q')} \right]_{l,l}} (\Delta x)^2 N. \tag{2.48}$$

The noise figure SNR_ρ^{full} corresponds to the SNR resulting from Roemer's optimal coil combination (also cf. Eq. 2.42). The SNR of SENSE reconstruction then reads:

$$SNR_\rho^{red} = \frac{SNR_\rho^{full}}{\sqrt{Rg_\rho}}.\tag{2.49}$$

In this formula, the g-factor has been introduced:

$$g_\rho = \sqrt{\left[(\mathbf{C}^{(q,q')})^H \mathbf{\Psi}^{-1} \mathbf{C}^{(q,q')}\right]_{l,l}^{-1} \left[(\mathbf{C}^{(q,q')})^H \mathbf{\Psi}^{-1} \mathbf{C}^{(q,q')}\right]_{l,l}} \geq 1.\tag{2.50}$$

The g-factor describes the spatial variations of loss of SNR caused by under-sampling. It is not below unity.[18]

d)   Ultimate SNR

In the previous section, it has been shown how the SNR in the image depends on the geometry of one certain RF-receiver coil array. This problem may be taken a step further: What is the best SNR that can be achieved with an optimal coil geometry? It turns out that an optimal coil geometry for one image voxel is generally sub-optimal for a different voxel. Nevertheless, it is useful to analyze the best possible SNR for each image voxel independently because this procedure allows one to define an upper bound of SNR for each image voxel. By comparing the optimal "ultimate" SNR with the SNR of a particular RF-receiver coil array, non-optimal properties of the coil can be identified.

The concept of ultimate intrinsic SNR was introduced to MRI in [117] and extended to parallel imaging a few years later [119, 200]. The solution found by Wiesinger et al. [200] shows that the ultimate SNR can be described simultaneously for fully sampled datasets as well as undersampled datasets. The main ideas are described in this section.

---

[18]This can be proven with the Cauchy-Schwarz inequality: For notational convenience set $\mathbf{A} := (\mathbf{C}^{(q,q')})^H \mathbf{\Psi}^{-1} \mathbf{C}^{(q,q')}$. It is to be shown that $(\mathbf{A})_{l,l} \cdot (\mathbf{A}^{-1})_{l,l} \geq 1$. Note that $\mathbf{A}$ is Hermitian. Therefore it only has real eigenvalues and can be diagonalized such that $\mathbf{A} = \mathbf{U}^H \mathbf{\Lambda}^2 \mathbf{U}$, where $\mathbf{\Lambda}^2$ contains the eigenvalues and $\mathbf{U}$ is a unitary matrix. Defining $\mathbf{u}$ as the l-th column of $\mathbf{U}$, it is straightforward to show that $(\mathbf{A})_{l,l} = \|\mathbf{\Lambda}\mathbf{u}\|^2$ and $(\mathbf{A}^{-1})_{l,l} = \|\mathbf{\Lambda}^{-1}\mathbf{u}\|^2$. With the Cauchy-Schwarz inequality it follows that $(\mathbf{A})_{l,l} \cdot (\mathbf{A}^{-1})_{l,l} = \|\mathbf{\Lambda}\mathbf{u}\|^2 \cdot \|\mathbf{\Lambda}^{-1}\mathbf{u}\|^2 \geq |(\mathbf{\Lambda}\mathbf{u})^H(\mathbf{\Lambda}^{-1}\mathbf{u})|^2 = |\mathbf{u}^H(\mathbf{\Lambda}\mathbf{\Lambda}^{-1})\mathbf{u}|^2 = |\mathbf{u}^H \mathbb{1}\mathbf{u}|^2 = \|\mathbf{u}\|^4 = 1$. The latter equality holds because $\mathbf{U}$ is unitary.

Recall that in SENSE the sensitivity weighting suppresses aliasing from reduced gradient encoding by ensuring that the constraint $c_\rho^{virt}(\vec{x}_{\rho'}) = \delta_{\rho,\rho'}$ (cf. Eq. 2.47) is satisfied, where ρ and ρ' are members of a group of aliased voxels at the locations $\vec{x}_\rho, \vec{x}_{\rho'}$. According to Eq. 2.46, c_ρ^{virt} is a linear combination of the individual sensitivities of the RF-receiver array. The weighting factors are determined in post-processing. The sensitivity c_ρ^{virt} is therefore not physically implemented; it is a sensitivity from a *virtual* coil. In the context of ultimate SNR, it is important to realize that the linearity of the coil combination entails that it would actually be possible - at least in principle - to physically construct a single coil which would have the very same sensitivity c_ρ^{virt}. This procedure would not be practical because a different coil configuration would be necessary for each reconstructed image voxel [145]. However, for the analysis of ultimate SNR it is sufficient to know that such a configuration could in fact be built. Thus, the constraint $c_\rho^{virt}(\vec{x}_{\rho'}) = \delta_{\rho,\rho'}$ has a concrete physical interpretation; according to the definition of the RF-coil sensitivity in Eq. 1.16, page 22, this constraint can be expressed in terms of the magnetic properties of the coil:

$$\left[\vec{\mathcal{B}}_x^{virt,\rho} - i\vec{\mathcal{B}}_y^{virt,\rho} \right](\vec{x}_{\rho'}) = \delta_{\rho,\rho'}. \tag{2.51}$$

The noise received with this virtual coil is, with Eqs. 1.17, 1.18, proportional to its sample resistance:

$$\psi_\rho \propto \int_V \sigma(\vec{x}) |\vec{\mathcal{E}}_\rho^{virt}(\vec{x})|^2 \, d\vec{x}. \tag{2.52}$$

The important result from the two latter equations is that noise and constraints imposed by the reconstruction are expressed in terms of electromagnetic quantities only: the noise by the coil's electric fields and the constraints by the coil's magnetic fields. The Maxwell equations couple the electric field with the magnetic field. Therefore, noise and the demanded magnetic constraints have to be treated simultaneously. There are many virtual coils which fulfill the constraint of Eq. 2.51 and it is the task of ultimate SNR to find that particular virtual coil which has the lowest noise resistance in the sample. But how can such a virtual coil be characterized? A virtual coil is characterized by the fact that a physical counterpart might exist. In order to keep the discussion simple, it is assumed that the virtual coils are represented by any current distribution outside of a spherical volume of radius r. The object to be imaged is assumed to (a) fill the sphere completely

(b) to be source-free and (c) to have scalar, homogeneous dielectric constant ϵ, magnetic permeability μ and conductivity σ. These assumptions are fairly well met under typical imaging conditions, more deeply discussed in [200]. Under these conditions, the set of all virtual coils is equivalent to the solution space of the source-free Maxwell equations:

$$\nabla \cdot \vec{\mathcal{E}}(\vec{x}, t) \;=\; 0, \quad \nabla \times \vec{\mathcal{E}}(\vec{x}, t) = -\frac{\partial \vec{\mathfrak{B}}(\vec{x}, t)}{\partial t},$$

$$\nabla \cdot \vec{\mathfrak{B}}(\vec{x}, t) \;=\; 0, \quad \nabla \times \vec{\mathfrak{B}}(\vec{x}, t) = \mu\epsilon\frac{\partial \vec{\mathcal{E}}(\vec{x}, t)}{\partial t} + \mu\sigma\vec{\mathcal{E}}(\vec{x}, t).$$

Considering that the solutions oscillate at the Larmor frequency, the spatial distribution can be separated from the temporal evolution leading to the following set of time-independent equations:

$$(\Delta + k_0^2)\vec{\mathfrak{B}}(\vec{x}) = 0, \quad \nabla \cdot \vec{\mathfrak{B}}(\vec{x}, t) = 0, \quad \text{where} \ \ k_0^2 = \omega\mu(\omega\epsilon + i\sigma),$$

$$\text{and} \ \ \vec{\mathcal{E}}(\vec{x}) = \frac{1}{\mu(\sigma - i\omega\epsilon)}\nabla \times \vec{\mathfrak{B}}(\vec{x}). \tag{2.53}$$

The solution space of these equations is a vector space. The basis functions that span the magnetic solution space are denoted here as $\vec{v}_j^M(\cdot)$ with $j \in \mathbb{N}$. The corresponding electric basis functions $\vec{v}_j^E(\cdot)$ can be calculated from their magnetic counterparts by virtue of the third formula in Eq. 2.53. Electric and magnetic sensitivity of the virtual coil are then described as a linear combination of those basis functions:

$$\vec{\mathcal{E}}_\rho^{virt}(\vec{x}) = \sum_j w_{\rho,j}\vec{v}_j^E(\vec{x}) \quad \text{and} \quad \vec{\mathfrak{B}}_\rho^{virt}(\vec{x}) = \sum_j w_{\rho,j}\vec{v}_j^M(\vec{x}).$$

Finding the optimal virtual coil is equivalent to finding an optimal weighting matrix $\mathbf{W}$ whose elements are the weights $w_{\rho,j}$. Ocali et al. [117] used a set of linear basis functions. Wiesinger et al. [200] later argued that many fewer basis functions (typically $< 10^5$) need to be considered for fairly accurate results when a multipole expansion of the fields is used.[19] With the basis functions, the constraint formulated above in Eq. 2.51 can be expressed in a form more suited for numerical treatment:

$$\mathbf{WS} = \mathbb{1}, \quad \text{where} \ \ S_{j,\rho} = \mu\left[(\vec{v}_j^M)_x - i(\vec{v}_j^M)_y\right](\vec{x}_\rho).$$

---

[19]Consult Appendix B in [200] for a detailed presentation of the multipole basis functions.

According to Eq. 2.52, the noise present in voxel ρ becomes:

$$\psi_\rho = (\mathbf{W}\boldsymbol{\Psi}\mathbf{W}^H)_{\rho,\rho}, \quad \text{where} \quad \Psi_{j,j'} \propto \sigma \int_V \vec{v}_j^E(\vec{x})\vec{v}_{j'}^E(\vec{x})^* \, d\vec{x}.$$

Following the same arguments that are used in section 2.1.5, page 56f, the optimal SNR can then be found for all voxels independently by solving the problem $\min_{\mathbf{W}} \mathrm{Tr}(\mathbf{W}\tilde{\boldsymbol{\Psi}}\mathbf{W}^H)$ subject to $\mathbf{WS} = \mathbb{1}$. This optimization problem has a structure that also is known from section 2.1.5, page 56f, with the solution:

$$\mathbf{W} = (\mathbf{S}^H\boldsymbol{\Psi}^{-1}\mathbf{S})^{-1}\mathbf{S}^H\boldsymbol{\Psi}^{-1}.$$

With the optimal weights, the quantity of interest can be calculated; for example, ultimate noise, SNR or g-factor. As an example, the solution to the ultimate g-factor is presented here:

$$g_\rho^{ult} = \sqrt{\left[(\mathbf{S}^H\boldsymbol{\Psi}^{-1}\mathbf{S})^{-1}\right]_{\rho,\rho}(\mathbf{S}^H\boldsymbol{\Psi}^{-1}\mathbf{S})_{\rho,\rho}} \geq 1.$$

Note that this formula is very similar to the formula found for the g-factor of a certain coil geometry in Eq. 2.50. In Fig. 2.14 ultimate g-factor maps are compared to g-factor maps of a typical industrial RF-receiver coil with eight elements.

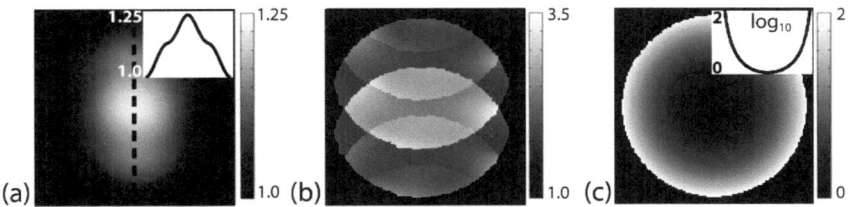

Figure 2.14: Ultimate g-factor for SENSE imaging at $3\,\mathrm{T}$. (a) For SENSE imaging with acceleration factor 4, the ultimate g-factor has values of only up to 1.25 with a maximum at the center. (b) Compared to the ultimate g-factor, a typical state-of-the-art eight-channel head receiver array has a g-factor of up to 3.5. Comparison with the ultimate g-factor can be useful to detect sub-optimal behavior in certain regions. (c) The ultimate SNR (normalized to unity), however, has a very sharp increase in feasible SNR toward the edge of the object. The reason for this increase is that higher-order field components vanish quickly toward the center of the object with increasing distance from the hypothetical conductors. Note the log-scale in (c) and the different scaling in (a-c).

e)   Superresolution Reconstruction

Recall from section 2.3.1b, page 79f, that, in Cartesian SENSE, the sensitivity weighting suppresses aliasing, but has no influence on image resolution. In SENSE, image resolution is uniquely determined by the gradient encoding scheme. Sánchez-González et al. [170] observed that an increase in image resolution (termed *"superresolution"* in [125]) is achieved when SENSE is replaced by a method called *minimum-norm reconstruction*.

Why is superresolution achieved with the minimum-norm reconstruction and not with SENSE? How can the superresolution effect be quantified? The goal of this section is to give answers to these questions and to draw some conclusions. An analysis of the quantification problem has been presented previously in [[160]].

Explanation of Superresolution   To understand why superresolution is achieved with the minimum-norm reconstruction and not with SENSE, it is useful to analyze the differences between both methods. Recall that SENSE reconstruction is based on the weak matrix approach. On the other hand, the minimum-norm reconstruction is basically a practical implementation of the strong matrix approach (cf. section 2.1.1b, page 45). The question to be answered is therefore rather: Why does the strong approach lead to superresolution and not the weak approach? In section 2.1.1c, page 45ff, it has been argued that the strong approach is more convincing than the weak approach. Whereas the strong approach determines the reconstruction weights by demanding an optimal SRF, the weak approach suffers from the problem that the weights are determined by simply predefining the SRF at a finite number of grid points.

Being based on the weak approach, in SENSE, the SRF is defined to be unity at its voxel center and zero at the centers of all neighboring voxel. The voxel size is chosen to match exactly the voxel size that would result from pure gradient encoding. In SENSE, sensitivity encoding is used to suppress aliasing, but it does not take into account that the variations in the RF-coil sensitivities can also be exploited to improve the SRF on a local scale. This is different when the strong approach is applied because this approach uses all available encoding information to optimize the SRF, thereby suppressing aliasing as well as improving image resolution as far as possible. SENSE may not lead to an improved resolution; however, this does not imply that superresolution could not be achieved with the weak approach. In fact, as shown in section 2.1.1c, page 45ff, weak and strong approaches converge if small voxels are chosen to reconstruct on. Otazo et al. [125] could recently show a superresolution effect for spectroscopic imaging data, if reconstructed with the weak approach onto a finer reconstruction grid than usual.

Quantification How can the superresolution effect be quantified? A good measure for image resolution is the SRF (cf. Eq. 2.16). In the context of superresolution, it is useful to analyze the Fourier-domain representation of the SRF:

$$\hat{f}_\rho(\vec{k}) = \sum_{\alpha,\kappa} F_{\rho,(\alpha,\kappa)}\hat{c}_\alpha(\vec{k} - \vec{k}_\kappa) = \sum_\kappa \hat{c}_{\rho,\kappa}^{eff}(\vec{k} - \vec{k}_\kappa).$$

The k-space representation of the SRF is a weighted sum of the RF-coil sensitivities represented in k-space and shifted by the k-space locations, encoded with the gradients. A wider k-space support of the SRF corresponds to a narrower SRF with improved resolution. Consider the 1D examples of Fig. 2.15. For Fourier encoding with a homogeneous coil the k-space extent is restricted to the acquired k-space grid (Fig. 2.15, left). In PI with non-homogeneous coil sensitivities, the finite k-space footprint of the sensitivities allows an extension of the k-space support of the SRF (Fig. 2.15, middle and right).[20] This is achieved by determining the reconstruction weights for example with the strong approach.

The plots of Fig. 2.15 clearly show that resolution (defined here as the distance between zero-crossings in the SRF) increases with increasing SRF k-space support. Moreover, there even is a decrease in sidelobe intensity corresponding to a reduced Gibbs ringing artifact. For the simulated finite-support sensitivity profiles, k-space support and image resolution both increase by exactly the same amount (50%). The k-space extent of the measured sensitivity profiles cannot be exactly determined because there is no clearly defined cut-off frequency. However, within the limits of accuracy of determining the k-space extent, the increase in image resolution (32%) matches well the increase in k-space ($> 25\%$) also for the measured sensitivity profiles. Considering the simplicity of the method - the k-space SRF only

---

[20]This k-space perspective allows a comparison of superresolution with GRAPPA (see section 2.3.2a, page 97ff): Whereas in GRAPPA, the finite k-space footprint of the receiver coil sensitivities is used to fill the space between acquired k-space lines, in superresolution, it is used to extrapolate the acquired k-space beyond its borders.

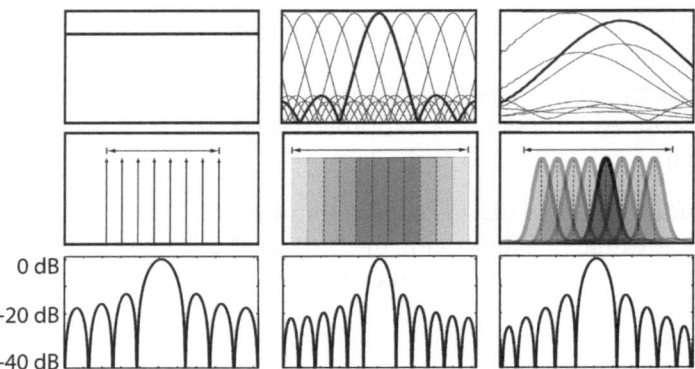

Figure 2.15: 1D Illustration of superresolution. Top row: Sensitivity maps. Central row: Corresponding SRF k-space support for 8 gradient encoding steps. Bottom row: Corresponding image space SRF. Left: Homogeneous profile. Middle: 8 simulated profiles with finite support in k-space. Right: 1D profiles of typical real-world sensitivity maps. The central row illustrates that the width of k-space support for the resulting SRF increases with higher variations of the sensitivity profiles. With the increase in spatial support of the corresponding SRF, the width of the main lobe and numbers of sidelobes scale accordingly. This results in a higher image resolution.

provides a global measure and ignores local properties of the sensitivities - this is a fairly good estimation.

Consider now Fig. 2.16, where 2D measurement results are shown. For the measurements, only a small voxel was excited and encoded with 8×8 and 16×16 k-space locations. The analysis of subfigure (b) illustrates the limitations of superresolution: For 8×8 k-space points, the resolution gain is 32.7%, for 16×16 points, the resolution gain is halved (16.2%). The reason for the decreased efficiency is that the ratio of k-space extension by sensitivity encoding and k-space support from gradient encoding decreases with more gradient encoding steps. For high-resolution imaging (256×256), the expected resolution increase is therefore not expected to be much higher than 1%. The effect is nearly negligible for high-resolution applications. Considering that the increased image resolution also comes at the expense of increased reconstruction time (and also increased noise [170]), it can be concluded that superresolution is restricted to low-resolution applications like spectroscopic imaging. The superresolution effect can be significant also in the context of PatLoc imaging (cf. chapter 7, page 235ff).

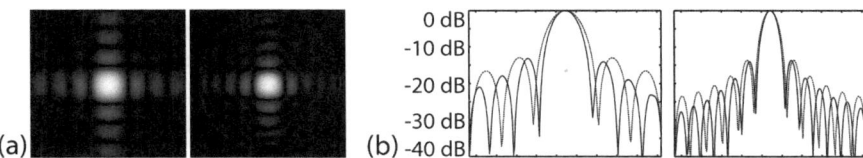

Figure 2.16: (a) Left: PSF for 2D conventional coil-by-coil reconstruction. Right: PSF for superresolution reconstruction. 8x8 k-space points were measured. There is some resolution improvement visible in the right image. (b) Left: 1D profiles through the center of the 2D PSF of subfigure (a). Right: Corresponding 1D profiles for a 16x16 acquisition. The superresolution effect on image resolution is higher for smaller k-space grids.

f) Non-Cartesian Methods

In contrast to Cartesian SENSE, where a regular sampling grid is acquired, non-Cartesian SENSE [134] is a method to reconstruct data encoded with non-Cartesian sampling trajectories. The non-Cartesian sampling destroys the coherent aliasing of Cartesian SENSE with the consequence that the encoding matrix does not have an MPPI which can be calculated sufficiently fast for practical image reconstructions. In Fourier imaging, the problem can be solved, for example, with the gridding method (cf. section 2.2.3, page 69ff). This method is not directly transferable to PI because, with gridding, only small gaps in k-space can be bridged [166]; gridding alone is therefore not suited for undersampled k-space data. Larger k-space shifts can be induced by combining data from several RF channels immediately in k-space. This technique is often used in combination with Cartesian trajectories and is discussed below in section 2.3.2, page 96ff; for non-Cartesian trajectories, such a k-space reconstruction is less efficient, but often still feasible [165].

In the present section, a different, well-established approach is taken, where maximum data consistency of measurement data and the reconstructed image in the l_2-norm sense is ensured. For numerical treatment, the signal equation (Eq. 1.31, page 38) is discretized resulting in the data-consistency constraint $s \approx Em$.[21] Depending on the accuracy of the discretization, this constraint can be fulfilled exactly or only approximately.[22]:

1. For coarse discretizations (i.e., $N_\rho < N_\kappa N_c$), data consistency cannot be ensured. In this case, an image vector m is sought, which minimizes the data-inconsistency $\|s - Em\|^2$. The first order necessary conditions to this minimization problem result in the equation $(E^H E)m = E^H s$.

2. For fine discretizations (i.e., $N_\rho > N_\kappa N_c$), an infinite number of image vectors is often consistent with the measurement data. Therefore, an image vector might be sought with minimum norm. Following equivalent arguments as used in section 2.1.5, page 56f, the solution would be found by first solving for the (redefined) Lagrange multipliers $(EE^H)\lambda = s$ and then using these to find the reconstructed image: $m = E^H \lambda$.

Even with fine reconstruction grids, data consistency is only ensured if full rank encodings E are considered. Well-chosen encoding schemes should have this property; however, very low eigenvalues often occur, and therefore poorly conditioned equations result. As a consequence, it is often useful to regularize the reconstruction [31]. A well-known regularization method is Tikhonov regularization, where the solution is found by minimizing $\|Em - s\|^2 + \zeta^2 \|m\|^2$. The parameter ζ is called *Tikhonov regularization parameter*. This approach is feasible for both coarse and fine discretizations and has the solution:

$$(A + \zeta^2 \mathbb{1})m = \tilde{s} \quad \text{with} \quad A = E^H E \text{ and } \tilde{s} = E^H s.$$

A very good presentation of Tikhonov regularization and the problem of finding adequate regularization parameters is found in [69].

Note that it can always be ensured that the matrix A is Hermitian and positive definite. Very well suited for the solution of large-scaled Hermitian, positive definite linear systems is the linear conjugate gradient method (CG method). The CG method was also used in this thesis several times and is briefly presented in the next section. Other methods are occasionally

---

[21] W. l. o. g. the matrix $\Delta V \cdot E$ is simply written as E here.
[22] This property is very similar to the different interpretations of the MPPI, cf. page 43f in section 2.1.1.

encountered in the MRI literature, among them a method called *algebraic reconstruction technique,* which makes use of the Kaczmarz iterations [19, 178].

Remark: There is a fundamental difference between the iterative method and the matrix approach: Whereas the matrix approach solves the reconstruction problem by *inverting* the encoding matrix (which can be problematic), the iterative method seeks to find a solution by several consecutive *forward evaluations* of the encoding model, an approach that is often less demanding. As a consequence, the reconstruction matrix $\mathbf{F}$ is actually never determined with the iterative approach. On the one hand, the matrix approach has the advantage that once the reconstruction matrix is determined reconstruction reduces to a mere matrix-vector multiplication: $\mathbf{m} = \mathbf{Fs}$. The iterative method on the other hand has the advantage that inversion of the very large matrix $\mathbf{E}^H\mathbf{E}$ is avoided by solving the least-squares problem $\|\mathbf{Em} - \mathbf{s}\|^2$. Note that for the matrix approach $\mathbf{F}$ is determined independent from the data $\mathbf{s}$. Therefore, an abstract approach involving the concept of voxel functions (see section 2.1.1, page 40ff.) is used to derive $\mathbf{F}$. The iterative method depends inherently on the data and therefore the approach taken is less abstract only involving the data-consistency constraint $\mathbf{s} \approx \mathbf{Em}$, whose meaning can easily be grasped.

In spite of the differences of the matrix approach and the iterative method, these methods are closely related to each other. Such a close relationship has already been declared in the *Remark* on page 44f in section 2.1.1. Concerning the data consistency, the relationship manifests as follows: Consider the first case above with $N_\rho < N_\kappa N_c$ and assume full rank encodings $\mathbf{E}$. Then $\mathbf{E}^H\mathbf{E}$ is invertible and the data-consistency constraint $(\mathbf{E}^H\mathbf{E})\mathbf{m} = \mathbf{E}^H\mathbf{s}$ has the unique solution $\mathbf{m} = (\mathbf{E}^H\mathbf{E})^{-1}\mathbf{E}^H\mathbf{s} = \mathbf{E}^+\mathbf{s}$. This is, however, also the MPPI solution found with the matrix approach. Similar arguments show the equivalence of the two approaches also for the case $N_\rho > N_\kappa N_c$.

Linear Conjugate Gradient Method The linear conjugate gradient method (CG method) was proposed by Hestenes and Stiefel in 1952 [65]. It is a conjugate direction method with interesting properties, well described in [169] and theoretically analyzed in [115] for real-valued quantities. Equivalent formulations exist also for complex-valued variables as already pointed out by Hestenes and Stiefel in [65].

The key point about the CG method is that minimization of the quadratic function $\phi(\mathbf{m}) := 1/2 \cdot \mathbf{m}^T \mathbf{A}\mathbf{m} - \tilde{\mathbf{s}}^T \mathbf{m}$ is equivalent to solving the linear system $\mathbf{A}\mathbf{m} = \tilde{\mathbf{s}}$. The square matrix $\mathbf{A}$ should be Hermitian and positive definite.

The rough procedure of the algorithm is the following: Starting from an initial guess $\mathbf{m}_0$, a series of intermediate solutions $\mathbf{m}_1, \mathbf{m}_2, \ldots$ is calculated. The next intermediate solution $\mathbf{m}_{k+1}$ is found by the vector sum of only the previous solution $\mathbf{m}_k$ and the previous conjugate direction $\mathbf{p}_k$, characterized by $\mathbf{p}_i^T \mathbf{A}\mathbf{p}_j = 0$ for all $i \neq j$:

$$\mathbf{m}_{k+1} := \mathbf{m}_k + \alpha_k \mathbf{p}_k.$$

The step length $\alpha_k \in \mathbb{R}$ is chosen to be the one-dimensional minimizer of $\phi(\mathbf{m}_k + \alpha_k \mathbf{p}_k)$ resulting in $\alpha_k = \|\mathbf{r}_k\| \cdot \|\mathbf{p}_k\|_{\mathbf{A}}^{-1}$.[23] The next conjugate direction $\mathbf{p}_{k+1}$ is constructed as a linear combination of the current steepest descent direction $-\mathbf{r}_{k+1} := -\nabla\phi(\mathbf{m}_{k+1}) = -\mathbf{A}\mathbf{m}_{k+1} + \tilde{\mathbf{s}} = -\mathbf{r}_k - \alpha_k \mathbf{A}\mathbf{p}_k$ and the last conjugate gradient direction: $\mathbf{p}_{k+1} = -\mathbf{r}_{k+1} + \beta_{k+1}\mathbf{p}_k$, where $\beta_{k+1} = \|\mathbf{r}_{k+1}\| \cdot \|\mathbf{r}_k\|^{-1}$. An efficient version of the linear conjugate gradient algorithm is given below in pseudo-code. For more details, refer to the textbook [115] or to the publication [134].

As initial conjugate direction $\mathbf{p}_0$, the steepest descent direction $\mathbf{r}_0$ is chosen. Without useful prior information, it is a good initial guess to set $\mathbf{m}_0 = 0$. In this case, the first iteration yields $\mathbf{m}_1 = \tilde{\mathbf{s}} = \mathbf{E}^H \mathbf{s}$, which represents the back-projection of the image and therefore an approximation to the solution of the problem.[24]

It is a well-known theoretical result that without noise the CG method converges at latest after N_ρ iterations. In MRI N_ρ is very large ($\approx 10^5$ for 2D imaging) and therefore the CG method seems to be unpractical. Even worse, convergence breaks down for noisy data, and MRI data are inherently noisy. In practice, however, the best result is typically found after about $20 - 40$ iterations already. The reason for this fast "practical convergence" is that the CG method has a self-regularizing property [138]: The low spatial frequencies converge faster than the high spatial frequencies, noise included.

---

[23]The expression $\|\cdot\|_{\mathbf{A}}$ represents a weighted norm, defined as $\|\mathbf{v}\|_{\mathbf{A}} := \mathbf{v}^H \mathbf{A}\mathbf{v}$ for an arbitrary vector $\mathbf{v}$. It is straightforward to verify that, for the matrix $\mathbf{A}$, assumed to be Hermitian and positive definite, $\|\cdot\|_{\mathbf{A}}$ is a well-defined vector norm.

[24]Another advantage of the zero image as initialization of the algorithm is that correct scaling of the initial image guess is not an issue.

Algorithm 2.1 Linear conjugate gradient algorithm

1: Choose the initial vector $\mathbf{m}_0 = \mathbf{0}$.
2: and set $\mathbf{r}_0 \rightarrow \mathbf{A}\mathbf{m}_0 - \tilde{\mathbf{s}}$, $\mathbf{p}_0 \rightarrow -\mathbf{r}_0$, $k \rightarrow 0$;
3: **for** $k = 0, 1, 2, \ldots$ **do**
4:      Set $\mathbf{q}_k = \mathbf{A}\mathbf{p}_k$;
5:      Set $\alpha_k \rightarrow \frac{\mathbf{r}_k^T \mathbf{r}_k}{\mathbf{p}_k^T \mathbf{q}_k}$;
6:      Set $\mathbf{m}_{k+1} \rightarrow \mathbf{m}_k + \alpha_k \mathbf{p}_k$;
7:      Set $\mathbf{r}_{k+1} \rightarrow \mathbf{r}_k + \alpha_k \mathbf{q}_k$;
8:      Set $\beta_{k+1} \rightarrow \frac{\mathbf{r}_{k+1}^T \mathbf{r}_{k+1}}{\mathbf{r}_k^T \mathbf{r}_k}$;
9:      Set $\mathbf{p}_{k+1} \rightarrow -\mathbf{r}_{k+1} + \beta_{k+1}\mathbf{p}_k$;
10:      Set $k \rightarrow k + 1$;
11:      **if** convergence test satisfied **then**
12:          **stop** with approximate solution $\mathbf{m}_{k+1}$.
13:      **end if**
14: **end for**

It is therefore useful to just stop the algorithm before noise accumulation occurs, be it after a certain number of iterations or based on the fulfillment of a suitable stopping criterion.[25] Refer to [134] to get more information on useful stopping criteria and practical ways of implementing adequate preconditioners to improve the convergence behavior. Fig. 2.17 illustrates the self-regularizing property of the CG method.

Practical Implementation of the CG Method for Iterative SENSE The bottleneck of the algorithm is the matrix-vector multiplication $\mathbf{q}_k = \mathbf{A}\mathbf{p}_k$ with $\mathbf{A} = \mathbf{E}^H \mathbf{E}$. The time-consuming and - depending on the actual implementation - also memory intensive operation is the matrix-vector multiplication of $\mathbf{E}$ and its adjoint $\mathbf{E}^H$ with the corresponding vectors. However, $\mathbf{E}$ is structured in SENSE imaging and the matrix-vector multiplication can be accelerated. In order to find an efficient implementation, consider that, according to Eq. 2.9, the encoding matrix separates into two sparse matrices,

---

[25]Note that early termination makes the *linear* CG method a *nonlinear* reconstruction; however, the introduced nonlinearities diminish with more iterations, and are typically almost negligible when the algorithm is terminated in practice, usually after $20 - 40$ iterations.

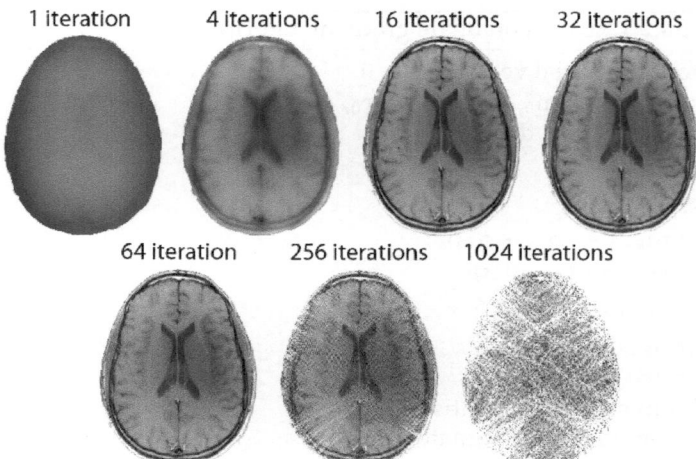

Figure 2.17: Self-regularizing property of the CG method. Shown are intermediate images for a non-Cartesian SENSE reconstruction. The brain imaging data have been acquired with a twofold undersampled radial trajectory. The first iteration corresponds to a simple back-projection resulting in a blurred image. It is clearly visible that the image resolution enhances with increasing iterations. After 32 iterations roughly, the blurring does not diminish any more, however, noise and reconstruction artifacts from setting the RF-sensitivity data to zero outside the object border (also cf. [170]) increase resulting in visibly degraded image quality after 64 iterations.

whose entries are easily calculated when delta functions are chosen as ideal voxel shapes:

$$\mathbf{E} = \mathbf{GC},$$
$$\text{with } G_{(\alpha,\kappa),(\alpha',\rho')} = \delta_{\alpha,\alpha'} e^{-i\vec{k}_\kappa \vec{x}'_\rho} \text{ and } C_{(\alpha,\rho'),\rho} = \delta_{\rho',\rho} c_\alpha(\vec{x}_\rho). \tag{2.54}$$

The matrix-vector multiplication of $\mathbf{C}$ with the corresponding vector is actually only an N_c-fold vector-vector multiplication and therefore very quick. The gradient encoding matrix $\mathbf{G}$ is sparse only in that sense that each coil image can be treated separately. For each single coil image, $\mathbf{G}$ is densely populated. However, fast algorithms exist at least for regular reconstruction grids $\mathcal{G}_{cart}$. One possibility are standard gridding algorithms (cf. the paragraph *Gridding Algorithm* on page 70f in section 2.2.3), which have been proposed to be used in the original publication dealing with non-Cartesian SENSE [134]. Other efficient implementations of the nuFFT such as the min-max interpolation method of Fessler et al. [36] may be used instead. The adjoint operation $\mathbf{G}^H$ can be performed in a similar manner [134, 36] and $\mathbf{C}^H$ is also effectively only a vector-vector multiplication. It can therefore be concluded that the structure of the encoding matrix in non-Cartesian SENSE imaging enables fairly quick implementations of the CG algorithm. Moreover, the presented algorithms are vastly parallelizable. This feature can be exploited to speed up the reconstruction even further. A practical reconstruction algorithm using linear CG and the nuFFT approach is depicted in Fig. 2.18.

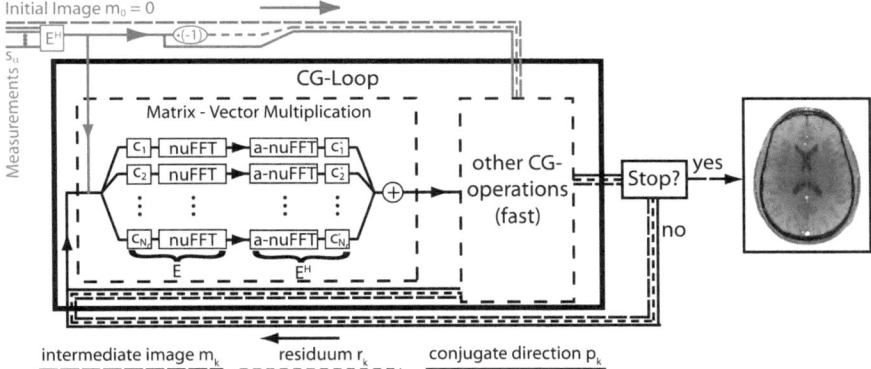

Figure 2.18: SENSE reconstruction for non-Cartesian trajectories with the CG method. The CG method is an iterative method. After initialization, the CG loop is iterated until a stopping criterion is met. The CG loop has three input variables: The first variable is the intermediate image $\mathbf{m}_k$. The second variable is the residuum $\mathbf{r}_k$, which measures the data consistency of intermediate image with the measurement data and the third variable is the current conjugate direction $\mathbf{p}_k$. There are some advantages to using a zero-image as the initial guess. In this case, the first conjugate direction is found by multiplying the signal measurement data with the Hermitian of the encoding matrix $\mathbf{E}$ and the initial residuum is calculated as its negative value. These initial variables are fed into the CG loop. Numerically the most demanding part of the CG loop is the matrix-vector multiplication of $\mathbf{E}^H\mathbf{E}$ with the conjugate direction $\mathbf{p}_k$. This matrix-vector multiplication can be accelerated by exploiting the structure of the SENSE encoding matrix. The matrix-vector multiplication reduces to $2N_c$ vector-vector multiplications comprising the vectorized RF-coil sensitivity data and N_c nuFFT operations plus the computation of their adjoints. At last, the individual vectors are summed up. The resulting vector together with the intermediate image $\mathbf{m}_k$, the residuum $\mathbf{r}_k$ and the conjugate direction $\mathbf{p}_k$ are then subject to additional fast vector-vector multiplications. Typical 2D image reconstruction require about $kmax = 20 - 40$ iterations until the stopping criterion is met and the final image is found by de-vectorizing $\mathbf{m}_{kmax}$.

2.3.2 k-**Space Reconstruction**

In 1997, at the 5th Scientific Meeting of the ISMRM[26], Daniel Sodickson presented (cf. [172]) a new imaging technique that marked a milestone in the history of MRI: He demonstrated cardiac in vivo images which were acquired very fast by replacing some of the sequential gradient encoding by parallel encoding with a multi-coil receiver array. His technique, which he gave the name SMASH (SiMultaneous Acquisition of Spatial Harmonics) [173], is based on the idea that low spatial harmonics can not only be generated by the gradients, but also approximately by a weighted sum of the RF-sensitivity profiles. Different weighting of the coil array signals can therefore induce small shifts in k-space; as a consequence, the sampling density of gradient encoding can be reduced with the advantage that the whole encoding process is accelerated.

It is evident that the RF coils cannot exactly mimic spatial harmonics, but only approximately. The original method therefore suffered from residual aliasing. These initial problems could be reduced significantly within the following years. An important improvement marked AUTO-SMASH [75, 58] where explicit acquisition of RF-coil sensitivity maps was avoided and replaced by the acquisition of a restricted amount of additional *auto-calibration k-space signal* (ACS) *lines*. This method was then improved even further and resulted in 2002 in GRAPPA (GeneRalized Autocalibrating Partially Parallel Acquisitions) by Griswold et al. [49]. GRAPPA and variants thereof are often used in the clinical routine today. Also in this thesis, GRAPPA plays a role and therefore the GRAPPA algorithm is presented in this section without going into the details.

GRAPPA [49] and SENSE are similar because both solve the same problem: image reconstruction from an undersampled Cartesian[27] trajectory. However, there are also fundamental differences between the two methods: In contrast to SENSE, which solves the problem in image space, GRAPPA is formulated in k-space. Another difference is that in SENSE RF-sensitivity profiles are explicitly determined, whereas in GRAPPA, sensitivity information is only used implicitly by the incorporation of additional ACS-lines. Also consider that the approximate approach taken with GRAPPA is re-

---

[26]International Society for Magnetic Resonance in Medicine

[27]Non-Cartesian GRAPPA is not treated here. Consult [48, 166, 165, 167] for more information on this topic.

Step One: GRAPPA Weight Determination

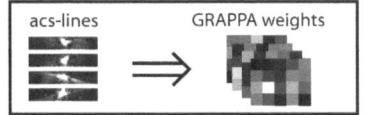

Step Two: Reconstruction

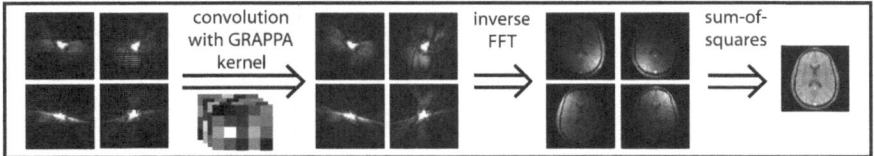

Figure 2.19: GRAPPA reconstruction algorithm. GRAPPA consists of two steps. In a first step, the GRAPPA weights are determined from the fully sampled auto-calibration lines. More details on how the weights are determined is found in the main text. In a second step, the magnetization is reconstructed. First, the missing k-space lines are filled in by convolving the measured signals with the precalculated GRAPPA weights. Then a coil-wise Fourier transform is performed and a root-sum-of-squares coil combination finalizes the reconstruction.

sponsible for (often beneficial) differences in image properties compared to the stringent SENSE-matrix approach. In spite of these differences both methods are closely related to each other and this chapter ends with linking both methods to one another by establishing a connection between the GRAPPA weights and the SENSE reconstruction matrix.

a) GRAPPA (GeneRalized Autocalibrating Partially Parallel Acquisitions)

GRAPPA uses a subsampled Cartesian imaging trajectory as input. Some additional, fully sampled k-space lines are acquired at the center of k-space (i.e., ACS-lines).[28] In a first step, so-called GRAPPA weights are calculated from the ACS lines. In a second step, the missing lines are filled in using the precalculated GRAPPA weights, then a coil-wise inverse 2D-FFT is performed and finally the coil images are combined, for example using a root-sum-of-squares (defined in fn. 10 on page 35). These reconstruction steps are illustrated in Fig. 2.19. The two decisive operations, reconstruction

---

[28]The optimal number of lines depends on many parameters (e.g. reduction factor, kernel size); typical are 24 ACS lines for 256×256-measurements (omitted k-space lines included). More on optimal selection of parameters for GRAPPA can be found in [114] or [6].

of the missing k-space lines and determination of the GRAPPA weights, are briefly described in the following two paragraphs. A detailed presentation of the GRAPPA algorithm is found for example in [5].

Reconstruction of Missing k-Space Lines The basic assumption in GRAPPA is that the signal s_α of each coil at a certain k-space position $\vec{k}_\kappa$ can be represented by a weighted sum of all coil signals at nearby k-space positions:

$$s_\alpha(\vec{k}_\kappa) = \sum_{\alpha',\beta} w_{\alpha',\beta}^{(\alpha)} s_{\alpha'}(\vec{k}_\kappa - \vec{k}_\beta). \tag{2.55}$$

The (shift-invariant) weighting factors are often called *GRAPPA weights*. In GRAPPA, this relation between the signals of neighboring k-space locations is exploited to accelerate Cartesian k-space trajectories by only acquiring each R-th k-space line. The $m = 1, \ldots, R - 1$ missing lines are then reconstructed based on the latter equation. Only the closest neighbors are considered, i.e., a small GRAPPA kernel $\mathcal{L}$ is chosen, for example 4 values along the y-direction and 5 along the x-direction. For further treatment, it is useful to write Eq. 2.55 in matrix-vector form:

$$\mathbf{s}_\alpha = \mathbf{w}_\alpha^{(m)} \hat{\mathbf{E}}_s^{(m)}, \quad \text{where} \quad (\hat{E}_s^{(m)})_{(\alpha',\beta),\kappa} := s_{\alpha'}(\vec{k}_\kappa - \vec{k}_\beta^{(m)}). \tag{2.56}$$

Here, the superscript m indicates that for each of the $m = 1, \ldots, R - 1$ missing k-space lines a separate set of GRAPPA weights needs to be considered: For $\beta = (\beta_x, \beta_y) \in \mathcal{L}$ the relative k-space shifts $\vec{k}_\beta^{(m)} = 2\pi\Delta k \cdot (\beta_x \vec{e}_x + (\beta_y R - m)\vec{e}_y)$ are different for each line.

Weight Determination The reconstruction is only feasible when the GRAPPA weights $\mathbf{w}_\alpha^{(m)}$ are known in advance. To this end, a sufficient number of ACS-lines s_α^{ACS} is acquired at the k-space center; these fully sampled lines are then used to estimate the weights $\mathbf{w}_\alpha^{(m)}$ by solving the following least-squares problem for each α and m independently:

$$\min_{\mathbf{w}_\alpha^{(m)}} \left\| \mathbf{w}_\alpha^{(m)} \hat{\mathbf{E}}_s^{(m,ACS)} - \mathbf{s}_\alpha^{ACS} \right\|^2. \tag{2.57}$$

In this equation, the matrix $\hat{\mathbf{E}}_s^{(m,ACS)}$ is formed for the ACS-lines only. Note that there is a fundamental difference to the reconstruction problem: In the reconstruction problem, the weights are known and the signal data are determined. In the weight determination step, the weights are not known and they are determined from known measurement data. The solution of the above minimization problem is given by:

$$\mathbf{w}_\alpha^{(m)} = \mathbf{s}_\alpha^{ACS} (\hat{\mathbf{E}}_s^{(m,ACS)})^+. \tag{2.58}$$

b) Relationship of GRAPPA and SENSE

The relationship of GRAPPA and SENSE has been a topic of discussion for quite a while and new aspects are still being discovered (e.g. [104]). In most publications, only specific aspects of the problem are analyzed; an overall picture is formed by bringing the different aspects together. The approach taken here merges ideas presented in [135, 49, 209, 147, 136, 104].

How can the problem of relating two methods to one another be approached? For an exact analysis, a mathematical point of view is often useful. Compare the latter equation (Eq. 2.58) with the solution of the matrix approach taken for SENSE, represented by Eq. 2.15. In both cases, GRAPPA and SENSE, a matrix is inverted. The reconstruction result is very similar, therefore also the involved matrices $\mathbf{E}$ for SENSE and $\hat{\mathbf{E}}_s$ for GRAPPA should be closely related to each other. But what is the exact relation between $\mathbf{E}$ and $\hat{\mathbf{E}}_s$?

First, it is useful to also describe the encoding matrix $\mathbf{E}$ in k-space by defining $\hat{\mathbf{E}} := \mathbf{E} \cdot \mathbf{iDFT}$. Interestingly, the k-space encoding matrix $\hat{\mathbf{E}}$ is built uniquely from the k-space representation of the RF-coil sensitivities $\hat{c}_\alpha(\cdot)$:

$$\hat{E}_{(\alpha',b),l} = (\hat{c}_{\alpha'})_{l-Rb}. \tag{2.59}$$

Here, only the index along the accelerated dimension is specified. The matrix $\hat{\mathbf{E}}$ is block-circulant. The inversion preserves the block-circulant property [104] and therefore many fewer reconstruction weights need to be determined than the reconstruction matrix $\hat{\mathbf{F}} = \hat{\mathbf{E}}^+$ has entries.[29] In

---

[29] A direct consequence of this block-circulant structure is that the reconstruction weights are shift-invariant. As a result of the effective weighting of the coil sensitivities with the object information in GRAPPA, the shift-invariance property is not exact in GRAPPA; notwithstanding, it is a useful assumption for image reconstruction. Also note that algorithms exist that invert a block-circulant very fast. Such algorithms typically make use of the fact that a square block-circulant matrix is block-diagonal in the Fourier-domain (cf. [104]); each block can then be inverted independently, thus accelerating the overall inversion. This is, however, exactly what is done in Cartesian SENSE reconstruction. Both approaches are in fact equivalent.

particular, it can be shown (see Appendix A.3.1, page 295f) that SENSE is equivalent to solving the expression

$$\mathbf{w}_\alpha^{(m)} = \hat{\mathbf{c}}_\alpha (\hat{\mathbf{E}}^{(m)})^+, \tag{2.60}$$

where the superscript $m = 0, \dots, R - 1$ indicates a shift of the index $l - Rb$ to $l - (Rb - m)$ in Eq. 2.59. The latter equation allows direct comparison of SENSE with GRAPPA. There are only two differences between this equation and Eq. 2.58:

1. In GRAPPA, fewer weights are considered compared to SENSE and less data are used for their determination (ACS-lines).

2. In GRAPPA, the weights are determined directly from the signal data, whereas in SENSE, the weights are determined from measured RF-coil sensitivity profiles.

The first difference is related to the discussion of an optimal (see e.g. chapter 2 in [114]) GRAPPA kernel. In Appendix A.3.2, page 297ff, it is proven that truncation of the SENSE encoding matrix does indeed not lead to significant loss of information if not driven too far. Often, the noise characteristics of the reconstructed images are even improved. It is shown that two factors are responsible that small kernels can be used in practice without image deterioration: the small k-space footprint of the RF-coil sensitivities, but also the fact that the SENSE g-factors are limited for high-quality coil designs and low acceleration factors.

The second difference gives rise to the question of how the usage of signal data in GRAPPA instead of RF-sensitivity data in SENSE for weight determination affects the reconstructed images. To answer this question consider that the signal of a particular RF channel can be interpreted as being the Fourier transform of the RF-coil sensitivity profiles weighted with the magnetization of the measured object, sometimes (e.g. in [171]) therefore termed *in vivo coil sensitivities* . With this interpretation, the only difference between GRAPPA and SENSE - apart from truncation of the encoding matrix - is that in GRAPPA, in vivo sensitivity data and in SENSE, pure sensitivity data are used.

It has been pointed out [183, 147] that there is a subtle difference between reconstruction with (low resolution) in vivo coil sensitivities or with pure sensitivities: When pure sensitivities are used, uniform reconstruction accuracy is ensured for each voxel. If in vivo sensitivities are used, the reconstruction accuracy is higher for voxels with increased image intensity. This means that aliasing from high-intensity voxels is suppressed, thus reducing the overall artifact power in the image.[30]

In summary, the close relationship between GRAPPA and SENSE has been reviewed in this section. The used matrix approach reveals that truncation of the SENSE matrix to the size of the GRAPPA problem is feasible without introducing significant errors. One difference between the two methods is that SENSE immediately yields a single reconstructed image, whereas in GRAPPA, unfolded images are determined for each RF channel first; finally, these images are combined with a root-sum-of-squares or other combination techniques. Another difference is that in SENSE, explicit information about the RF-sensitivity profiles is required, whereas in GRAPPA, this information is used only implicitly, thus eliminating problems associated with inaccuracies of the sensitivity determination. In contrast to SENSE, not pure sensitivity data, but in vivo sensitivity data are effectively used in GRAPPA with the effect of reduced artifact power in the images. This is beneficial in the context of PI because aliasing poses a particular problem with subsampled trajectories.

---

[30]To be precise: The "in vivo" weighting only has an influence on the images if an overdetermined system of equations is solved for image reconstruction, as for example done in SENSE after matrix truncation (or implicitly also in GRAPPA). For the standard SENSE reconstruction, the weighting has in principle no influence. This is closely related to the fact that the condition $\mathbf{FE} = \mathbb{1}$ can be satisfied exactly in situations where this condition represents an underdetermined system of equations.

Chapter 3

Overview of PatLoc Imaging and Presentation of Initial Hardware Designs

THE acronym *PatLoc* = <u>*Pa*</u>*rallel Imaging* <u>*T*</u>*echnique using* <u>*Loc*</u>*alized Gradients* covers the two main aspects of this novel imaging modality: In PatLoc, signals are encoded with a *new type of gradient system* and received with several RF-receiver coils *in parallel*. The acronym implies that the PatLoc project included significant efforts in hardware development. This is certainly an important aspect, but the primary relevance of PatLoc for MRI is a conceptually new approach to MRI signal encoding with the ultimate goal of providing new means to generate innovative applications for medical diagnosis. The concept of PatLoc and arising applications are illustrated in this section and two hardware implementations are presented, which were developed during the course of the PatLoc project.

This chapter is special in that the presented material is based on work that has been performed by several members of the PatLoc team. The emphasis is placed on topics with significant own contributions, documented through (co-)authorship in various publications, among the most relevant to this chapter are [[61, 156, 42, 207, 63, 199, 24]].

3.1 The Concept

Since the advent of MRI, gradients were built with preferably linear field geometries. The PatLoc approach breaks with this tradition by intentionally introducing *nonlinear and non-bijective spatial encoding magnetic fields* (NB-SEMs). This conceptual extension of the signal encoding process has dramatic consequences for MRI signal localization.

Interestingly, some of the most fundamental effects of non-bijective encoding can be understood with a simple 1D example. Consider Fig. 3.1. In this example, a magnetic encoding field with quadratic geometry $\psi(x) \propto x^2$

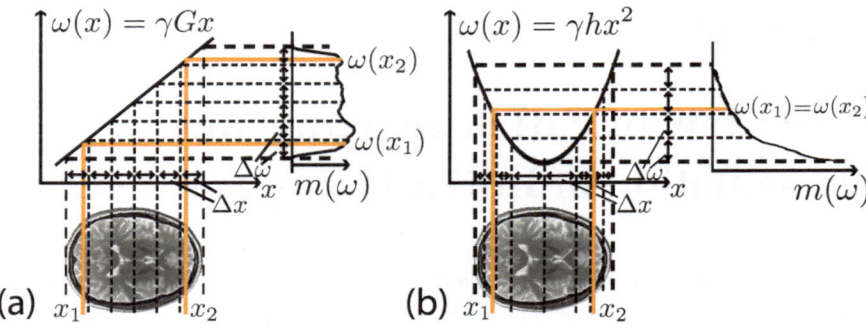

Figure 3.1: Concept of PatLoc imaging. (a) Conventional gradient encoding (cf. Fig. 1.7). (b) PatLoc encoding with a quadratic field. It is shown how the frequency content of the MR signal is linked to the location of origin via the magnetic encoding fields. The notation conforms to the main text. The comparison reveals differences to conventional encoding: First, as indicated by the thin dashed lines, the nonlinearity of the encoding field has the consequence that the voxel size (Δx) and therefore also image resolution is not homogeneous. Second, as indicated by the orange lines, the non-bijectiveness of the encoding fields has the consequence that different locations of the image are encoded with the same frequency. One advantage is a doubling of image resolution (on average). However, it is not possible to unambiguously determine the source location of the signal if encoding is solely done with such a non-bijective field.

instead of the traditional linear geometry $\psi_{grad}(x) \propto x$ is considered. The quadratic function differs in two ways from the linear function:

First, it is nonlinear. This nonlinearity has the consequence that image resolution is spatially dependent in PatLoc. The resolution increases with increasing steepness of the SEM. More subtle is the observation that the SNR is expected to decrease, where the encoding fields are steeper. This can be concluded from the low signal energy resulting from those steep regions as indicated by the $m(\omega)$-plots in Fig. 3.1. This behavior is in agreement with conventional Fourier imaging (cf. Eq. 2.36, page 65), where increased image resolution comes at the expense of loss of SNR.

The second property of x^2 is that it is non-bijective. This means that, except for $x = 0$, there are always two locations, which are mapped onto one single frequency. A measurement from a single coil is therefore not sufficient to uniquely determine the location of the signal origin. This ambiguity is similar to what is known from conventional accelerated parallel imaging (cf. for example Fig. 2.10, page 76). In PatLoc, the encoding ambiguities are resolved with the help of several receiver coils with different sensitivity at the ambiguous locations. Note that after unfolding twice as many voxels are reconstructed. Correspondingly, the average image resolution is doubled. Fig. 3.2 motivates that signal discrimination is feasible with several RF-receiver coils.

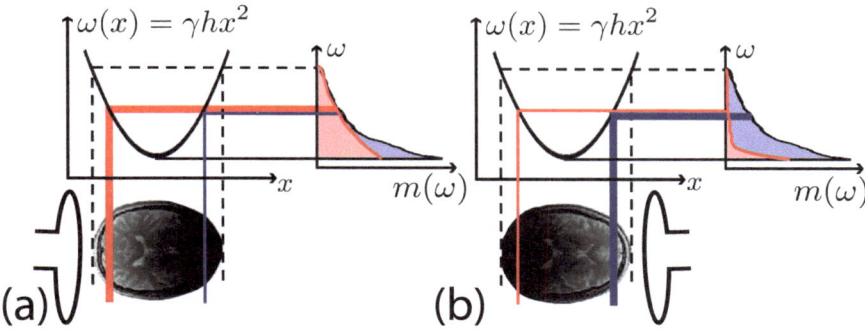

Figure 3.2: Determination of source locations with parallel acquisition. (a) and (b) show the situation for two RF-receiver coils with different spatial sensitivity. Coils (a) and (b) are sensitive on opposite sides of the example object. The signal paths are in red or blue color depending on from which side of vertex of the parabolic encoding field the signal emanates. The highlighted signal paths in (a) show that almost the complete signal energy originates from the left of the vertex, whereas the signal paths in (b) show that the opposite is the case for the second coil. For this particular frequency, the difference in RF-coil sensitivities therefore allows one to uniquely determine the locations of the signal sources. The signal plots indicate that this is also true for most frequencies. At the center, however, there is a significant sensitivity overlap and more insight into the problem is necessary to answer the question to what extent signal discrimination is possible.

These properties – non-homogeneous, but on average increased image resolution, spatially varying SNR, and the necessity to supplement encoding with RF arrays – are also inherent to 2D imaging with two NB-SEMs (see e.g. chapter 5.1, page 155ff), and typical if more than two SEMs are used for signal encoding (see e.g. chapter 7.2.2, page 255ff). These and other properties of NB-SEMs offer new degrees of freedom for MRI signal encoding. The next section gives examples how these new degrees of freedom can be exploited to develop interesting new applications for MRI.

3.2 Applications

3.2.1 Background: New Encoding Options

There are very good arguments to use linear gradient fields in MRI. These fields allow signal encoding in the Fourier domain of the object. For single-channel Cartesian acquisitions, image reconstruction is fast (FFT) and results in images with constant spatial resolution (cf. Eq. 2.33) and optimal, homogeneous SNR (cf. Eq. 2.36). These properties are very advantageous in many ways, yet not the only measure for diagnostic usability.

A good example is parallel imaging, where the homogeneous and optimal SNR properties of the reconstructed images are sacrificed in favor of imaging speed; many other useful applications have evolved with the development of PI. The main reason for this tremendous impact of PI has been the extension of encoding capabilities compared to single-channel acquisitions.

In this sense, PatLoc has a similar target: extending the encoding capabilities of current imaging hardware. This task is achieved by making the gradient system itself more flexible. This approach is promising because the gradients provide the major part of the overall encoding information. A PatLoc encoding system offers new encoding options by not restricting encoding to linear SEMs; curvilinear and non-bijective SEMs are also available for signal localization.

The relevance of PatLoc is augmented by the availability of parallel reception on many modern scanners. Reconsider that the additional information provided by an array of RF coils has shown that gradient encoding can be reduced to an extent, which would normally lead to non-unique encoding. PI therefore allows incomplete gradient encoding that can also be a consequence of non-bijective SEMs. Despite the various possibilities that PI offers to use non-complete gradient encoding strategies, the existing gradient hardware has remained the same, while the research concentrated on modifying k-space sampling schemes. In PatLoc it is reviewed whether modifications of the gradient system lead to more efficient signal encoding especially in the context of PI. Novel encoding strategies are investigated, adequate reconstruction methods are developed and new applications in medical diagnostics are explored.

Potential benefits of PatLoc were already discussed in the initial conceptual publication [[61]]. It was motivated therein that PatLoc is useful because it allows customization of the encoding fields to the underlying anatomical structures. Also, it has been hypothesized in [[61]] that the problem of peripheral nerve stimulation (PNS) could be reduced with PatLoc. Soon, it has been realized that PatLoc can be efficient in the context of RF reception [[156]] (low g-factor) as well as in the context of RF transmission [54, 152], [[191]] (shorter pulses, more efficient acquisitions of functional MRI data). Particularly interesting are the options, which PatLoc offers for reduced field-of-view imaging [[213, 207]]. One example is the elimination of balanced SSFP[1] banding artifacts [[206]]. PatLoc is still a very new technology. The wide range of possible applications is promising and the increasing interest in PatLoc and related approaches [178, 80, 98, 97, 93], [[100, 101]], will undoubtedly lead to many new and creative ideas for medical diagnosis. I have selected a few interesting applications, which are described in the following three sections in more detail.

3.2.2 Improved Encoding Efficiency

With modern gradient hardware a linear SEM can be switched fast and accurately. Moreover, the three available channels allow arbitrary spatial orientation of the linear SEM. However, there is no possibility to deviate from the linear geometry. One of the major incentives for the development of a PatLoc system has been the observation that alternative SEM geometries are often better adapted to the anatomical shapes of the measured objects. Also, alternative field geometries have different effects on technical as well as physiological restrictions. It is therefore to be expected that improvements in encoding efficiency can be achieved with PatLoc resulting in reduced scan times or increased diagnostic information. This aspect is further motivated in this section by discussing situations with increasing flexibility; a single SEM, then two SEMs and finally more than two SEMs are considered.

Encoding with One SEM   As an example, consider the MR-Encephalography project [64, 69, 211]. The aim of this project is to map brain physiology with a maximum temporal resolution. Image resolution on the other hand

---

[1]Acronym for *Steady-State Free Precession*. More information on balanced SSFP imaging sequences can be found in [53], page 796.

is not of major interest. In this context, the idea came up to encode with only one gradient coil and replace the encoding of the second gradient coil entirely by RF-sensitivity encoding (also cf. [[61]]). This approach would significantly lower the achievable image resolution. On the other hand, the signal acquisitions would be much faster because slow sequential gradient encoding would be replaced by fast simultaneous RF-sensitivity encoding. In this situation, the question arose if a linear encoding field is really always the optimal choice; in cortical imaging for example, information is required from the periphery of the brain only. However, linear gradient fields also encode the center of the brain and, due to the rectangular shape of the fields, also significant parts outside of the brain are encoded. In this situation, elliptical encoding fields would be better suited because the geometrical shape of these fields would cause magnetic field variations to be significant almost exclusively within the region of interest. This claim is supported by Fig. 3.3.

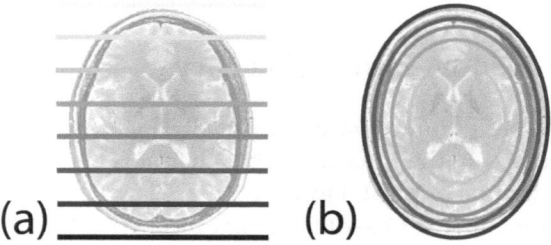

Figure 3.3: Encoding with one SEM. An example for cortical imaging. (a) Encoding with a conventional linear gradient field (field isolines are shown). (b) Efficient depth-encoding with elliptical SEMs having a high spatial derivative at the periphery. For cortical imaging, it is important to retrieve information from the periphery of the brain. In fast imaging modalities, where a gradient is used only for depth-encoding, and encoding along the circumferential direction is done with RF coils, elliptically-shaped encoding fields are better adapted to the anatomy of the cortex than linear fields.

Encoding with Two SEMs Not only ultra-fast imaging modalities, where a single gradient field is used, would profit from optimized field designs. Also encoding modalities, where two SEMs are used for in-plane imaging profit from the additional flexibility that PatLoc offers. In the 1D example of Fig. 3.1, it is motivated that image resolution depends on the spatial derivative of the encoding fields. The dependency of image resolution to the field derivatives can be exploited in the following way: Suppose that not the

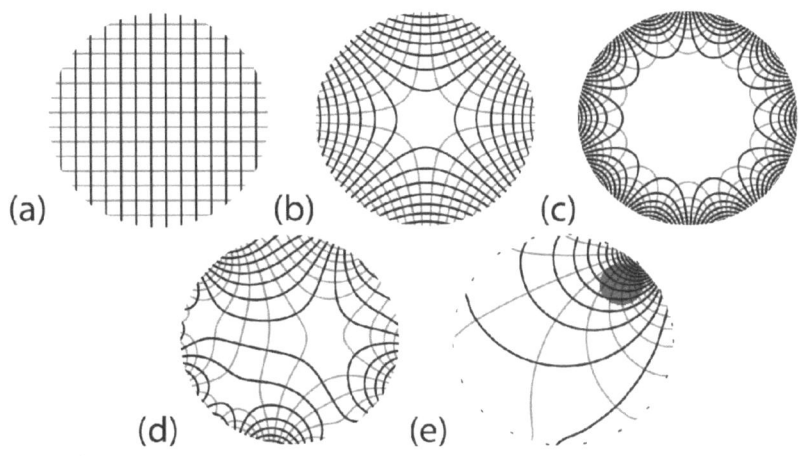

Figure 3.4: Contour plots of several orthogonal hypothetical SEMs. Size and shape of the small areas between the contour lines reflect the local image resolution. (a) Standard linear SEMs have homogeneous resolution. (b) For quadrupolar SEMs, there is a clear resolution gradient toward the periphery. Note that with the same number of isocontour lines (i.e., for the same amount of acquired data), there are twice as many voxels compared to linear encoding fields. (c) For multipolar SEMs with even higher polarity, the number of voxels is higher, however, also the resolution gradient is more pronounced. (d) Shown is an arbitrary SEM. It has an almost arbitrary resolution pattern. At the periphery, a tendency toward an increased image resolution is visible. (e) Especially for ROIs at the periphery (gray circle), encoding can be highly efficient if optimized for those ROIs only.

whole object, but only a sub-volume is important for a certain measurement. Then, fields with strong spatial derivatives are required for this sub-volume and outside of this region it is sufficient to have flat field geometries. PatLoc can be used to design SEMs such that encoding is more efficient in the ROI while restricting loss of encoding efficiency to regions of minor interest. For more homogeneous resolution inside the ROI, a method has been developed, which allows one to partially homogenize image resolution by sacrificing some of the abundant SNR of the low-resolution image parts [[190]]. A nice way of visualizing image resolution is to plot contour lines of both encoding fields on top of each other. Some theoretical examples of different orthogonal field geometries are shown in Fig. 3.4.[2] These examples show

---

[2]Consult Appendix A.4, page 299ff, for an elegant way of describing orthogonal fields in 2D with complex-valued analysis. More information is found in [[159]].

that there is a high flexibility in field design. Even more flexibility exists when the requirement of orthogonality is relaxed.

The quadrupolar field design, which corresponds to Fig. 3.4b, has been realized experimentally (see section 3.3, page 121ff). If those fields are used instead of the linear encoding fields, the encoding efficiency differs throughout the image. Because of the nonlinearities, almost no information of the image is encoded at the center, whereas at the periphery, a high resolution results (cf. Fig. 3.5). Analogous to the 1D example of section 3.1, page 103ff, the non-bijectiveness of the fields is responsible for a doubling of the average image resolution compared to standard gradient encoding for the same amount of acquired data.

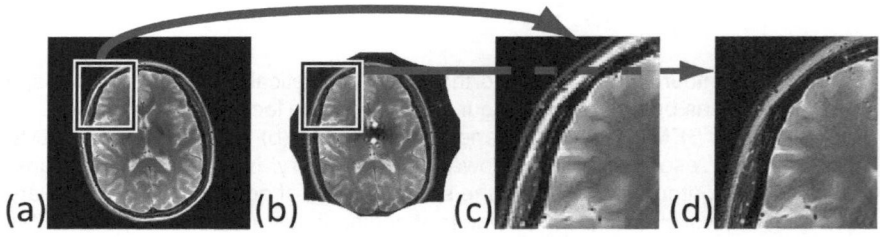

Figure 3.5: Image resolution with quadrupolar SEM encoding. (a) With standard linear gradient fields image resolution is homogeneous. (b) With quadrupolar SEMs, almost no image information is available at the center. Image resolution improves however toward the periphery. Some pronounced streaking artifacts are visible, which originate from the center. (c) and (d) Comparison of two similar zoomed-in sections show that image resolution is indeed higher with PatLoc within the peripheral region. Both images have been acquired with the same imaging parameters to allow fair comparison.

The contour plots shown in Fig. 3.4 and the experimental results shown in Fig. 3.5 reveal that encoding is typically more efficient near the coil surfaces (at the periphery). The reason for this property is obvious: The influence of the currents in the coils decreases with increasing distance. Especially at the periphery, there is room to improve the encoding efficiency as indicated by Fig. 3.4e.[3] Hence, a more flexible field design would profit from coil arrangements, which can be adapted to the anatomical shape of the imaged

---

[3]The example shown in subfigure (e) has been found using complex-valued analysis (cf. Appendix A.4, page 299ff) by minimizing $|f'(s)|$ (f and s are defined here as in Appendix A.4) outside of the ROI under the constraint that $(\sum_{s \in ROI} |f'(s)|^2)^{1/2}$ is constant within the ROI. Note that $|f'(s)|$ is equivalent to the Jacobian determinant of the corresponding

part of the body. In summary, an encoding system with two NB-SEMs of adequate geometry is useful to locally improve image resolution or to accelerate image acquisitions. The effects are enhanced considering that an intrinsic acceleration is associated with non-bijective encoding.

Encoding with More than Two SEMs   It is clear that effective field design is only possible with a flexible encoding system. Such a system would preferably consist of a large amount of coil channels. In Freiburg, a six channel system has recently been established, which allows simultaneous switching of the three linear channels and the two quadrupolar SEMs [[42]]. Also, a planar three-channel coil is currently being tested [[103]]. In the future, efforts will be focused on the development of a much more flexible multi-channel system.

The variations in image resolution resulting from such multi-channel systems depend not only on the field geometry, but also on the chosen time courses of the coil currents. The impact of such multi-dimensional encoding strategies on image properties like image resolution is therefore much more complex than if only two SEMs are involved. The local k-space concept, developed by Dr. Daniel Gallichan, has proven very helpful in this regard. The idea of local k-space has fruitfully been used to design and analyze complex multi-dimensional trajectories [[42]]; moreover, it is useful in related topics like GradLoc [[207]]. A discussion of this important concept should therefore not be spared, and is explained with further detail at the end of this section.

An interesting example in the present context is the 4D-RIO[4]-trajectory [[42]] that makes use of linear SEMs as well as NB-SEMs. On the one hand, images encoded with this multidimensional (4D) trajectory have properties that resemble those which are typically associated with linear gradient fields; for example, an extended portion of the image exhibits a homogeneous resolution (cf. Fig. 7.12, page 265). On the other hand, fundamental differences to conventional imaging arise; for example, image contrast is heavily affected by the 4D encoding.

---

two-dimensional real-valued vector field and thus approximates image resolution very well (cf. chapter 5.1.1e, on page 169, in combination with Eq. 5.8).

[4]Acronym for _4-Dimensional Radial In/out vs. Out/in_. This trajectory is briefly presented in chapter 7.2.1b, page 254f.

4D-RIO illustrates the capabilities of multi-dimensional trajectories to create new imaging effects, made possible by the additional spatial and temporal degrees of freedom that become available to redefine the magnetic field evolution within the measured object. These additional degrees of freedom may also be exploited to reduce scan time; to understand this, it is crucial to note that any encoding strategy is subject to many different limitations. There are restrictions of technical nature. For example, the SEMs cannot be switched infinitely fast because the coils that generate the SEMs have a finite inductivity. Also, there are restrictions of physiological nature, notably peripheral nerve stimulation caused by switched magnetic fields. These technical and physiological restrictions have the effect that there is a minimum execution time associated with a particular encoding strategy. One encoding strategy can be faster, i.e., more efficient, than a different strategy. Multi-dimensional PatLoc trajectories offer the possibility to design fast encoding strategies that are less demanding for certain restrictions than if encoded with purely linear SEMs, without necessarily having to cut back on relevant image information (like for example image resolution in the ROI).

The relationship between restrictions and encoding strategy is very complex and far from being understood. A thorough analysis of this important topic is still to be undertaken. In the following section, after a short note on local k-space, at least qualitative arguments are presented which show that NB-SEMs have the potential to reduce the problem of peripheral nerve stimulation.

The Concept of Local k-Space   The concept may be understood by comparing it to standard k-space. Recall that k-space corresponds to the space of encoded *spatial frequencies*. When k-space is sampled, different spatial frequencies of the object are acquired. The achieved image resolution is related to the highest sampled spatial frequencies, and aliasing occurs if the distance between the sampled spatial frequencies is too high (cf. paragraph *Field-of-View* on page 62ff in chapter 2.2.1c). In contrast to conventional imaging, where the spatial frequencies of the encoding functions do not change throughout the image, in PatLoc, each location encounters modulations with different spatial frequencies during the acquisition process. Therefore, each position has its own local distribution of encoded spatial frequencies; these local spatial frequencies define the spatial information that is available about the measured object at each location; in other words:

the encoded information at location $\vec{x}_\rho$ is defined by the distribution of the *local k*-space variable:

$$\vec{k}_{loc}(\vec{x}_\rho, t) := (\nabla\phi)(\vec{x}_\rho, t). \tag{3.1}$$

Here, $\phi(\cdot)$ represents the encoded phase distribution at location $\vec{x}_\rho$ at time-point t, and $\nabla\phi$, the corresponding local spatial frequency distribution. Some examples of local k-space distributions are depicted in Fig. 3.6.

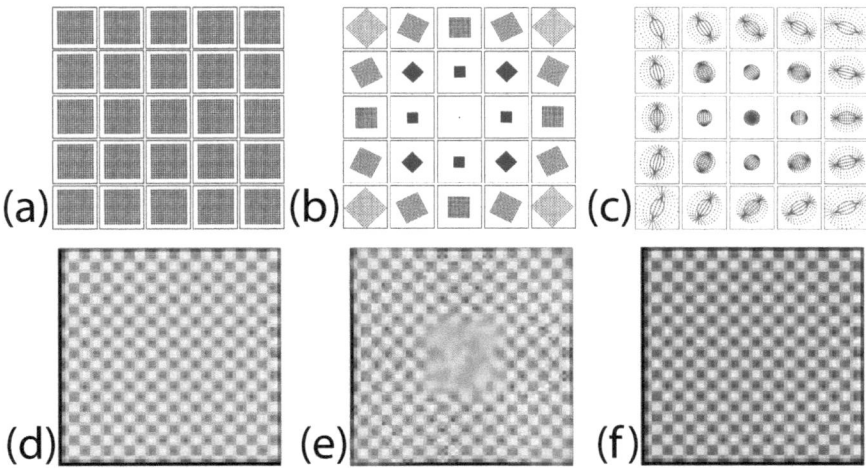

(a) (b) (c)

(d) (e) (f)

Figure 3.6: Local k-space (a-c) and examples of corresponding reconstructed images (d-f). (a,d) Conventional imaging. Local k-space is the same everywhere. Therefore, image resolution is constant throughout the image. (b,e) PatLoc imaging with two orthogonal quadrupolar SEMs. At the periphery, local k-space is enlarged, whereas it collapses to a single point at the center. Correspondingly, image resolution is high at the periphery, whereas it degrades toward the center. (c,f) Complex 4D trajectory, where linear and quadrupolar fields are involved. The trajectory is the 4D-RIO trajectory presented in [[42]]. The extent of local k-space is more evenly distributed compared to the pure quadrupolar PatLoc example. Therefore, also image resolution does not deteriorate toward the center (also see Fig. 7.13, page 267). The images are courtesy of Dr. Daniel Gallichan. Similar images have been published in [[42]].

The figure also illustrates that the extent of local k-space is closely related to the local image resolution. This observation can also be substantiated by theoretical means as shown in Appendix A.5.1, page 303ff. This shows that the relation between k-space extent and image resolution, that is well-known from conventional imaging, can immediately be adopted on a local level as well. Interestingly, this is not possible for the aliasing artifact: From the local sampling density alone no precise conclusions concerning aliasing at a certain location can be drawn because the aliasing artifact is not a local effect. Also note that, in the basic formulation of the concept, supplementary RF encoding is disregarded.

In the context of PatLoc imaging, it is particularly useful to link local k-space to what is actually done in the experiment. The exact relationship between the user-defined PatLoc acquisition trajectory and local k-space distribution is presented in Appendix A.5.2, page 305f, and illustrated for the three examples of Fig. 3.6.

3.2.3   Reduction of Peripheral Nerve Stimulation

A problematic side-effect of gradient switching is the possibility of peripheral nerve stimulation. PNS is a physiological reaction often perceived as a tingling sensation. It can, however, also cause significant pain and in the worst case, cardiac arrest might be triggered [46]. Gradient technology has advanced significantly in terms of field strength and switching rate, such that PNS has become a patient safety issue on many modern MR systems. This implies that nowadays gradient trajectory performance is often not restricted by gradient technology, but rather by physiological restrictions. The PatLoc approach offers possibilities to speed up the encoding process without exceeding the PNS limits. To understand this, a quick review of the causes for PNS is given in the next two paragraphs. A detailed presentation of this topic with further references is found in [46].

The term *peripheral nerve stimulation* correctly reveals that involuntary *nerve activation can be triggered* by switched gradients, i.e., by magnetic fields, which vary in the audio-frequency range. PNS is not a direct magnetic effect because it is a well-known fact from electrophysiology that nerve activation is triggered by the electric field and not the magnetic field itself [46]. However, basic electromagnetic theory states that an electrical field is generated by a time-varying magnetic field and therefore also a switched gradient field can cause nerve stimulation. More concretely, the integral of the electric field along a certain path (= voltage) is proportional to the time derivative of the magnetic flux flow through an enclosed area (Faraday's law): $\oint \vec{E} d\vec{l} = \iint \dot{\vec{B}} d\vec{A}$. Consider now a simple an idealistic situation

[144], where the human body is modeled as a cylinder with homogeneous tissue parameters and where the encoding field is assumed to have a pure constant gradient in the z-direction.[5] It can easily be shown that under these assumptions, the above equation has the solution: $E \propto r \cdot dB/dt$, where r is the distance from the z-axis. From this equation, it can be concluded that the current flows inside the human body are proportional to dB/dt. And indeed, stimulation occurs primarily at the periphery of the body like shoulders and arms [33], where dB/dt is typically very high. However, the currents are also proportional to the size r of the current loops. This is the main reason, why patients should avoid folding their hands during a scan [38].

The model is especially useful to predict current flows in the human body. These current flows can lead to nerve stimulation. It has been observed and analyzed a long time ago by Weiss and Lapicque [195, 89] that currents must flow for a certain amount of time τ to build up sufficient potential differences to cause cell depolarization. Irnich et al. have shown in [71] that the stimulation model of Weiss and Lapicque can be combined with the model presented in the previous paragraph. They derive a formula (Eq. 9 in [71]), which is of particular interest also in the context of PatLoc imaging, for the minimum magnetic field strength $B(\tau)$ required to cause nerve stimulation: $B(\tau) = B_{min} \cdot (1 + \tau/\tau_c)$. In this formula, τ can be interpreted as the pulse duration, τ_c is the chronaxie [89], a tissue dependent time constant, and B_{min} is the minimum, physically not realizable, instantaneous field change required to cause stimulation. Apart from the dependency on pulse duration, the formula is very interesting because it suggests that it is rather the absolute value of the peak-to-peak magnetic field change, which matters and peak dB/dt is not of primary interest. This result has been substantiated in [71] and also the results evaluated from different publications [33] support the claim that it might be reasonable for legal regulations to determine switching limits rather on B itself than on dB/dt.

Why is this interesting in the context of PatLoc? Consider Fig. 3.7. In this figure, a switched quadratic gradient is compared to a switched linear gradient. The comparison of Fig. 3.7a with Fig. 3.7b shows that the non-bijectiveness of the fields can indeed lead to reduced peak-to-peak magnetic field variations during switching. Note that the reduction depends on

---

[5]In reality, a gradient field is necessarily accompanied by concomitant field components (cf. e.g. [9]; also see chapter 1.2.2, on page 28).

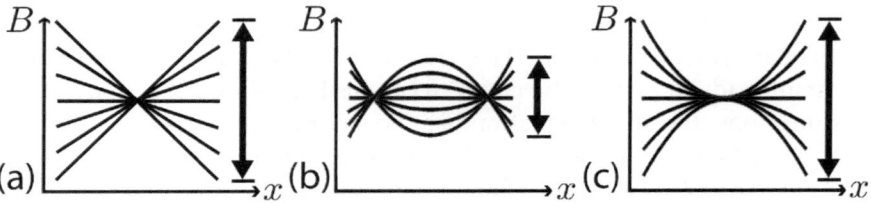

Figure 3.7: PNS in PatLoc: a 1D example. (a) Shown is a linear gradient field, which is switched from one extreme to the other. (b) The peak-to-peak variation is halved for a quadratic encoding field. This has beneficial consequences for PNS. Note that the average encoding efficiency, given by the derivative of the SEM, is preserved. (c) Care must be taken how the switching is performed, otherwise no gain might result.

how the fields are actually switched. If they are switched as indicated in Fig. 3.7b, the amplitude is halved; if, however, switched as in Fig. 3.7c, the amplitude is the same! It is clear that the 1D example of Fig. 3.7 can only give a rough understanding about the PNS capabilities of practical PatLoc measurements. Concomitant fields must be considered and, what is even more intricate, it is important to consider that the different geometric shapes of the encoding fields influence the non-local effects (for example current loops, influence of differing tissue properties), which are important for PNS. Initial investigations have been performed to ensure that safety margins are not exceeded by the used experimental setup [[24]]. This was necessary to get ethical approval from the Ethics Commission of the University of Freiburg. Further investigations with more flexible SEM systems are indispensable to evaluate the PNS capabilities of PatLoc under realistic conditions. This will also involve patient studies and therefore safety considerations will be of primary importance in this regard.

3.2.4 Applications Involving Nonlinear Phase Preparation

Particularly promising are applications with nonlinear phase preparation added to conventional gradient encoding. Nonlinear phase preparation is a method, where a nonlinear PatLoc-SEM is switched before signal reception. The nonlinearity of the SEM causes signal echoes to be formed at different time points, depending on the location of the signal source. This spatio-temporal correlation of echo formation is exploited by a method that has been termed *GradLoc* to perform reduced FOV-imaging [[213, 207]] and by

STAGES[6] [[206]] to enhance the homogeneity of the B_0 field during signal acquisition. The lion's share for the development of these two applications can be attributed to Dr. Walter Witschey. Relevant prior art is referenced and briefly discussed in the above publications. The basic ideas and initial results are reviewed in this section. For simplicity, only SEMs with quadratic terms are considered for phase preparation.

a) GradLoc: Reduced Field-of-View-Imaging

In conventional imaging, the k-space signal energy is typically focused at the center of k-space (echo). This behavior changes dramatically, when a quadratic SEM is applied during phase encoding in addition to the linear gradients: The k-space echo spreads out over a region that becomes larger with increasing field strength of the quadratic field. This effect is often denoted as *phase-scrambling* (also see [131]) and is illustrated in Fig. 3.8. This figure also reveals an astonishing property of quadratic phase preparation: With increasing quadratic phase, the k-space progressively resembles the actual image. When the quadratic field is increased even further, parts of the echoes leave the acquired region and, consequently, peripheral parts of the image are cropped (also visible in Fig. 9d in [72]), whereas the central part of the image remains almost unaffected.

What is the reason for this strong correlation between image space and k-space? Recall that in conventional imaging, the gradients impose a phase $\phi \propto kx$ onto the magnetization, where k is the k-space variable and x is the source location.[7] The quadratic SEM is responsible for an additional phase accumulation proportional to αx^2 resulting in the overall phase of $\phi \propto (k + k_q(x))x$, where $k_q(x) = \alpha x$. Quadratic phase preparation therefore leads to a splitting of the echo into individual components, where the echo of each source location x is not centered around $k = 0$, but shifted to $-k_q(x) = -\alpha x$. Most signal energy of each individual component is therefore located at $-\alpha x$ in k-space. This is the reason for the one-to-one correspondence of k-space signal echo shift and image space source location and why (a) k-space and reconstructed image look similar and why (b) for large values of α, those parts of the reconstructed image vanish which correspond to k-space values that have been shifted outside of the acquired

---

[6]Acronym for *Steady-STAte Gradient Echo Shimming*.
[7]The explanation is in 1D. It can be extended to 2D and 3D in a straightforward manner [[207]].

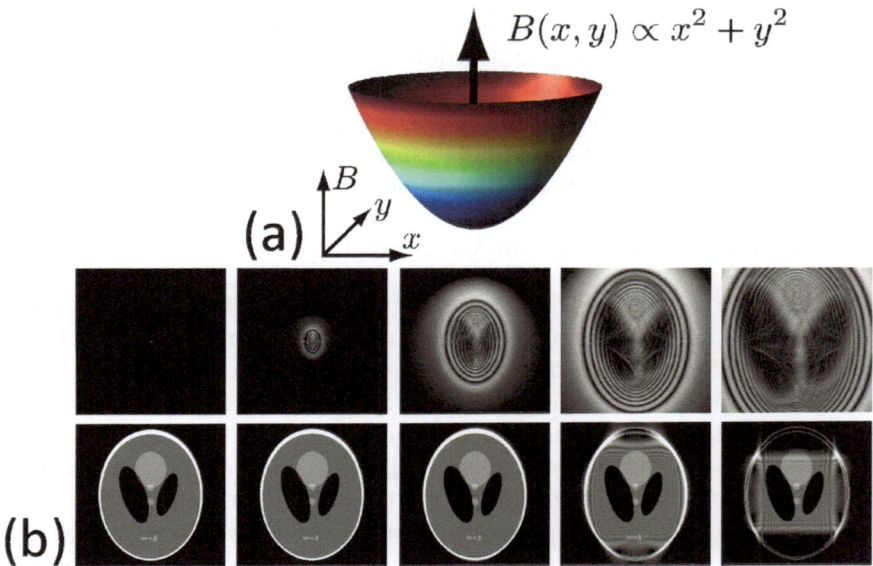

Figure 3.8: Effect of quadratic phase preparation. (a) Geometry of a 2D quadratic encoding field. (b) Bottom: Reconstructed image. Top: Corresponding k-space signal. From left to right: Without phase preparation, there is a single central k-space echo. With increasing quadratic phase, the echoes originating from different parts of the object separate. For large quadratic phase, peripheral echoes are not acquired anymore and signal loss in the reconstructed images occurs. According to the square-shaped acquisition window, the shape of the localized image is also square-shaped. Some residual aliasing from high-frequency components remains visible.

k-space region. More precisely, if the k-space region K has been acquired, only those parts of the image are visible, which lie in the region $V \propto \alpha K$.

This relation is also valid in 2D and 3D [[207]] and has a direct application: The user can select a ROI V within the object, perform standard imaging supplemented with quadratic phase preparation, and acquire the k-space region with the same shape as the ROI: $K \propto V/\alpha$. This procedure allows reduced FOV-imaging because the fold-over artifacts otherwise encountered along the phase encoding direction (Fig. 3.9a) are avoided. A similar result may be found with selective excitation pulses. Such pulses are, however, typically long and often a significant amount of energy is deposited in the measured objects. These negative effects are avoided with GradLoc.

Note that the localized boundary in V is not perfectly sharp. The reason for this unwanted effect is that most, but not all signal energy is located at the center locations of the individual echoes. High-frequency information may result in artifacts, for example some residual artifacts are visible outside of the localized square in Fig. 3.9a. Surprisingly, these artifacts do not seem to be problematic under in vivo imaging conditions (see Fig. 3.9b).

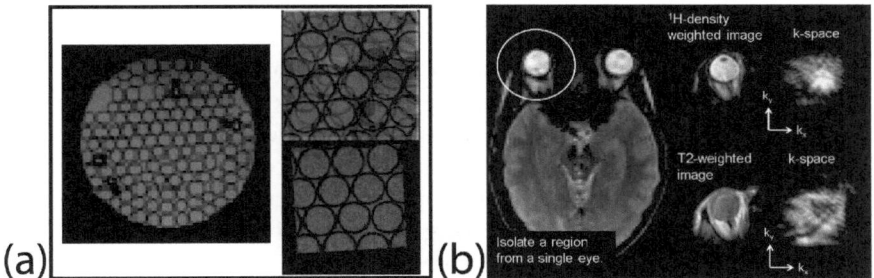

Figure 3.9: GradLoc measurement results. (a) Phantom measurements. Left: No aliasing occurs with full k-space sampling. Right, top: Undersampling along the vertical direction results in the typical fold-over artifact. Right, bottom: With a quadratic phase, a high-resolution image without aliasing results. (b) These advantages are also visible under in vivo conditions. Note the comparably weak high-frequency artifact compared to the simulations in Fig. 3.8. The images are courtesy of Dr. Walter Witschey. The images in (a) have been taken from [[205]] and the image in (b) was part of the corresponding poster presentation at the ISMRM conference 2011 in Montreal. The phase of the acquired data was prepared with a quadrupolar SEM provided by the available PatLoc hardware. This SEM and the quadratic SEM used in Fig. 3.8 both result in linear k-space echo shifts and are therefore equivalent in the context of GradLoc [[205]].

b) STAGES: Dynamic Intra-Slice Shimming

STAGES [[206]] is a novel dynamic shim updating technique; similar to GradLoc, it is based on the localization properties resulting from nonlinear phase preparation. Shimming comprises methods to enhance the homogeneity of the B_0-field, which is perturbed by susceptibility differences between tissue borders. Active shimming is typically performed with a set of shim coils that are designed to generate the lowest orders of solid harmonics. Shimming may be divided into static shimming and dynamic shimming methods. In static shimming, B_0-inhomogeneity maps are acquired and the currents in the shim coils are adjusted before the actual measurement to optimize the shim for the whole excited region or also for a particular ROI. In dynamic shimming, several shim updates are performed during the acquisition. A problem with existing shimming methods is that they are restricted to shimming between successive excitations; i.e., the shims may be updated from slice to slice. It is however not possible to shim during the acquisition of a single slice if encoding is done with only linear gradients. That is, where STAGES comes into play: It is possible to perform not only *inter*-slice shimming, but also *intra*-slice shimming.

This is possible because of the k-space relocalization properties of the non-linear phase preparation. Recall that k-space is actually traversed in the temporal domain along a user-defined k-space trajectory (cf. chapter 1.2.2, page 27ff). Relocalization of MR signals in k-space is therefore, from the perspective of the concrete measurement, a temporal rearrangement of the individual MR echoes, which originate from different locations of the measured object. In the previous section, where GradLoc is explained, it is shown that a quadratic SEM leads to a one-to-one correspondence of k-space and source location. In the temporal description this means that at each instant of time, signal echoes are recorded, which originate from a very localized region *within* the excited slice. Thus, it is possible to optimize the shim for that localized region only. While traversing k-space, the region that contributes signal changes. It is therefore possible to update the shims to the currently contributing region with the consequence of significantly enhanced image quality. Note that such an *intra*-slice shim updating protocol requires a nonlinear SEM. With linear SEMs, the signal echoes occur all at the same time. Therefore all image parts are equally affected by the shimming parameters. If these are optimized at one instant for a certain region, the quality may be enhanced at that location, however, only at the expense of image deterioration elsewhere. This problem is avoided with nonlinear phase preparation.

The dynamic shimming capabilities have been demonstrated for a problem, which is known to result from B_0-inhomogeneities: In balanced SSFP sequences (cf. [53], page 796), banding artifacts with unwanted signal loss occur (see Fig. 3.10a). Fig. 3.10b shows that these banding artifacts could be eliminated with STAGES. More information about the concrete update scheme and the used sequence parameters is found in [[206]].

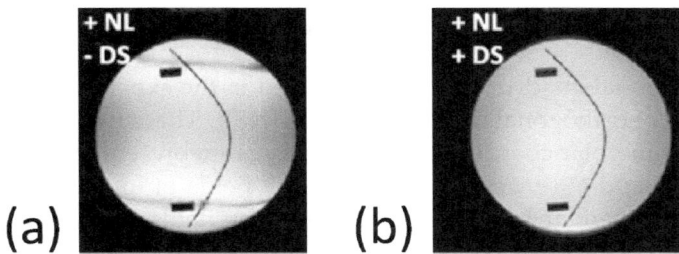

Figure 3.10: Banding artifact suppression with STAGES. (a) Images acquired with balanced SSFP sequences are typically corrupted with such a banding artifact. (b) With STAGES this artifact is eliminated. The images are courtesy of Dr. Walter Witschey and have been taken from [[206]].

3.2.5 Summary

These examples show that PatLoc has potential benefits in various areas of MRI. Some of these benefits could already be verified with the current PatLoc hardware, others still wait for ethical approval to be evaluated. Some benefits like improved encoding efficiency call for a more flexible gradient system. PatLoc is still a young imaging modality with many open questions. It is very probable that further investigations will create new ideas about how the gained flexibility in signal encoding can be used to solve current problems in MRI and generate new applications for medical imaging.

3.3 Initial Experimental Setups

In this section, the first two hardware designs of a PatLoc imaging system are presented that were constructed during the course of the PatLoc project. Another, high-performance system is currently being installed and is not presented here. The first PatLoc prototype coil has been built to fit into a $9.4\,\text{T}$ BioSpec research system for small animal MRI (Bruker BioSpin MRI GmbH, Ettlingen, Germany). The second PatLoc coil was constructed significantly larger as an insert coil for human head imaging on a MAGNETOM Trio, A Tim System $3\,\text{T}$ (Siemens Healthcare, Erlangen, Germany). Both PatLoc gradient coils were designed to generate two orthogonal quadrupolar encoding fields. These fields are introduced in the following section before the animal and the human systems are presented in more detail.

3.3.1   Multipolar Encoding Fields

The orthogonal quadrupolar SEMs realized in the experiments form special types of orthogonal multipolar SEMs [[63]]. These two fields are best
described in polar coordinates, where they are represented by $\psi_1(r, \varphi) \propto$
$r^L \cos(L\varphi)$ and $\psi_2(r, \varphi) \propto r^L \sin(L\varphi)$. The fields of lowest order $L = 1$
are just the standard x- and y-gradients. The fields with $L = 2$ are the
quadrupolar fields which are generated with the custom-made PatLoc hardware. The field geometry of the two quadrupolar fields is shown in Fig.
3.11; it is equivalent to the geometry of the fields generated by shim coils of
order $(L := 2, L := 2)$.

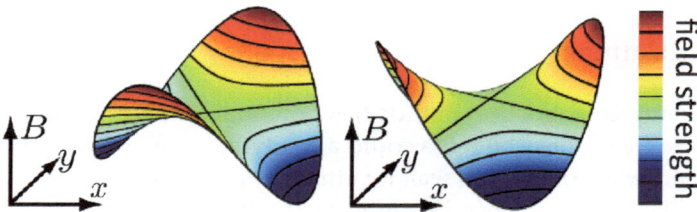

Figure 3.11: Quadrupolar SEMs. The two orthogonal quadrupolar SEMs form
hyperbolic paraboloids, which are rotated against each other by 45°. They are flat
at the center and the field strength increases quadratically in the radial direction.
Along the circumferential direction, the field changes sinusoidally with two poles on
opposite sides of the center.

Both fields are also orthogonal to the z-gradient $\psi_3(\cdot) \propto z$. Orthogonality
means in this case that the gradients of the magnetic fields are perpendicular.
The orthogonality of the fields can easily be computed by verifying that
$(\nabla \psi_i) \cdot (\nabla \psi_j) = 0$ for all $i \neq j$. Orthogonal multipolar SEMs have the
remarkable property that appropriate combinations of them generate *all
feasible* magnetic encoding fields under the condition that the gradients of
these two fields plus the z-gradient are globally orthogonal to each other.
This statement is proven in Appendix A.4, page 299ff. One important result
of the proof is that it identifies the linear gradient fields as the most basic
encoding fields, followed by orthogonal quadrupolar SEMs. From this
mathematical point of view, the realized PatLoc hardware is the first and
most basic step toward encoding fields with a virtually arbitrary geometry,
and PatLoc imaging can be regarded as a natural generalization of standard
Fourier imaging.

The requirement of orthogonality is not a necessary condition for imaging, however, it ensures maximal encoding efficiency because encoding along orthogonal directions adds complementary information, whereas encoding along the same direction does not yield new information. Fig. 3.12 illustrates that the angle of encoding directions has consequences for the shapes of the voxels and therefore also for image resolution. Within the accuracy of the voxel model as used in the figure, the voxels form parallelograms for linear SEMs whose area is given by $f = |(\nabla\psi_1)| \cdot |\nabla\psi_2)|/\sin(\phi)$, where ϕ is the angle between the gradient fields of the two SEMs. For given field strengths, image resolution is therefore maximized when the field gradients approach orthogonality. Another advantage of orthogonal SEMs is that the voxels form compact squares instead of anisotropic parallelograms. For small voxels, the same is true for nonlinear SEMs.

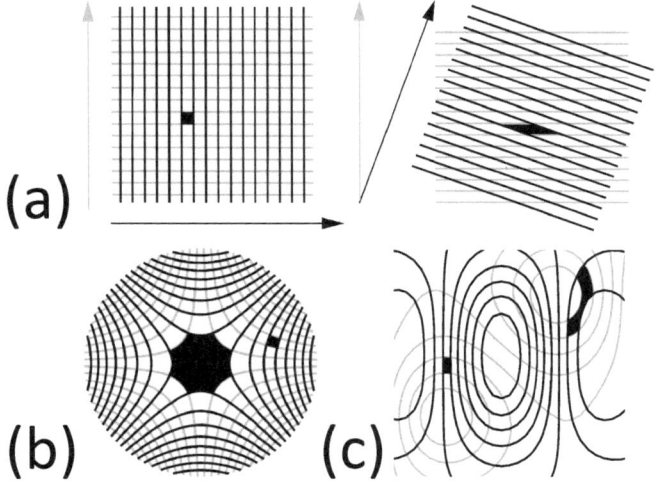

Figure 3.12: Voxel shapes and local encoding directions. (a) Two linear SEMs. Left: Orthogonal SEMs. Right: Non-orthogonal SEMs. The areas enclosed by the contour lines roughly approximate size and shape of the voxels within the reconstructed images. Within this approximation, voxels have the highest quality with orthogonal encoding directions. (b) At the periphery, an optimal voxel shape is preserved with quadrupolar orthogonal SEMs. Only at the center, deviations from the optimal shape are visible. (c) The shown example of two nonlinear SEMs illustrates that the angle of the encoding directions is an important parameter in determining the image quality also for the case of general nonlinear SEMs.

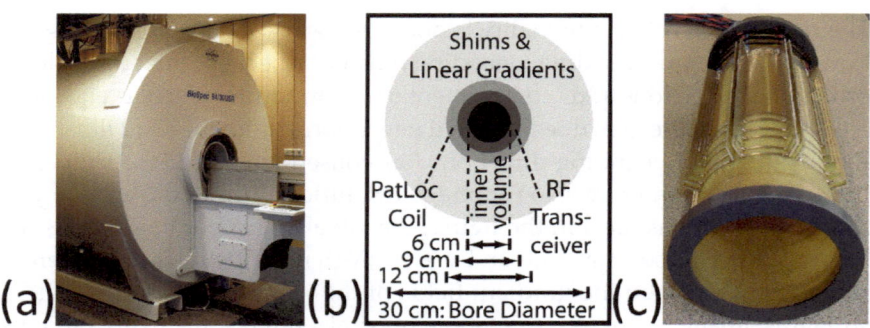

Figure 3.13: Experimental setup of the first PatLoc measurements. (a) The measurements were performed on a Bruker BioSpec 94/30 USR system. (b) From the $30\,cm$ of the scanner bore only $12\,cm$ could be used for the PatLoc insert and $6\,cm$ were available for the measurements. (c) The PatLoc coil was manufactured manually based on an optimized octagonal wire topology. The optimal field geometry was between the 3rd and 4th rung at the opposite side of the cabling.

Note, however, that the voxel volume is for example only diminished by $13\,\%$ when the field directions form an angle of only $60\,°$ with each other: The sinusoidal relationship of voxel size and angular encoding directions has the consequence that fairly large deviations from orthogonality can be tolerated in practice without a strong impact on encoding efficiency and image quality. Deviations from exact orthogonality can even be useful; for engineering reasons, but also from a theoretical perspective. For example, it might be useful to flatten out the multipolar fields toward the edges because the volume very near to the coil surface can often not be used for imaging and strong gradients in regions not being covered by the object should be avoided in order to guarantee a high level of encoding efficiency.

3.3.2 Animal System

The very first PatLoc experiments were performed on a $9.4\,T$ BioSpec system for preclinical MRI (Bruker BioSpin MRI GmbH, Ettlingen, Germany, see Fig. 3.13a). The basic experimental setup has been presented in [[199]]. The results relevant to this thesis are reviewed here and information is added where necessary. The scanner bore had a diameter of $30\,cm$, but only a volume of $6\,cm$ in diameter could be used for phantom measurements because several hardware components like standard gradient hardware and

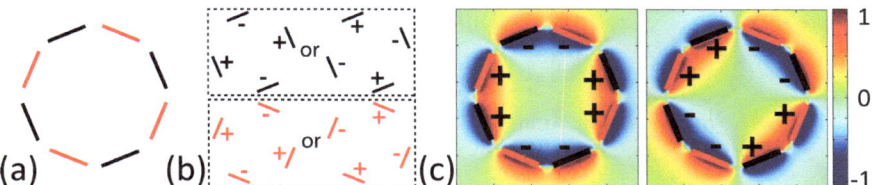

Figure 3.14: Generation of quadrupolar SEMs with the small-bore PatLoc prototype coil. (a) Two times four elements were connected with each other. (b) The four elements from each group were driven with alternating currents, which could flow in both directions. (c) One quadrupolar SEM was generated by driving both groups with equal currents. The second, orthogonal SEM was produced by reversing the current direction in one of the two element groups (shown is a slice at $z = 0$). The two quadrupolar fields could therefore be switched independently with the same controller normally used for the x- and y-gradients.

PatLoc coil insert used up the space in between. A cross section through the coil arrangement inside the scanner bore is depicted in Fig. 3.13b.

The PatLoc coil itself is shown in Fig. 3.13c. The coil was constructed manually with a length of 35 cm from which only about 6 cm could be used for imaging. The wire arrangement was based on a topology that had already been used for PatLoc simulations before [[61]]. The coil consisted of eight identical elements, arranged in an octagonal structure. In the simulations, the individual elements had imitated the symmetric design published in [21]. For the prototype coil, this design was optimized based on the method presented in [[105]] and for practical reasons, an asymmetric design was chosen for the individual elements with the current return paths all on the same side of the coil (cf. Fig. 3.13c).

In order to get two orthogonal quadrupolar SEMs, the eight elements were divided into two groups. Each group consisted of four elements, which were connected as shown in Fig. 3.14a. The first quadrupolar field was generated by applying equal currents in both element groups. The second quadrupolar field was generated by applying currents with reversed direction through the second element group. This procedure is depicted in Fig. 3.14b,c. The PatLoc coil could therefore be integrated into an existing hardware environment and the two channels, normally used for the switching of the x- and y-gradients were used to switch the two orthogonal quadrupolar SEMs instead. Fig. 3.15 shows that the design of the PatLoc prototype coil generated SEMs that were fairly similar to the exact quadrupolar coun-

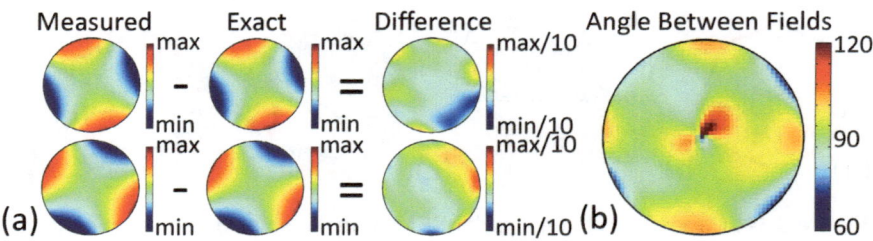

Figure 3.15: PatLoc SEMs generated by the small-bore prototype coil. (a) Top row and bottom row show the two different quadrupolar SEMs. On the left, measured PatLoc fields are shown. From these fields, exact hyperbolic paraboloids are subtracted resulting in a difference map. This map indicates that the true SEMs deviate from the exact counterparts by up to 10 % referred to the maximum field strength at the edge of the FOV. (b) Distribution of the angles between the two encoding directions. Note that all angles are between $60°$ and $120°$ indicating fairly high encoding efficiency.

terparts, at least in the central slice. In the relevant volume, the encoding directions were always between $60°$ and $120°$, which is sufficient to ensure efficient encoding in the whole volume of interest (see last paragraph of the latter section 3.3.1, on page 124).

One of the first images acquired with this hardware is shown in Fig. 3.16a. Signal data of a kiwi fruit were acquired with a 128×128 spin echo sequence ($TE = 50$ msec, $TR = 2$ sec). For the reference measurement the same parameters were used. The most obvious difference between the two images is the resolution gradient toward the outer parts of the kiwi fruit in the PatLoc image. Considering that the PatLoc prototype coil could only be driven with a maximum of 8.25 A, which is two orders of magnitude smaller than what modern gradient amplifiers achieve, the image quality is not perfect, but surprisingly good. The image quality could be improved significantly with an industrially manufactured high-performance gradient coil integrated into a comparable Bruker system [120]. One 256×256 image is shown in Fig. 3.16b.

3.3.3   Human System

After the initial PatLoc measurements on the Bruker hardware, a second PatLoc coil was developed and integrated into a MAGNETOM Trio, A Tim System 3 T (Siemens Healthcare, Erlangen, Germany). The goal was to

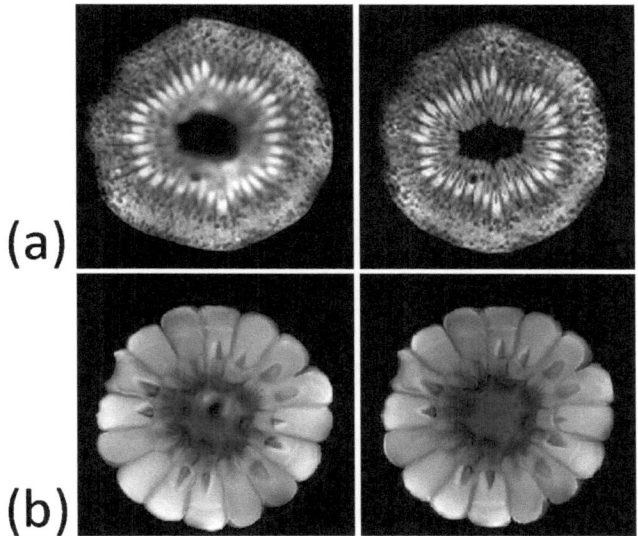

Figure 3.16: Measurement results with the small-bore system. (a) On the left, one of the very first reconstructed images is shown acquired with the PatLoc prototype coil. Shown is the image of a kiwi fruit. On the right, a reference image is shown acquired with the standard gradient system. The same imaging parameters were chosen. (b) With the second-generation small-bore PatLoc coil, the image quality could be improved significantly. Shown is a cross-section of a corn cob acquired with a spin echo sequence. On the left, the PatLoc image, and on the right, a reference image. The images in (b) were produced by Stéphanie Ohrel at Bruker BioSpin MRI GmbH, Ettlingen, Germany, and presented at the Annual Meeting of the ISMRM 2010 in Stockholm. The presentation was directly related to the abstract [120].

perform in vivo imaging of the human head with a PatLoc gradient coil having a reasonable performance.

The intended design was first described in [198]. Coil design and coil characteristics are described in [196, 197] and some information about coil integration into the scanner hardware is given in [[42]]. The safety considerations, evaluated in [[24]], formed the basis for obtaining formal ethics approval for research measurements on human volunteers by the institutional review board of the University of Freiburg. Written consent was obtained from each volunteer prior to all in vivo measurements performed for this thesis.

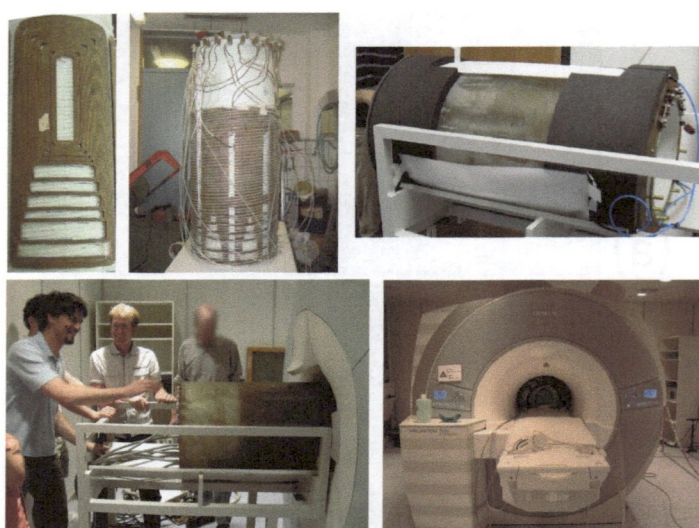

Figure 3.17: Construction of the PatLoc human head insert coil. From left to right, top row: The new coil consisted of several identical wire elements, which differentiated significantly from the elements of the PatLoc prototype coil. These elements were mounted on a cylindrical former, water cooling was added and the components were fixed with epoxy resin. Bottom row: With the RF coils inside, the coil was then introduced into the scanner bore.

The basic construction steps of the PatLoc coil are depicted in Fig. 3.17 and described in the figure caption. Although the shape of the SEMs, which could be generated with the new coil, was very similar to the fields of the initial PatLoc prototype coil, the approach to achieve this was different. The first PatLoc coil was equipped with a single layer of eight elements. With this design, all eight elements had to be used to generate both quadrupolar SEMs (cf. Fig. 3.14). The new design consisted of two layers, each with four elements. This is depicted in Fig. 3.18a, b. Each layer directly represented one of the quadrupolar SEMs. Fig. 3.19 shows that the generated fields were very similar to exact quadrupolar encoding fields. Note that not only the arrangement of the coil elements, but also the single elements were redesigned. More on the optimization of the design of the elements and the coil itself can be found in [196, 76], [[105]].

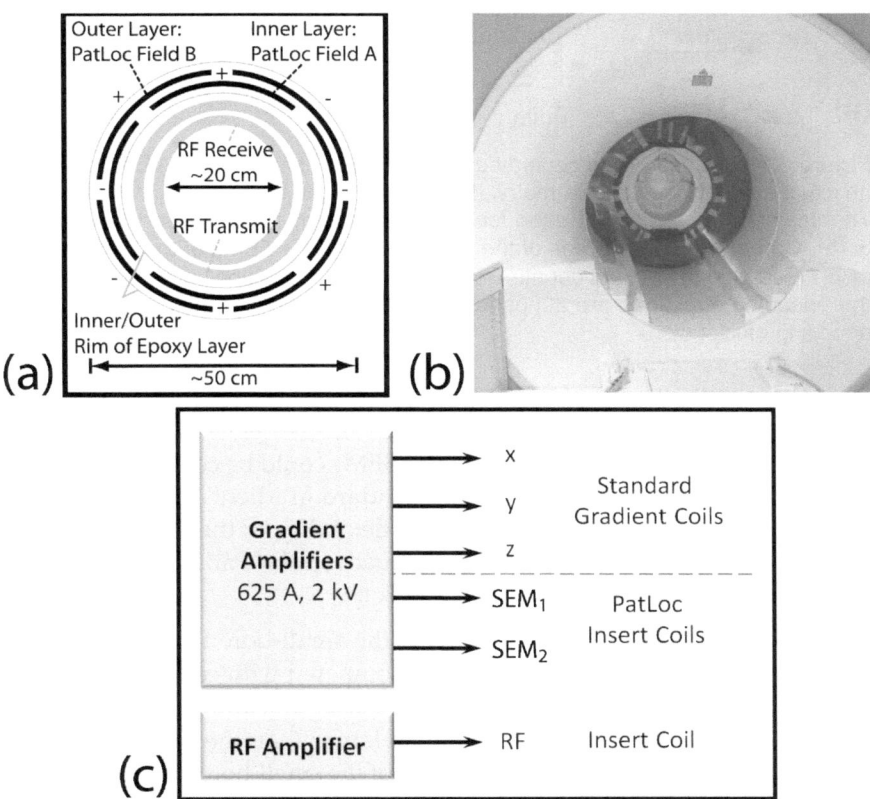

Figure 3.18: The PatLoc human head insert and its integration into the scanner environment. (a) Design of the PatLoc insert. The two-layer structure, with one layer for each SEM, was constructed to generate two orthogonal quadrupolar SEMs by alternating the current directions between adjacent elements. Placed inside, RF-transmit and receiver coils were sized to provide enough space for a human head. (b) The main components of the insert are visible in this photograph. (c) The standard gradient system was complemented with additional channels for independent operation of the gradient coils and the PatLoc head insert.

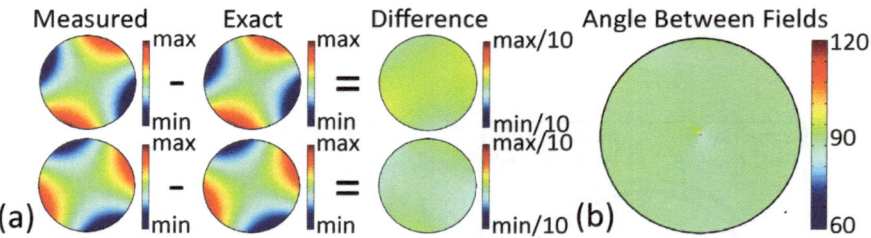

Figure 3.19: PatLoc SEMs generated by the human head insert. (a) Deviation from an exact quadrupolar field geometry. (b) Angle between the two encoding directions. The scaling is the same as used for the prototype small-bore insert coil (cf. Fig. 3.15). Compared to the SEMs of the prototype coil, the SEMs of the human head insert resemble their exact counterparts even more. Deviations are below 2% and the encoding directions are almost everywhere close to $90°$ indicating very high encoding efficiency.

In contrast to the first PatLoc prototype coil, the standard functionality of the scanner was not restricted during PatLoc measurements. The hardware was modified such that the quadrupolar SEMs could be controlled simultaneously and independently from the standard gradient system. The new coil integration approach enhanced the flexibility of the system because more channels were available (with the quadrupolar PatLoc coil, 5 instead of 3) for signal encoding (also cf. Fig. 3.18c).

The most important coil parameters for the small-bore PatLoc prototype coil and the large human head insert are compared with each other in Table 3.1. The comparison of the two coils reveals significant differences. Most obvious, the human head insert is much larger than the prototype insert coil. This explains the better performance of the small-bore prototype coil in terms of resistance, inductance and rise time. More important, however, is that larger objects (like the head) could be measured with the human head insert. Larger objects provide more signal with positive consequences for SNR. Despite the much higher field sensitivity of the small-bore prototype coil, the maximum gradient strength and especially the maximum magnetic field strength achievable with the human head insert is higher; these properties of the head insert are beneficial for image quality, but are still not optimal because the design of the coils allowed only a maximum current of 80 A, much less than the amplifiers could have provided (625 A). Problematic with the measurements on the small-bore system was that the PatLoc prototype coil could only be driven with a low current of 8.25 A. Therefore,

Table 3.1: Comparison of important coil parameters of the first small-bore prototype insert and the human head insert.

Parameter	Insert: Small-Bore	Human Head
usable diameter (with RF inside) [cm]	6	20
usable length [cm]	6	> 20
maximum current [A]	8.25	80
inductance [μH]	30	2200
resistance [mΩ]	400	510
rise time [μs]	24	200
dwell time [μs]	100	10
field sensitivity[8] [mT/Am^2]	26.1	1.44/1.36
max. gradient at the periphery [mT/m]	12.9	22.5
max. field strength at the periphery [mT]	0.2	1.1

the dwell time had to be chosen fairly large, setting a considerable lower bound on the choice of the echo time. Also, the large dwell times and SNR restrictions hindered the acquisition of high-resolution images with the first small-bore prototype coil.

The overall assessment of these parameters reveals that measurements with the human head insert should be more flexible and a higher image quality is to be expected. Measurements performed with the human insert confirm this assessment. As an example, an image of a fruit basket, which has been acquired with the head insert, is compared in Fig. 3.20 to the PatLoc prototype kiwi image shown in Fig. 3.16a.

Once the system had been set up correctly, it was not problematic to acquire high-resolution images with the human head insert. The image of the fruit basket has no geometric distortions; only some residual aliasing artifacts are visible, which are related to inaccuracies in the determination of the RF-sensitivity profiles. These artifacts are tolerable because they appear only at the low-resolution center.

---

[8]Field sensitivity of the outer and inner layer (cf. Fig. 3.18). With a different method, 1.42 mT/Am^2 was measured for the inner layer and 1.30 mT/Am^2 for the outer layer.

PatLoc

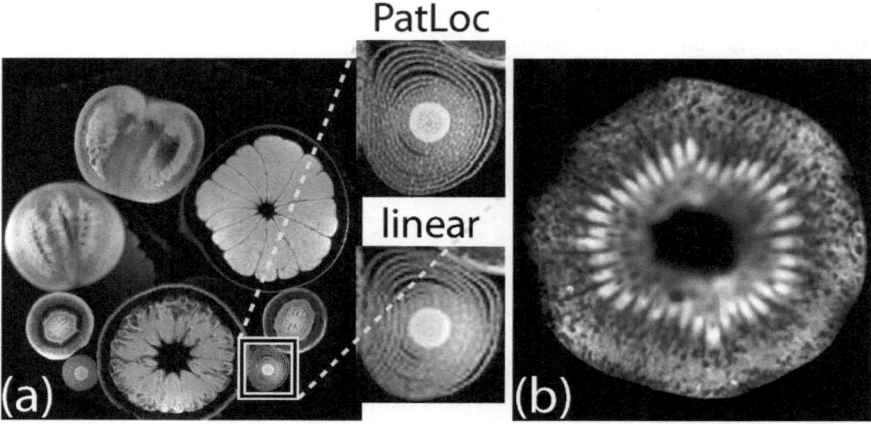

Figure 3.20: Comparison of PatLoc images acquired with the human head insert (a) and with the older small-bore prototype coil (b). The fruit basket was reconstructed from 384^2 data points. In compliance with the specifications of the prototype coil, only 128^2 data points were acquired for the kiwi fruit. The comparison of the zoomed-in sections of the PatLoc acquisition and an identical measurement, but encoded with the standard gradient system, shows that the image quality could be enhanced significantly compared to the first prototype system.

The problems associated with the first small-bore prototype coil could be solved with the second-generation small-bore PatLoc coil [120] and an image quality was achieved that is in no way inferior to the images found with the human head insert (cf. Fig. 3.16b). Currently, a high-performance coil is being manufactured also for the human system. The new coil will allow detailed assessment of image quality and fair comparison with conventional state-of-the-art gradient systems integrated into human systems.

Contributions of this Thesis and Current State of Research

THIS is a brief overview. More details about the major findings of this thesis are found in the summary, chapter 8.1, page 277ff, and important literature is presented where it seems most appropriate.

Contributions of This Thesis   Before this thesis was conducted conceptual ideas about PatLoc imaging had existed, and initial numerical simulations had substantiated the feasibility of MRI with NB-SEMs if combined with parallel image acquisition techniques [62]. A simplified encoding model had been used with non-overlapping RF-coil sensitivities that allowed straightforward image reconstruction. PatLoc measurement hardware had not yet been designed.

The main goal of this thesis was to elaborate the theoretical basis of PatLoc signal encoding, to develop efficient image reconstruction methods, and to evaluate these with numerical as well as experimental data, including in vivo measurements. In chapter 4 common principles of PatLoc encoding and reconstruction are presented. In chapters 5 to 7, reconstruction algorithms and imaging results are analyzed in detail for several PatLoc encoding strategies. The subsequent chapters therefore reflect the scientific outcome that is in line with the main focus of this thesis; also, the two primary own publications [[156, 158]] concern this part of the thesis.

A significant part of the scientific output also concerns other topics; among others, hardware, methods, applications. However, the main responsibility for these topics rested with other members of the PatLoc team; the PatLoc overview in chapter 3 is presented with a focus on topics that have resulted in (co-)authorship[1] contributions, for example [[61, 156, 42, 207, 63, 199, 24]].

Also the introductory chapter 2 contains material of scientific value. Its main impact lies on the conceptual level; some of the most important state-of-the-art MR image reconstruction methods are related to a common principle,

---

[1] It is repeated here that double brackets, [[·]], indicate own (co-)authorship.

thereby establishing interesting connections between them - as well as between existing methods and PatLoc image reconstruction, as shown in chapter 4. Moreover, in chapter 2.3.1e the superresolution effect of RF encoding is quantified. Further contributions are found in the appendix, sections A.3 to A.5.

A full list of own publications is included below on page 329ff.

Current State of Research   Prior to the PatLoc project, benefits from using NB-SEMs had rarely been discussed in the literature; among the few publications are [193, 110, 208, 131, 128, 126]. Each of these publications presents very interesting ideas; however, only specific aspects with very special field geometries are discussed therein. No attempt had been undertaken to develop a general imaging concept - like PatLoc imaging. These publications have had an impact on this thesis in some places; the major influence, however, comes from literature that deals with standard parallel image acquisition, most notably [173, 135, 134, 49].

In the meantime, several research groups have contributed important ideas to the growing field of imaging with NB-SEMs. Especially the group of Todd Constable (for example [22, 178, 41, 181]) from Yale university, USA, has to be mentioned, and Fa-Hsuan Lin (for example [97], [[101]]) from the Massachusetts General Hospital, USA. Recently, Layton et al. [93] from the university of Melbourne, Australia, have published interesting research results; actively involved is the research group of Rudolf Stollberger from the University of Graz, Austria, [[86]]. Noteworthy is also [87] by Kopanoglu et al. from Bilkent University, Ankara, Turkey, and the excellent work of Peter Jakob's group from the University of Würzburg, Germany, [203, 1].

Chapter 4

Basics of Signal Encoding and Image Reconstruction in PatLoc Imaging

TWO topics are treated in this chapter. On the one hand, it is discussed how the PatLoc imaging process can be modeled; on the other hand, the chapter deals with the problem of how images can be reconstructed in PatLoc. A common treatment of both topics in one chapter is useful because an approach of image reconstruction is taken here that makes immediate use of the imaging model. This chapter is based on work published in [[156]].

After derivation of the PatLoc signal equation, an introductory 1D reconstruction example is presented. Then, the matrix approach of chapter 2 is analyzed in the context of PatLoc imaging and extended to non-Cartesian reconstruction grids. After discussing how basic image properties can be investigated, the adaptation of iterative CG reconstruction to PatLoc imaging is discussed.

In the present chapter, a general perspective is adopted and the introduced material is the starting point for the development of efficient reconstruction algorithms for specific imaging modalities like Cartesian (chapter 5) or radial (chapter 6) PatLoc imaging and more general modalities (chapter 7).

4.1 The Fundamental Signal Model for PatLoc Imaging

A physical model should map the relevant information and ignore what can be neglected in a particular context. In this thesis, the context is PatLoc imaging; in other words, spatial encoding with nonlinear SEMs. From a theoretical point of view, the description of signal encoding in PatLoc is certainly interesting; from a practical point of view, it is also necessary because the reconstruction algorithms that are developed in this thesis rely on signal models which adequately describe the spatial encoding properties of PatLoc SEMs. In the first section of the present chapter a minimal model is presented; i.e., it maps only those features of the imaging process which are absolutely essential for the development of basic and useful reconstruction algorithms for PatLoc imaging. Model refinements are only briefly discussed.

In chapter 1 fundamental models were presented, which have proven to be useful and sufficient to describe the basic characteristics of Fourier imaging and parallel imaging. Many established reconstruction algorithms have been developed based on those models of signal encoding. The fundamental signal equation is Eq. 1.21; it is repeated here:

$$s(t) = \int_V m(\vec{x})c(\vec{x})e^{-i\phi(\vec{x},t)} \, d\vec{x}. \tag{4.1}$$

This equation expresses the fact that the recorded signal $s(t)$ results from an ensemble of non-interacting spins with density $m(\cdot)$ excited within a volume V. The equation also takes into consideration that the spin density is modulated by the sensitivity $c(\cdot)$ of the RF-receiver coils and by a phase factor $\phi(\cdot)$, which is normally influenced by the linear gradient fields. Other effects are ignored here. Particularly, in Eq. 1.22 it has been shown that the phase of the r-th readout is influenced by phase encoding and then by frequency encoding:

$$\phi(\vec{x},t;r) = \phi(\vec{x},0;r) + \gamma \int_{\tilde{t}=0}^{t} B_{enc}^{z}(\vec{x},\tilde{t};r) \, d\tilde{t}. \tag{4.2}$$

In this formulation, *the only difference of PatLoc to standard imaging is that the magnetic encoding field B_{enc} does not result from the linear gradient fields, but from SEMs with arbitrary[1] geometry.* It can be concluded from this observation that this model of signal encoding is also useful in the context of PatLoc imaging.

Recall that (cf. chapter 1.2.2, page 27ff), with the introduction of a k-space variable, signal and magnetization can be expressed by a simple Fourier relation, as long as a maximum of three orthogonal linear SEMs are involved. This Fourier relation is no longer valid in PatLoc, where nonlinear SEMs are

---

[1]In practice, fundamental restrictions exist, like for example compatibility with Maxwell's equations, and practical issues like wire topology, power consumption, thermal limitations, acoustic noise or nerve stimulation must be considered.

applied, and, what makes things even more complicated, where more than three SEMs might be available for signal encoding. It is shown here that the introduction of a "k-space" variable is also useful in the context of PatLoc imaging. The formal structure of this section follows the presentation on page 29f in chapter 1.2.2, and a comparison of the two sections clarifies that the "PatLoc k-space" variable, as it is defined here, is analogous to the standard k-space variable. It is shown here that, with this analogous definition of k-space, the signal equation for PatLoc imaging formally generalizes the signal equation known from conventional PI (cf. Eq. 1.31, page 38).

Comparable to conventional imaging, also in PatLoc, the magnetic encoding field $B_{enc}^z(\vec{x})$ can be a superposition of several SEMs. Depending on the experimental setup, the number of SEMs is, however, not necessarily restricted to three. In the general case, N_g SEMs are used for encoding. Each coil j generates a different SEM with field strength $B_j^z(\vec{x}, \tilde{t}; r) = I_j(\tilde{t}; r)b_j(\vec{x})$. It consists of the spatially varying SEM sensitivity $b_j(\mathbf{x})$ and the time-varying current $I_j(\tilde{t}; r)$ through coil j, which can be influenced according to the dynamic restrictions of the hardware. For such an experimental setup, the effective encoding field is then given by:

$$B_{enc}^z(\vec{x}, \tilde{t}; r) = \sum_{j=1}^{N_g} B_j^z(\vec{x}, \tilde{t}; r) = \sum_{j=1}^{N_g} I_j(\tilde{t}; r)b_j(\vec{x}). \tag{4.3}$$

The important result from Eq. 4.3 is that the magnetic field decomposes into the user-defined time-courses of the coil currents and a spatial component which is defined by the geometries of the SEMs. As a consequence, the phase distribution in Eq. 4.2 can be specified with the introduction of an N_g-dimensional PatLoc k-space variable analogous to the conventional k-space variable and with the definition of an N_g-dimensional encoding function $\psi(\cdot)$:

$$\phi(\vec{x}, t; r) = (\mathbf{k}_r + \mathbf{k}(t; r))^T \psi(\vec{x}), \tag{4.4}$$

where the components $j = 1, \ldots, N_g$ of the initial PatLoc k-space position $\mathbf{k}_r$ - with τ_r being the duration of phase encoding belonging to the r-th signal readout - and the k-space traversal during readout $\mathbf{k}(t; r)$ are defined as:

$$(k_r)_j := \beta \int_{\tilde{t}=0}^{\tau_r} I_j(\tilde{t}; r) \, d\tilde{t} \quad \text{and} \quad k_j(t; r) := \beta \int_{\tilde{t}=0}^{t} I_j(\tilde{t}; r) \, d\tilde{t}. \tag{4.5}$$

and where the components of the encoding function $\psi(\cdot)$ are proportional to the applied SEMs:

$$\psi_j(\vec{x}) := \gamma/\beta \cdot b_j(\vec{x}). \tag{4.6}$$

β is a scaling factor, which can be chosen freely. In conventional imaging with linear gradient fields, for practical reasons, β is set to be γg, where g is the gradient strength with unit coil current (cf. Eq. 1.25, page 29). This definition is problematic in the context of PatLoc, where the gradient strength is a quantity that varies along the spatial dimensions. If - as done here - the PatLoc k-space variable is defined to vary only along the temporal dimension, it is not advisable to refer to any spatial property of the SEMs in the definition of β, including the gradient strength (or its average). However, as β is just a scaling factor, it can be defined as unity or 2π, as in Eq. 5.15, or by any other value, depending on what is most convenient in a particular situation. For simplicity, when scaling is not of particular interest, the term "SEMs" is also used to denote the individual components ψ_j of the encoding function.

Introducing the k-space notation (Eqs. 4.4, 4.5) into the signal equation (Eq. 4.1) leads to:

$$s(t;r) = \int_V m(\vec{x})c(\vec{x})e^{-i(\mathbf{k}_r + \mathbf{k}(t;r))^T \psi(\vec{x})}\,d\vec{x}. \tag{4.7}$$

For the determination of image contrast, the temporal order of data sampling along the imaging trajectory is important. However, just like in the linear case presented above (chapter 1.2.2, on page 30), explicit time-dependent effects like relaxation are ignored here. Under these assumptions, the exact time of data sampling can be disregarded, and it is sufficient to define the set of acquired PatLoc k-space locations $\mathcal{K} = \{\mathbf{k}_r + \mathbf{k}(t;r); \tilde{t} \in [0;T], r = 1, \ldots, N_{pe}\}$.[2] Thus, also in the context of PatLoc imaging, it is

---

[2]Note that in the general case and in contrast to conventional imaging, it is no longer possible to densely sample (PatLoc) k-space (cf. the paragraph *Excursion: Completeness of k-Space Encoding* on page 64); only a sparse trajectory through a high-dimensional PatLoc k-space is traversed. Therefore, the trajectory $\mathcal{K}$ cannot be treated as a subset of the potentially very large vector space $\mathbb{R}^{N_g}$. For multi-dimensional encoding the PatLoc k-space trajectory loses its meaning as the Fourier analogue of the image in favor of the local k-space with consequences for image reconstruction. Adequate reconstruction methods are presented in chapters 7.1.1 and 7.1.2, page 237ff.

useful to simplify the signal equation by only considering the signal values
at the sampled k-space locations $\mathbf{k}_\kappa \in \mathcal{K}$. The signal is then given by:

$$s(\mathbf{k}_\kappa) = \int_V m(\vec{x})c(\vec{x})e^{-i\mathbf{k}_\kappa^T \psi(\vec{x})}\, d\vec{x}. \tag{4.8}$$

Depending on the PatLoc k-space trajectory and the encoding function $\psi(\cdot)$,
encoding might be insufficient for non-ambiguous reconstruction. In this
case, it is necessary to complement SEM encoding with parallel acquisition
using N_c receiver coils with sensitivities $c_\alpha(\cdot)$. The acquired signals $s_\alpha(\cdot)$
are then given by:

$$s_\alpha(\mathbf{k}_\kappa) = \int_V m(\vec{x})c_\alpha(\vec{x})e^{-i\mathbf{k}_\kappa^T \psi(\vec{x})}\, d\vec{x}. \tag{4.9}$$

In the subsequent chapters derivations of reconstruction algorithms will be
presented which are based on this fundamental signal equation of PatLoc
imaging.

Consider the comparison of the signal equation in standard parallel imaging
(Eq. 1.31) with the corresponding equation in PatLoc imaging:

$$\underbrace{s_\alpha(\vec{k}_\kappa) = \int_V m(\vec{x})c_\alpha(\vec{x})e^{-i\vec{k}_\kappa \vec{x}}\, d\vec{x}}_{\text{Standard PI}} \qquad \underbrace{s_\alpha(\mathbf{k}_\kappa) = \int_V m(\vec{x})c_\alpha(\vec{x})e^{-i\mathbf{k}_\kappa^T \psi(\vec{x})}\, d\vec{x}}_{\text{PatLoc}}$$

$$\tag{4.10}$$

The two equations differ only in the phase factor. The phase $\vec{k}_\kappa \vec{x}$ must be
replaced by $\mathbf{k}_\kappa^T \psi(\vec{x})$. There are basically two differences:

1. The spatial variable $\vec{x}$ is replaced by a general encoding function $\psi(\vec{x})$,
   thereby introducing new *spatial* degrees of freedom to MRI signal
   encoding.
2. The dimensions of $\mathbf{k}$ and ψ correspond to the number N_g of SEMs
   used for imaging. In conventional imaging N_g is 2 for in-plane encoding and 3 for volume encoding. In PatLoc, N_g can be any natural
   number. The possibility to use multi-dimensional trajectories also
   adds new *temporal* degrees of freedom to MRI signal encoding.

Remark: The term *nonlinear and non-bijective SEMs* may be misleading because it is rather the combination of the used SEMs, which can make encoding ambiguous. It is therefore clearer to say that the encoding function ψ has

the property of being nonlinear and non-bijective. For multi-dimensional trajectories, it also seems appropriate to simply use the term *nonlinear SEMs*.

The signal model represented by Eq. 4.9 is very basic; only the most fundamental implications are reflected by the model that PatLoc encoding has on MR images. Two effects are considered: SEM encoding, supplemented by RF-receiver sensitivity encoding. All other factors that may influence the acquired signals are disregarded. For example, when, in PatLoc, more than three SEMs are used for signal encoding, $T1$ and $T2$ relaxation can have unusual effects on image contrast. Not considered is the possibility to encode information into the phase of the magnetization with adequate RF-transmit pulses. Hardware imperfections are ignored and it is not discussed that the spins do not form, in reality, an isolated mono-nuclear ensemble of non-interacting spins.

The list of important effects that are not considered is actually very long and research in this regard is still in the early stages. One example in this context is [[121]], where it has been shown that it is possible to integrate B_0-inhomogeneities into the signal equation without the necessity to significantly modify image reconstruction. In this thesis, these and other model refinements are usually disregarded.

4.2   Basics of Linear Image Reconstruction in PatLoc Imaging

Based on the signal equation for PatLoc imaging, derived in the previous section, general approaches to linear image reconstruction are treated here. Nonlinear image reconstruction methods are excluded from the discussion. Before the general theory is presented, a basic introductory example of image reconstruction is discussed.

4.2.1   A Simple 1D Example

Reconsider the simple introductory example of chapter 3.1, page 103ff, with the idealized assumption that the sensitive volume of different RF coils do not overlap. This example is very simple and most probably not useful in practice; nevertheless, the reconstruction from this example already shares important aspects with the reconstruction algorithms which are derived in the subsequent chapters with the help of the general matrix theory of the present chapter, without the use of restrictive and unrealistic assumptions. The introductory example of chapter 3.1 may not be particularly practical, but, in theory, it may result from a feasible experiment with the following assumptions:

- The excitation volume V is a very thin and long bar-shaped region, which extends along the x-axis.
- Only one readout of very long duration and continuous sampling is acquired with the echo formed at $t = 0$.
- A single SEM with field strength $B(x) = hx^2$ along the excited x-axis is used.[3] W. l. o. g. assume $h = \gamma^{-1}$.
- The encoding field remains constant during readout.

With these assumptions, the signal equation (Eq. 4.7) can be specified accordingly:

- Similar to the formal reduction from 3D to 2D for slice selection (cf. chapter 1.2.3, on page 33), the present problem with a bar-shaped excitation volume can be reduced to 1D. Therefore the variable $\vec{x} \in \mathbb{R}^3$ can be replaced by $x \in \mathbb{R}$.
- There is only a single readout; therefore, the dependency of the signal $s(t; r)$ on r, which normally marks different readouts, can be neglected.
- In the phase factor $(\mathbf{k}_r + \mathbf{k}(t; r))^T \psi(\vec{x})$, the first summand can be ignored because it is assumed that no additional phase encoding is performed ($\mathbf{k}_r = 0$).
- With the definitions of Eqs. 4.5, 4.6, the phase $\mathbf{k}(t; r)^T \psi(\vec{x})$ reduces to $x^2 t$.

Incorporating these issues into the signal equation yields:

$$s(t) = \int_{-\infty}^{\infty} m(x)c(x)e^{-ix^2 t}\,dx. \tag{4.11}$$

Consider now two RF-receiver coils with idealized coil sensitivities. The first coil shall have a homogeneous sensitivity on the positive part of the x-axis, and no sensitivity on the negative part of the axis (i.e., $c_1(x) = 1$ for

---

[3]Such a field is for example generated by a quadrupolar encoding field for $y = 0$ and $z = 0$, cf. chapter 3.3.1, page 122ff.

$x > 0$ and $c_1(x) = 0$ otherwise). As opposed to this, the second coil shall be sensitive to the negative part of the axis and insensitive to the positive part (i.e., $c_2(x) = 1$ for $x \leq 0$ and $c_2(x) = 0$ otherwise). It is therefore assumed that the coil sensitivities do not overlap and complementarily cover the whole object. Consider now the signal of the first coil:

$$s_1(t) = \int_{-\infty}^{\infty} m(x)c(x)e^{-ix^2t}\,\mathrm{d}x = \int_{0}^{\infty} m(x)e^{-ix^2t}\,\mathrm{d}x. \qquad (4.12)$$

This equation can be transformed with the variable transformation $\omega = x^2$. This transformation is *bijective* because x is restricted to the positive arc of the parabola. The transformed equation is then given by:

$$s_1(t) = \int_{0}^{\infty} \frac{\tilde{m}(\omega)}{\sqrt{\omega}} e^{-i\omega t}\,\mathrm{d}\omega. \qquad (4.13)$$

As presumed above, the readout is of very long duration. For simplicity, the assumption is made here that the readout is even of infinite length. Therefore, signal data is available for all $t \in \mathbb{R}$. With this assumption, multiplication of the Fourier transform of the signal data with $\sqrt{\omega}$ yields:

$$\tilde{m}(\omega) = \sqrt{\omega} \cdot \mathcal{FT}\{s_1\}(\omega). \qquad (4.14)$$

Finally, the spin density $m(x)$ is recovered for $x > 0$ by transforming $\tilde{m}$ back to the image space variable $x = \sqrt{\omega}$. The signal of the second coil can then be used to reconstruct the spin density for $x \leq 0$: For the second signal, the variable transformation $\omega = x^2$ is also bijective because only the left arc of the parabola is considered. By first calculating $\tilde{m}(\omega) = \sqrt{\omega} \cdot \mathcal{FT}\{s_2\}(\omega)$ and then back-transforming $\tilde{m}(\omega)$ with $x = -\sqrt{\omega}$, the spin density is indeed regained for all $x \leq 0$. The results from the first signal and the second signal can then be combined to find the spin density $m(x)$ for all locations x. This reconstruction procedure is visualized in Fig. 4.1.

The three reconstruction steps - Fourier transformation, intensity correction and variable transformation - also form fundamental steps for a more practical situation, where a 2D slice is encoded with two NB-SEMs (see next chapter). The similarity of the 1D example and the more practical 2D problem of the following chapter becomes even more obvious when the assumptions of the 1D example are formulated more realistically.

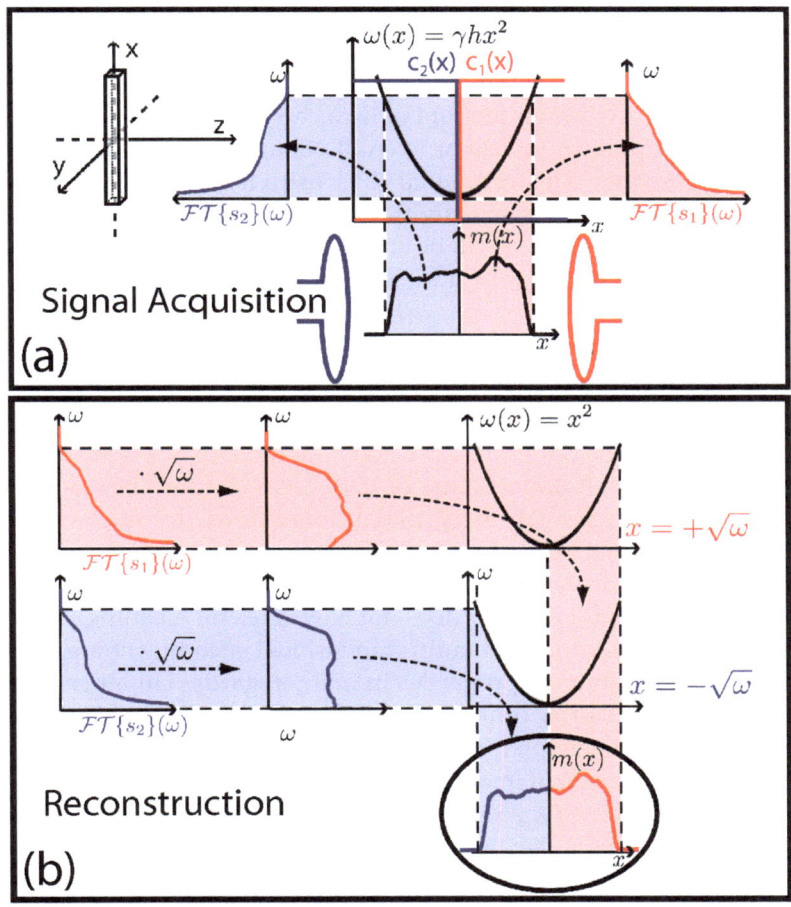

Figure 4.1: Signal acquisition (a) and reconstruction (b) for a simple 1D example. (a) A thin bar-shaped volume is excited and signals are recorded with two RF-receiver coils. One RF coil has a sensitivity only at those positions which correspond to the right arc of the quadratic SEM (red). The other RF coil is sensitive only on the left arc of the SEM (blue). The signal recorded with the RF coil on the right therefore contains only image information from the right half of the spin density $m(x)$, whereas the signal recorded with the other RF coil results from the left side of the spin density. (b) First, the recorded signals are Fourier transformed. After that, the signal is intensity-corrected by multiplication with $\sqrt{\omega}$. Then, the signal from the right RF coil is mapped back to the positive x-axis and the signal from the other coil is mapped to the negative x-axis. Finally, the two reconstructed signals are pieced together.

First, consider that in practice, readouts have a restricted duration; consequently, image resolution is finite and the variable transformation leads to a non-homogeneous distribution of image resolution. Second, take into account that only a discrete amount of data can be acquired. This problem is especially important for 2D or even 3D imaging. Aliasing can result that can be resolved with additional RF-sensitivity encoding. And third, observe that in reality, the sensitivities of the RF coils overlap with each other. In the next chapter, it will be shown that an additional SENSE-like matrix inversion step must be added to the reconstruction to cope with these overlaps.

The 1D example and the more practical 2D reconstruction of the following chapter share many characteristics with each other. The main reason for the similarity is that in the 1D example a single SEM is used to encode a single spatial dimension. In the 2D reconstruction two SEMs are available to encode two spatial dimensions. In both cases, the number of SEMs is equal to the number of encoded spatial dimensions. More complicated is the situation when more than two SEMs are used to encode a 2D slice. The problem with such multi-dimensional encoding strategies is that the 2D Fourier transform generally does not have a useful meaning. Notwithstanding, the 1D example and multi-dimensional encoding strategies also have similar fundamental properties in many regards. Under certain circumstances a 1D Fourier transform along the temporal dimension has a useful meaning (cf. chapter 7.1.2, page 240ff); also for the most general case of multi-dimensional imaging, image resolution is typically not a homogeneous property of the reconstructed images (cf. e.g. Fig. 7.11, page 264). Despite these similarities, the 1D example cannot explain all properties of PatLoc imaging, especially not the possibilities that PatLoc offers in the temporal domain; the example should not be overinterpreted and care should be taken when generalizations to higher dimensions are made without further examination.

4.2.2   Matrix Inversion Approaches in PatLoc

A general framework for linear reconstruction methods was presented in chapter 2.1, page 40ff. Recall that two approaches were discussed in chapter 2.1.1, page 40ff: the weak and the strong approach. Both require the inversion of a large matrix, thus explaining the term *matrix inversion approaches* in the section title. The framework had originally been proven useful in the context of parallel imaging with linear SEMs; however, the theory is not restricted to standard PI. Of central importance in the context of this reconstruction framework are the encoding functions $\text{enc}_{\alpha,\kappa}(\vec{x})$. These functions map the spatial distribution of any encoding scheme that can be described by a finite amount of values; nothing more is demanded; also PatLoc falls under this imaging category, which shows that the matrix approaches can also be applied to PatLoc imaging data. According to Eq. 4.9, the encoding functions in PatLoc are given by:

$$\text{enc}_{\alpha,\kappa}(\vec{x}) = c_\alpha(\vec{x})e^{-\mathrm{i}\mathbf{k}_\kappa^T \psi(\vec{x})}. \tag{4.15}$$

With these encoding functions, the encoding matrix $\mathbf{E}$ and the correlation matrix $\mathbf{B}$ can be built following Eqs. 2.9, 2.14. W. l. o. g. assuming normalized voxel volumes ($\Delta V := 1$), the weak reconstruction matrix is found, according to Eq. 2.11, by taking the MPPI solution $\mathbf{F} = \mathbf{E}^+$, and the strong reconstruction matrix is given by $\mathbf{F} = \mathbf{E}^H\mathbf{B}^+$, according to Eq. 2.13. The image is reconstructed by calculating the matrix-vector product

$$\mathbf{m} \overset{(2.4)}{=} \mathbf{F}\mathbf{s}. \tag{4.16}$$

The presented mathematical framework is therefore in principle applicable to PatLoc. It has, however, one restriction, which should be relaxed to permit a flexible development of reconstruction methods in PatLoc imaging: In PatLoc, it can be useful under certain conditions to reconstruct images onto non-equidistant reconstruction grids. There is typically no need to take such irregular grids into consideration when linear SEMs are used for encoding. This can be different in PatLoc, where nonlinear SEMs are applied. For example, a non-regular grid is chosen in the fundamental Cartesian reconstruction method, presented below in chapter 5.1, page 155ff. The extension to irregular reconstruction grids requires some changes in the general theory; these are delineated here, and it is discussed separately that a precise definition of the term *nominal voxel volume* is important in this regard. Also, it is presented how image properties, such as image resolution or SNR, can be determined in PatLoc imaging.

a)   Extension to Non-Rectilinear Reconstruction Grids

The consequences for the weak (cf. chapter 2.1.1a, page 42ff) and the strong (cf. chapter 2.1.1b, page 45) reconstruction approach are discussed here.

Weak Reconstruction   As was already pointed out in chapter 2.1.1a, page 42ff, the size of the reconstructed voxels is typically ignored in the calculations even though correct mathematical treatment has to consider the voxel size. This imprecision is acceptable and harmless for regular reconstruction grids, which are typically chosen. Non-regular reconstruction grids necessitate a more exact treatment.

Reconsider the condition of weak reconstruction, given by Eq. 2.8, page 42. It has been argued why it is necessary to introduce the voxel volume ΔV on the right hand side of Eq. 2.8. When non-regular reconstruction grids are considered, this voxel volume can vary from voxel to voxel. Therefore, ΔV should be replaced by a different symbol (v_ρ) to indicate this dependency. Equation 2.8 then becomes:[4]

$$\int_V i_\rho^*(\vec{x}) f_{\rho'}(\vec{x}) \, d\vec{x} = v_\rho^{-1} \delta_{\rho,\rho'}. \tag{4.17}$$

The encoding matrix can still be defined in the same way as before (cf. Eq. 2.9). Similar to the conventional case, the shape of the ideal voxel function is of minor interest if, for all data points (α, κ), the encoding functions $\text{enc}_{\alpha,\kappa}(\vec{x})$ do not vary significantly over the size of a voxel. This criterion is fulfilled for sufficiently dense reconstruction grids. The local nominal voxel volume (defined in the next section on page 148) should be chosen smaller than an oscillation of the encoding function with the highest spatial variation at the corresponding location. If done so, it is sufficient to simply consider delta functions $i_\rho^*(\vec{x}) := \delta(\vec{x} - \vec{x}_\rho)$ as ideal voxel shapes. With delta functions and Eqs. 2.9, 4.15, the entries of the encoding matrix are given by:

$$E_{(\alpha,\kappa),\rho} := c_\alpha(\vec{x}_\rho) e^{-i\mathbf{k}_\kappa^T \psi(\vec{x}_\rho)}. \tag{4.18}$$

---

[4]The equation is valid for reconstructions that aim at finding the average density of the magnetization within a voxel; if the total magnetization within the reconstructed voxels is of interest, the values v_ρ must be replaced by their inverses v_ρ^{-1} and in subsequent equations, also the matrix $\mathbf{V} := \text{diag}(v_1, \ldots, v_{N_\rho})$ must be replaced by its inverse $\mathbf{V}^{-1}$.

With this definition and Eq. 2.7, the condition of weak reconstruction can be rewritten as a matrix equation:

$$\mathbf{F}(\mathbf{EV}) = \mathbb{1}, \qquad (4.19)$$

where $\mathbf{V}$ is a diagonal matrix $\mathbf{V} = \mathrm{diag}\,(v_1, \ldots, v_{N_\rho})$, which deviates from a multiple of the unity matrix if non-equidistant reconstruction grids are chosen. The MPPI solution of this equation is then given by:

$$\mathbf{F} = (\mathbf{EV})^+. \qquad (4.20)$$

According to the discussion following Eq. 2.11, page 43, the MPPI solution covers overdetermined as well as underdetermined situations. Nevertheless, it is useful to analyze two special cases in more detail.

1. Consider a coarse grid such that the condition of weak reconstruction can be satisfied. Moreover, assume that $\mathbf{E}$ has full rank. Then, the reconstruction matrix is given by:

$$\mathbf{F} = \mathbf{V}^{-1}(\mathbf{E}^H\mathbf{E})^{-1}\mathbf{E}^H = \mathbf{V}^{-1}\mathbf{E}^+. \qquad (4.21)$$

   After multiplication of the signal with the MPPI of the encoding matrix, the intermediate image must therefore be multiplied with $\mathbf{V}^{-1}$. This multiplication corresponds to an intensity correction as final reconstruction step, which is necessary whenever non-rectilinear reconstruction grids are used.

2. Next, consider a fine grid such that the condition of weak reconstruction cannot be satisfied everywhere. Again assume a full rank encoding matrix. Then, a feasible solution is found by minimizing the least-squares problem $\|[\mathbf{F}(\mathbf{EV}) - \mathbb{1}]\mathbf{W}\|_F^2$. Set $\mathbf{W} := \mathbb{1}$ to ensure equal weighting for all image voxels (cf. page 44 in chapter 2.1.1a). Then the explicit solution is given by:

$$\mathbf{F} = \mathbf{V}\mathbf{E}^H(\mathbf{E}\mathbf{V}^2\mathbf{E}^H)^{-1}. \qquad (4.22)$$

Strong Reconstruction   The usage of non-rectilinear reconstruction grids has no effect on the formal structure of the solution from the strong reconstruction because the correlation matrix $\mathbf{B}$ is determined by integration along the spatial dimension. The solution is therefore also given by Eq. 2.13, which is repeated here:

$$\mathbf{F} = \mathbf{E}^H \mathbf{B}^+. \tag{4.23}$$

As already pointed out before, the integration has to be discretized in practice. Typically, a Riemann sum with equidistant node locations is chosen. If the integration is approximated by the usage of the encoding matrix with entries on non-equidistant locations along the spatial dimension, the correlation matrix should rather be approximated by $\mathbf{B} \approx \mathbf{EVE}^H$. Then, the solution of this discretized version of the strong reconstruction approach is given by $\mathbf{F} = \mathbf{E}^H (\mathbf{EVE}^H)^{-1}$. This reconstruction is the solution to $\min_{\mathbf{F}} \left\| [\mathbf{F}(\mathbf{EV}) - \mathbb{1}] \mathbf{V}^{-1/2} \right\|_F$. Such a reconstruction would therefore weight errors in small voxels more than in large voxels. This should be avoided by introducing the weighting matrix $\mathbf{V}^{1/2}$. That solution then conforms exactly to the solution from weak reconstruction, presented in Eq. 4.22.

b)   Nominal Voxel Volume

According to Eqs. 4.17 - 4.20, the reconstruction depends on the quantities v_ρ. In the previous section, these quantities were treated as being identical to the nominal voxel volume, which simply describes the volumes that are actually covered by the reconstructed image voxels. The validity of this approach is examined in this section. In a first step, several methods are presented that show how the nominal voxel volume can be determined. In a second step, it is shown that it is reasonable to use the nominal voxel volume to describe v_ρ. For simplicity, the presentation is restricted to 2D; notwithstanding, pixels are denominated as "voxels", in conformity with the rest of this dissertation. Extension to 3D does not require major modifications.

Methods for the Determination of the Nominal Voxel Volume   There is no unique way of determining the nominal voxel volume. However, an appropriate method is required for non-homogeneous distributions of image voxels because, typically, only the voxel centers are given, not the corresponding voxel volumes. Three methods are described here.

- Voronoi diagrams [2]. The same method is used to determine the density compensation function in non-Cartesian MRI (also cf. chapter 2.2.3 on page 70f).

- Contour plots. This method can be used if a continuous function $\vec{\psi} : \mathbb{R}^2 \to \mathbb{R}^2$ is known that transforms the non-rectilinear grid to a rectilinear grid. The enclosed area formed by the contour lines of the two components $\psi_1(\cdot)$ and $\psi_2(\cdot)$ gives similar results than the Voronoi method. These two first methods are illustrated in Fig. 4.2 for a homogeneous and a non-homogeneous distribution of image voxels.

- Local volumetric deformation. The voxel volumes can also be approximated by the local volumetric deformation induced by the function $\vec{\psi}(\vec{u})$ at the voxel centers. This approximation is typically fairly accurate except for extreme cases, for example in the vicinity of local extrema, where very large voxels occur (also cf. the *Remark* on page 166).

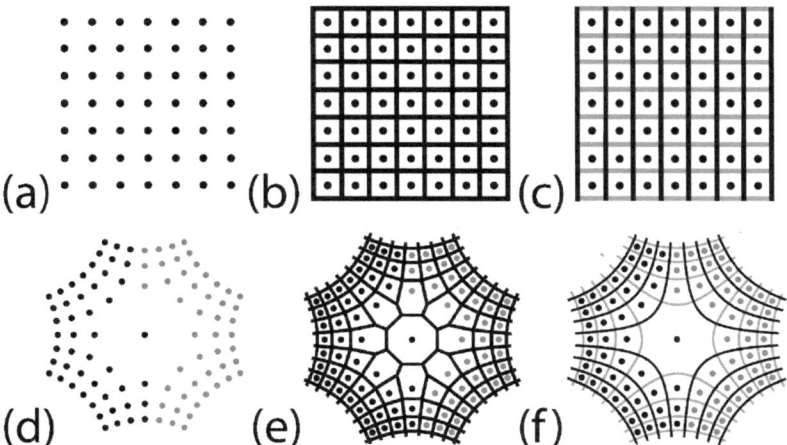

Figure 4.2: Determination of the nominal voxel volume. (a) Locations of a rectilinear reconstruction grid. (b) The Voronoi diagram can be used to define the nominal voxel volume. (c) Also the enclosed area of the contour lines can serve to determine the nominal voxel volume. For rectilinear grids both methods produce the same result. (d-f) The analogous situation is depicted for a non-rectilinear grid. Deviations of the two methods are visible for the large voxels at the center.

The Jacobian determinant describes the deformation,[5] and transforms a voxel with volume ΔU according to:

$$\text{Vol}(V_\rho) \approx \left| \det\left(\frac{\partial \vec{\psi}^{-1}(\vec{u}_\rho)}{\partial \vec{u}} \right) \right| \cdot \Delta U. \tag{4.24}$$

Here, $\text{Vol}(V_\rho)$ denotes the nominal voxel volume. Keep in mind that the voxel volume solely depends on the chosen reconstruction grid.

Relationship Between v_ρ and the Nominal Voxel Volume   It rests to be shown that v_ρ is closely related to the nominal voxel volume $\text{Vol}(V_\rho)$. To show this, assume an ideal voxel shape that is zero except for all $\vec{x} \in V_\rho$, where it is given by $i_\rho(\vec{x}) = 1/\text{Vol}(V_\rho)$, according to Eq. 2.5. Consider first a coarse reconstruction grid such that the weak condition of Eq. 4.17 can be satisfied. In this case $f_\rho(\cdot)$ is localized in relation to the voxel volume V_ρ and most signal energy results from within V_ρ. According to Eq. 2.6, page 42, it is reasonable to assume that the integration of the SRF over the object volume V is approximately unity. Therefore, it is plausible to conclude that

$$1 \approx \int_V f_\rho(\vec{x}) \, d\vec{x} \approx \int_{V_\rho} f_\rho(\vec{x}) \, d\vec{x} = \text{Vol}(V_\rho) \int_V i_\rho(\vec{x}) f_\rho(\vec{x}) \, d\vec{x} = \text{Vol}(V_\rho) v_\rho^{-1}.$$

It follows immediately that $v_\rho \approx \text{Vol}(V_\rho)$. For coarse grids, it is therefore useful to define v_ρ by the nominal voxel volume. For fine grids, the same is true: Based on Eqs. 2.6, 2.7, it can be shown that a useful reconstruction is found by approximating the unity matrix by **FEV** and not by **FE** to get the correct intensity and a balanced weighting for all voxels. Also very convincing is the argument that the solution obtained from the data-consistency constraint and the matrix approach solutions should be consistent with each other. From the *Remark* presented below on page 153, it can be concluded that consistency is ensured if v_ρ is defined equivalent to the nominal voxel volume.

It is not critical that the nominal voxel volume cannot be determined in a unique way; for coarse grids, a bad guess of v_ρ will have an effect on the intensity of the reconstructed images only and minor intensity variations generally do not affect the diagnostic usability of an image. For fine grids,

---

[5]With complex-valued notation (see Appendix A.4, page 299ff), the fields can be represented by a holomorphic function $f(s)$. The deformation is then simply described by the magnitude of the complex derivative $|f'(s)|$.

a bad guess of v_ρ will also affect optimal balance of the voxel weighting, which is, however, not crucial either.

Remark: In general, the nominal voxel volume is not related to image resolution; by definition, it is a property of the chosen image reconstruction grid only. It can be useful, however, to define a reconstruction grid with a density proportional to the effective spatial resolution of the reconstructed images. This is done in standard Fourier imaging as well as in the Cartesian PatLoc reconstruction algorithm, presented below in chapter 5.1, page 155ff.

c) Analysis of Fundamental Image Properties

In chapter 2.1.3 and 2.1.4, page 50ff, methods were described that can be used to determine fundamental image properties for any linear reconstruction method. The matrix inversion approaches are linear, and applicable to imaging with NB-SEMs; therefore, the described methods are also useful for PatLoc imaging. For example, image SNR can be calculated with the help of Eq. 2.22, page 55, or spatial resolution can be analyzed with the SRF based on Eq. 2.16, page 50. The approaches require evaluation of the reconstruction matrix **F** and are therefore only useful in situations, where **F** can be calculated accurately and fast enough. This is not often possible, an example is the Cartesian PatLoc reconstruction method presented in chapter 5.1, page 155ff.

For linear reconstruction algorithms it is also possible and usually faster to simply rely on reconstructions based on simulated input data. SNR may be determined by evaluating the statistics of several reconstructions from pure noise data. Image resolution might be determined by evaluating several PSFs (cf. Eq. 2.17, page 50), reconstructed from data with signal from single source locations. Such an analysis requires repeated application of the reconstruction algorithm and may still be very time-consuming. Matters are aggravated because these methods provide only a descriptive picture of the image properties making it difficult to systematically analyze their causes.

A third and fast option is to rely on approximate methods. For two nonlinear SEMs image resolution may be estimated from the extent of the acquired PatLoc k-space in combination with the deformation induced by the field nonlinearities (cf. e.g. paragraph *Resolution – Sampling Window Approach* in chapter 5.1.1e on page 168ff). When more than two SEMs are applied, image resolution is still determined by the PatLoc k-space trajectory and the spatial derivatives of the SEMs; the local k-space combines these two effects (cf. Eq. A.23, page 305), and from its extent the spatial resolution may directly be estimated (cf. Appendix A.5.1, page 303ff). The distribution of image resolution can also serve as a quick estimate for SNR variations (cf. e.g. Fig. 7.12); another approximate method for SNR is described in [93].

4.2.3   Consequences of Non-Rectilinear Reconstruction Grids for Iterative Reconstruction

Similar to non-Cartesian PI, where reconstruction with the CG method has proven to be useful, iterative methods are also of interest in the context of PatLoc imaging as an alternative to the matrix inversion approaches. Also for such CG-based algorithms the usage of non-rectilinear reconstruction grids requires modifications of the standard approach. Recall that the iterative CG method is based on the compliance to the data-consistency constraint, which is given by $s \approx Em$. This is true for rectilinear reconstruction grids. If, however, non-equidistant locations are chosen for the reconstruction, the data-consistency constraint must be modified. Remember that the constraint results from the discretization of the signal equation. In PatLoc, the signal is given by Eq. 4.9, page 139. Typically, the discretization is described by a Riemann sum with equidistant nodes, whose positions are given by the reconstruction grid. The same is true for non-rectilinear reconstruction grids. Note that, in this case, the integrand evaluated at the nodes must be multiplied by the nominal voxel volume v_ρ:

$$s_{\alpha,\kappa} = \int_V m(\vec{x}) \mathrm{enc}_{\alpha,\kappa}(\vec{x}) \, \mathrm{d}\vec{x} \approx \mathrm{enc}_{\alpha,\kappa}(\vec{x}_\rho) v_\rho m(\vec{x}_\rho). \qquad (4.25)$$

In matrix notation, the data-consistency constraint then reads $s \approx EVm$, where V is the diagonal matrix as introduced above. In the iterative reconstruction, the matrix E therefore has to be replaced by EV. For example, for $N_\rho < N_\kappa N_c$,[6] the l_2 minimization of the data-consistency error then results in the matrix equation

$$(E^H E)Vm = E^H s. \qquad (4.26)$$

---

[6]For $N_\rho > N_\kappa N_c$ and/or Tikhonov regularization, the modifications presented in chapter 2.3.1f, page 89ff, apply correspondingly.

This equation represents a matrix equation which can be solved for example with the CG method described on page 93 in chapter 2.3.1f. The computation time is almost not affected by the additional multiplication with $\mathbf{V}$ because this matrix is diagonal. On the contrary: In chapter 7.1.3, page 247ff, it is shown that under certain circumstances image reconstruction can be speeded up significantly because non-rectilinear reconstruction grids can lead to faster computations of $\mathbf{E}$.

Remark: The discretization approach is also consistent with the weak matrix inversion method presented above. Assume $N_\rho < N_\kappa N_c$ and full rank encodings $\mathbf{E}$. Then $\mathbf{E}^H\mathbf{E}$ is invertible and the minimization of the data-consistency constraint $(\mathbf{E}^H\mathbf{E})\mathbf{V}\mathbf{m} = \mathbf{E}^H\mathbf{s}$ has the unique solution $\mathbf{m} = \mathbf{V}^{-1}(\mathbf{E}^H\mathbf{E})^{-1}\mathbf{E}^H\mathbf{s} = \mathbf{V}^{-1}\mathbf{E}^+\mathbf{s}$. This is, however, also the MPPI solution $\mathbf{F} = \mathbf{V}^{-1}\mathbf{E}^+$ found with the weak matrix approach (see Eq. 4.21, page 147). Similar arguments show the consistency of the two approaches also for the case $N_\rho > N_\kappa N_c$.

4.2.4 Tailoring Reconstruction to Specific Encoding Strategies: An Outline

In the present chapter, two different approaches to reconstruct images from general PatLoc-encoded datasets were presented (matrix inversion, iterative solution) and it was shown how fundamental image properties like SNR or image resolution can be analyzed. With these methods – at least in principle – all tools necessary for image reconstruction in PatLoc are available.

Yet, whether NB-SEMs are applied or linear gradient fields, the problem remains that, under practical conditions, the matrix inversion approach is usually not an option without further acceleration because the matrix to be inverted is just too large. To be useful, also the iterative method needs to be speeded up. Fortunately, a profound analysis of the structure of the encoding matrix reveals that algorithmic improvements are possible for all PatLoc encoding strategies.

The following three chapters are devoted to the problem of finding and analyzing fast and accurate reconstructions for several specific encoding strategies. The most basic situation of 2D Cartesian encoding with two NB-SEMs is the topic of the next chapter. A non-Cartesian radial encoding strategy with two NB-SEMs is discussed in chapter 6. For such acquisitions, performed with two NB-SEMs, direct reconstruction algorithms are practical and it is often not necessary to rely on iterative algorithms. Iterative methods are analyzed in chapter 7, where it is shown that these methods are especially useful for subsampled as well as for multi-dimensional encoding strategies.

Chapter 5

Direct Reconstruction for Cartesian PatLoc Imaging

$\mathbf{F}$OR good reason, Cartesian sampling trajectories are the most important acquisition strategies in MRI: Robust acquisition and reconstruction go hand in hand with this Cartesian method. In this chapter, it is shown that the same is true in PatLoc imaging. Though being applicable to only a particular encoding strategy, the methods developed in this chapter may be regarded as the most fundamental methods in PatLoc imaging. Special emphasis is placed on an image space oriented reconstruction. The presentation is based on work published in [[155, 161, 162, 156]]. The shorter, second part of this chapter sheds light on the possibilities of k-space oriented image reconstruction in PatLoc imaging by editing the work presented in [[154]].

5.1 Direct Image Space Reconstruction

The Cartesian image space method introduced in this section is of particular relevance for this thesis. The first PatLoc measurements were performed with Cartesian trajectories encoded with two NB-SEMs and, consequently, various images are depicted in this thesis which were reconstructed with the Cartesian image space method (see e.g. Figs. 3.5, 5.13 or 7.7). In chapter 3.2.2 it was argued on page 108f that such Cartesian PatLoc encoding strategies are useful to enhance the image quality for example in cortical imaging. Cartesian trajectories were also used in chapter 3.3, page 121ff, to test and evaluate the performance of the different imaging hardware designs. One reason was the high reproducibility of the Cartesian PatLoc imaging sequence, but also its straightforward implementation, which can be based on a conventional sequence.

Also from a purely algorithmic point of view the Cartesian image space method has advantages over other reconstructions. It turns out that the Cartesian image space reconstruction is a very fast, robust and simple implementation of the weak matrix approach presented in the previous chapter. The matrix approach is non-iterative and it is beneficial because it can accurately be analyzed; for example, image properties are clearly defined and can readily be calculated.

Noteworthy is the similarity of the Cartesian image space reconstruction with Cartesian SENSE (see chapter 2.3.1a, page 74ff). The nonlinearities of the SEMs are, however also responsible for some differences compared to what is known from SENSE image reconstruction. An intensity-correction step must be added to the reconstruction and distortions have to be corrected. Another important feature of the Cartesian PatLoc approach is that aliased voxels are not equidistantly distributed as in SENSE imaging. In PatLoc, the aliasing pattern depends on properties of the SEMs. For two orthogonal quadrupolar fields, pairs of aliased voxels exist and they are rotated by $180°$ around a common center. The reason for this different property is that aliasing in PatLoc and SENSE have different physical sources. In PatLoc, it is the non-bijectiveness of the encoding fields that causes aliasing, whereas in SENSE, k-space undersampling is responsible for the observed behavior. Nonetheless, this difference does not affect the standard theoretical model of signal encoding. Both effects can be treated alike in the reconstruction and it is possible to reconstruct subsampled PatLoc datasets by combining PatLoc and SENSE reconstruction in a straightforward manner.

In this section, the theoretical background of the Cartesian method is thoroughly described. Simulation and experimental results are presented and discussed, demonstrating the effectiveness of the proposed reconstruction.

5.1.1   Theory

The Cartesian image space reconstruction is applicable to an encoding strategy that has the following two assumptions:

1. Two nonlinear and non-bijective SEMs for 2D imaging are applied; i.e., the z-gradient is used for slice selection, and the two NB-SEMs, for in-plane encoding.[1]
2. Cartesian sampling trajectories are used.

---

[1]The calculations can easily be extended to 3D imaging.

Based on these assumptions, the Cartesian reconstruction is derived with two different approaches. First, the weak matrix approach of the previous chapter is analyzed by taking into account the above assumptions. It is shown that the encoding matrix becomes very structured with the consequence that this matrix can be inverted with low computational cost. Second, an intuitive approach is taken by referring directly to the PatLoc signal equation.

In order to clarify fundamental implications of nonlinear and non-bijective encoding to the reconstructed images, the two NB-SEMs are specialized to orthogonal quadrupolar SEMs in accordance with the realized PatLoc hardware design. By describing the two NB-SEMs as a non-bijective vector field, it becomes obvious that the Cartesian image space method indeed represents a generalized version of SENSE image reconstruction. The vector field description also facilitates investigation of image properties like image resolution and SNR, and the similarity to SENSE also shows that the ultimate g-factor can be calculated with the same method that is used in chapter 2.3.1d, page 82ff.

a) General Matrix Inversion Approach

For the matrix approach the relevant information about signal encoding is collected in the encoding matrix $\mathbf{E}$. Its general form (Eq. 4.18) is repeated here:

$$E_{(\alpha,\kappa),\rho} := c_\alpha(\vec{x}_\rho)e^{-i\mathbf{k}_\kappa^T\psi(\vec{x}_\rho)}. \tag{5.1}$$

With the two assumptions (Cartesian sampling, two SEMs), this matrix has a special structure. The first assumption, application of exactly two NB-SEMs, results in a vector field description of ψ, where ψ is of the kind $\psi : V \longrightarrow U$ with both $U, V \subset \mathbb{R}^2$; i.e., the encoding space U has the same dimension (i.e. 2) as the excited region V, which represents a 2D area after integration along the direction of slice selection. Also the PatLoc k-space vector $\mathbf{k}$ is then in $\mathbb{R}^2$. It is therefore useful to use the same symbols for the image space variable $\vec{x}$ and the vector field, as well as for the k-space variable, by writing $\vec{k}$ and $\vec{\psi}$ instead of $\mathbf{k}$ and ψ. The elements of the encoding matrix then become:

$$E_{(\alpha,\kappa),\rho} = c_\alpha(\vec{x}_\rho)e^{-i\vec{k}_\kappa\vec{\psi}(\vec{x}_\rho)}. \tag{5.2}$$

The second assumption means that a trajectory is chosen which is also typical for conventional Fourier imaging. According to Eq. 2.28, $\vec{k}_\kappa \in \mathcal{K} = 2\pi\Delta k \cdot (\mathcal{I}_N \times \mathcal{I}_N)$, where Δk is the PatLoc sampling distance, which can be found with Eq. 4.5, and where $\mathcal{I}_N$ is a discrete interval as defined on page 291 in Appendix A.1.[2] Again, it is helpful to identify the index κ with the ordered pair $(p, p') \in \mathcal{I}_N \times \mathcal{I}_N$. The encoding matrix then has the following entries:

$$E_{(\alpha,p,p'),\rho} = c_\alpha(\vec{x}_\rho)e^{-2\pi i\Delta k(p\psi_1(\vec{x}_\rho)+p'\psi_2(\vec{x}_\rho))}. \tag{5.3}$$

These entries differ from the conventional analogue only in one aspect: The equidistant image space variables x and y are replaced by the locations given by $\psi_1(\vec{x}_\rho)$ and $\psi_2(\vec{x}_\rho)$. Typically, the set of locations $\vec{x}_\rho$ form a rectilinear grid Σ_{cart} with the consequence of a non-rectilinear distribution of the target set $\vec{\psi}(\Sigma_{cart})$. The problem with this non-rectilinear distribution is that the SEM phase term of the encoding matrix does not consist of pure planar waves as in conventional imaging. Note however, that it is not compulsory to use a rectilinear reconstruction grid Σ_{cart}. The locations where the magnetization is reconstructed can be chosen freely. The idea of accelerating the reconstruction is to use a non-rectilinear grid Σ_{nrec} such that **E** consists of planar waves. The imposed structure allows fast inversion of the encoding matrix with the FFT. From a numerical point of view, this is beneficial because calculation of the FFT is fast, accurate and has a condition number of unity, therefore it does not enhance the noise level.

The special structure of the encoding matrix is found by choosing a rectilinear grid not in image space V, but in a different space representation, termed here the *PatLoc encoding space U*, defined by $U := \vec{\psi}(V)$. The problem with this approach is that the function $\vec{\psi}(\cdot)$ is not necessarily bijective in PatLoc imaging. Nevertheless, knowing the shape of the SEMs, it is possible to find a partition $\{V_l; l = 1, \ldots, L\}$ of V with the property that $\vec{\psi}$ is bijective on each subregion V_l.[3] In this context, it is useful to define the bijective

---

[2] For simplicity, it is assumed here that an $N \times N$ dataset with equal PatLoc k-space sampling distance along both dimensions is acquired. The calculations can easily be generalized to unequal parameters.

[3] From a strictly formal mathematical perspective $\vec{\psi}$ can be regarded as a covering map; i.e., a map whose inverse has the property of mapping an open set onto a number of disjoint open sets bijectively and continuously [40]. For magnetic fields the number of disjoint open sets is in general low. This interpretation is possible by defining $\vec{\psi}_O := \vec{\psi}|_{V_O}, V_O := V \backslash O$, where $O := \{x \in V, |\det(\partial\vec{\psi}/\partial\vec{x})| = 0\}$. The restriction onto V_O is unproblematic in non-degenerate situations, where O is of lower dimensionality than V.

functions $\vec{\psi}^l := \vec{\psi}|_{V_l}$ for all $l = 1, \ldots, L$. Note that $\vec{\psi}^l \neq \psi_l$. Each image space location $\vec{x}_\rho$ then belongs to exactly one region V_l. Therefore, it is also useful to introduce a new index l to indicate the subregion to which the image space location belongs, so $\vec{x}_\rho \to \vec{x}_{(l,\rho)}$. Let $\vec{u}_{(l,\rho)} := \vec{\psi}(\vec{x}_{(l,\rho)})$. With this notation, the inverse function is well-defined: $\vec{x}_{(l,\rho)} := (\vec{\psi}^l)^{-1}(\vec{u}_{(l,\rho)})$ and a bijective mapping from image space grid locations to encoding space grid locations can be constructed. If now all locations $\vec{u}_{(l,\rho)}$ are chosen the same for each $l = 1, \ldots, L$, the index l can be dropped from the encoding space variable: $\vec{u}_{(l,\rho)} \to \vec{u}_\rho$.

This approach shows that it is indeed possible to choose a rectilinear reconstruction grid $\Sigma_{cart}^{PatLoc} := \Delta u \cdot (\mathcal{I}_N \times \mathcal{I}_N)$ in the PatLoc encoding space instead of the image space with the consequence that the FFT can immediately be applied for image reconstruction. Figure 5.1 visualizes the transformation from image space locations to PatLoc encoding space locations for the example of orthogonal quadrupolar fields (also cf. Fig. 5.5 for a visualization of the corresponding continuous transformation).

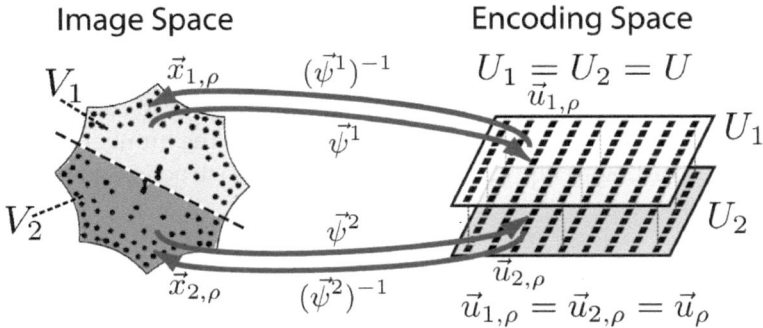

Figure 5.1: Reconstruction grid in image space and PatLoc encoding space. The example corresponds to the situation encountered with orthogonal quadrupolar SEMs. The image space is subdivided into two regions (V_1, V_2). Each region is mapped bijectively ($\vec{\psi}^1$, $\vec{\psi}^2$) to a corresponding region in PatLoc encoding space (U_1, U_2). The regions V_1, V_2 have a characteristic shape, that depends on the used SEMs if both U_1 and U_2 are chosen to have the same rectilinear geometry. Instead of choosing a rectilinear reconstruction grid in image space, a rectilinear grid is chosen in PatLoc encoding space, with coinciding regions U_1 and U_2. Therefore the grid locations $\vec{u}_{1,\rho}$ and $\vec{u}_{2,\rho}$ are the same and the first index can be dropped. With the back-transformation, it is then possible to map each location $\vec{u}_\rho$ onto two corresponding locations $\vec{x}_{1,\rho}$ and $\vec{x}_{2,\rho}$ in image space. The resulting grid of reconstruction locations is non-rectilinear.

Similar to the conventional analogue (Eq. 2.30) the distance Δu is chosen such that

$$\Delta u \Delta k = 1/N. \qquad (5.4)$$

For rectilinear grids, it is useful to identify the index ρ with the ordered pair (q, q'), and, by defining $\tilde{c}_\alpha^l := c_\alpha \circ (\vec{\psi}^l)^{-1}$ for all $l = 1, \ldots, L$, the encoding matrix of Eq. 5.3 reads:

$$E_{(\alpha,p,p'),(l,q,q')} = \tilde{c}_\alpha^l(q\Delta u, q'\Delta u)e^{-\frac{2\pi i}{N}(pq+p'q')}. \qquad (5.5)$$

The latter equation rewritten in matrix form results in:

$$\mathbf{E} = \widetilde{\boldsymbol{DFT}} \cdot \tilde{\mathbf{C}}, \text{ with } \widetilde{\boldsymbol{DFT}} = \boldsymbol{DFT} \otimes \mathbb{1} \text{ and } \tilde{\mathbf{C}} = \sum_{q,q'} \mathbf{I}_{q,q'} \otimes \mathbf{C}^{(q,q')}, \quad (5.6)$$

and where $C_{\alpha,l}^{(q,q')} = c_\alpha^l(q\Delta u, q'\Delta u)$. Exactly this formal structure is known from Cartesian SENSE image reconstruction (cf. Eqs. 2.39, 2.40, page 75). There is only one difference compared to SENSE: The PatLoc reconstruction grid is non-rectilinear in image space variables. Therefore, the nominal voxel volume $v_{l,q,q'}$ (and therefore the intensity correction) is not the same for all voxels with consequences for the calculation of the reconstruction matrix $\mathbf{F}$ (see chapter 4.2.2a, page 146ff). It is reasonable to assume $N_c > L$ because the number of receiver coils should exceed the number of bijective regions. According to Eq. 4.21 and Eq. 5.6 the reconstruction matrix is then given by:

$$\mathbf{F} = \mathbf{V}^{-1}\mathbf{E}^+ = \mathbf{V}^{-1}\tilde{\mathbf{C}}^+ \cdot \widetilde{\mathbf{iDFT}}, \text{ where } \tilde{\mathbf{C}}^+ = \sum_{q,q'} \mathbf{I}_{q,q'} \otimes (\mathbf{C}^{(q,q')})^+. \quad (5.7)$$

The structure of $\mathbf{F}$ is depicted in Fig. 5.2. Also compare this figure to Fig. 2.11 on page 77, where the Cartesian SENSE reconstruction matrix is depicted.

b)   Cartesian PatLoc Reconstruction Algorithm

For the reconstruction each matrix factor of $\mathbf{F}$ (i.e., $\widetilde{\mathbf{iDFT}}$, $\tilde{\mathbf{C}}^+$ and $\mathbf{V}$) is successively applied to a vector. Each of these matrix-vector multiplications are fast operations:

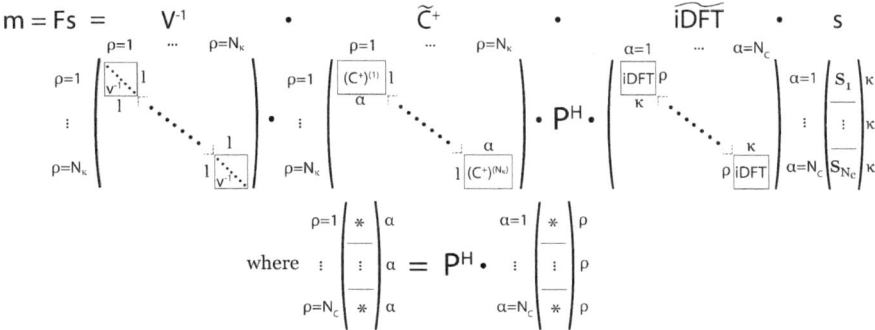

Figure 5.2: Structure of the reconstruction matrix of the Cartesian PatLoc method. The reconstruction matrix is decomposable into two block-diagonal matrices, a permutation matrix and a diagonal matrix. One block-diagonal matrix represents coil-wise inverse 2D-DFTs. The second block-diagonal matrix is formed by inverting a matrix which contains the sensitivity profiles of the receiver coils represented in PatLoc encoding coordinates. It is very sparse and can be structured voxel-group-wise. The block-diagonal structures of the matrices occur along different dimensions. Therefore, it is necessary to permute coil dimension and spatial dimension in between. The diagonal matrix contains the volumetric correction factors. The occurrence of this matrix is the only difference to Cartesian SENSE what the structure of the reconstruction matrix is concerned.

1. Equivalent to Cartesian SENSE, the reconstruction begins with a coil-wise inverse 2D-FFT ($\widetilde{\mathbf{iDFT}}$) applied to the signal data s_α resulting in N_c coil images η_α represented in PatLoc encoding space.

2. The aliased images are unfolded by inverting the sensitivity matrix $\widetilde{\mathbf{C}}$ and by applying $\widetilde{\mathbf{C}}^+$ to the coil images η_α. The matrix $\widetilde{\mathbf{C}}$ is sparse with small blocks of dimension $(N_c \cdot L)$ on its diagonal, which can be inverted quickly and independently from each other. Note that the sensitivity matrix $\widetilde{\mathbf{C}}$ is constructed from sensitivity maps transformed to PatLoc encoding space coordinates, for example by bicubic interpolation.

3. In contrast to Cartesian SENSE, a voxel-wise intensity correction ($\mathbf{V}^{-1}$ is diagonal) must be performed. In chapter 4.2.2, page 144ff, it is shown that the intensity correction is given by the nominal voxel volume of the reconstruction grid. In chapter 4.2.2b, page 148ff, several methods are discussed how the nominal voxel volume can be

determined. Here, the approximate continuous method could simply be used because, by definition, the encoding function $\vec{\psi}(\cdot)$ maps the non-rectilinear reconstruction grid onto a rectilinear grid. By formulating the induced deformation (also cf. Eq. 4.24) not with the inverse, but with the forward function, the entries of $\mathbf{V}$ are given by:

$$v_{l,q,q'} = |\det(\partial\vec{\psi}/\partial\vec{x})|^{-1} \cdot (\Delta u)^2, \tag{5.8}$$

where $\vec{x}$ is evaluated at $\vec{x} = (\vec{\psi}^l)^{-1}(q\Delta u, q'\Delta u)$.

In order to finally visualize the reconstructed magnetization, the image must be interpolated onto a Cartesian grid because the magnetization $\mathbf{m} = \mathbf{Fs}$ is reconstructed on non-equidistant image locations $\vec{x}_{l,\rho}$. Bicubic interpolation might be used or other methods like the multilevel b-spline approach [94]. For the interpolation, a grid (with grid locations $\vec{x}_{rc}$) should be chosen fine enough to capture the highest local resolution within the image. The algorithm, with the three reconstruction steps plus the final interpolation step, is illustrated in Fig. 5.3. The images shown after the coil-wise inverse 2D-FFT are represented in PatLoc encoding space where the grid locations $\vec{u}_\rho$ form a rectilinear grid. These locations are distributed differently in image space following the relation $\vec{x}_{l,\rho} = (\vec{\psi}^l)^{-1}(\vec{u}_\rho)$. The final interpolation step can therefore also be interpreted as rewarping the image from PatLoc encoding space back to image space (cf. Fig. 5.3e).

The numerical complexity of the Cartesian PatLoc method is of the order $\mathcal{O}(N_c N_\kappa \log N_\kappa + N_\rho(N_c L^2 + 1))$. It is much lower compared to a complexity of[4] $\mathcal{O}(N_c N_\kappa N_\rho^2)$ for direct computation without exploiting the structure of $\mathbf{E}$ or of $\mathcal{O}(N_c N_\kappa N_\rho)$ for each loop of the iterative CG method. This represents an improvement in computation time by several orders of magnitude. As an example, with $N_c = 8$, $L = 2$, $N_\kappa = 256^2$ and $N_\rho = N_\kappa$ untreated direct inversion would require more than 10^{15} operations, one loop of the iterative CG method more than 10^{10} operations whereas the structured inversion requires only about 10^7 operations.

---

[4]For $N_c N_\kappa \geq N_\rho$.

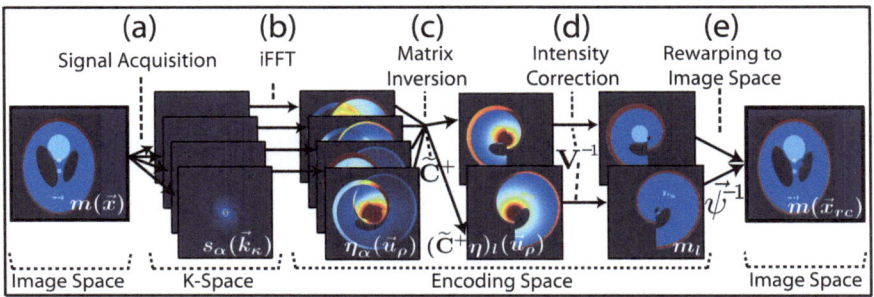

Figure 5.3: Cartesian image space PatLoc reconstruction algorithm. (a) Based on a numerical phantom, data acquisition is simulated. (b) The first reconstruction step consists in a coil-wise application of the 2D-FFT resulting in aliased, intensity-modulated and highly distorted coil images. (c) The matrix inversions remove the aliasing. (d) An intensity correction is performed. (e) The object is visualized in image space. The basic reconstruction steps are depicted based on simulated data with quadrupolar SEMs and profiles of a real-world RF-surface coil array. The simulated signal data were filtered with a Kaiser-Bessel window to remove Gibbs ringing. Images and reconstruction steps are labeled with the variables as they occur in the text. Compare with Fig. 2.12, page 78, where the SENSE algorithm is depicted, to see that the Cartesian PatLoc algorithm generalizes SENSE.

c) Equivalent Fourier Transform Approach

Consider here an equivalent, more intuitive, approach. The starting point of this Fourier transform approach is the expression for individual coil data (Eq. 4.9), represented for the time being for a continuous k-space variable:

$$s_\alpha(\vec{k}) = \int_V m(\vec{x}) c_\alpha(\vec{x}) e^{-i\vec{k}\vec{\psi}(\vec{x})} \, \mathrm{d}\vec{x}. \tag{5.9}$$

As above (cf. Eq. 5.2), the variable **k** is written as $\vec{k}$ and ψ as $\vec{\psi}$ in this equation to indicate that for the case of two SEMs, the dimension of these vectors conforms to the dimension of the image space variable $\vec{x}$. According to the discussion following Eq. 5.3 on page 158, the region of integration V can be split into L different subregions V_l, on which $\vec{\psi}$ is bijective. The integration over V can then be described as a sum of integrations over the individual subregions. For each individual integral, the variable transformation to

$\vec{u} = \vec{\psi}^l(\vec{x}), l = 1, \ldots, L$ can be performed. After swapping the summation and the integral one finds:

$$s_\alpha(\vec{k}) = \int_U \left[\sum_{l=1}^{L} \tilde{m}^l(\vec{u}) \tilde{c}_\alpha^l(\vec{u}) \tilde{v}^l(\vec{u}) \right] e^{i\vec{k}\vec{u}} \, d\vec{u} \qquad (5.10)$$

$$= \int_U \tilde{\eta}_\alpha(\vec{u}) e^{i\vec{k}\vec{u}} \, d\vec{u}. \qquad (5.11)$$

Here $U := \vec{\psi}(V_l)$ has been set, where, w. l. o. g. , U does not depend on the choice of a subregion V_l. Depending on the method used to determine the nominal voxel volume (see chapter 4.2.2b, page 148ff), the geometric distortion factors $\tilde{v}^l(\vec{u}) = |\det(\partial(\vec{\psi}^l)^{-1}/\partial \vec{u})|$ are equivalent or at least very similar to the intensity correction used in the matrix inversion approach (cf. Eq. 5.8, page 162). In the latter equation (Eq. 5.11), the Fourier transformed coil image $\tilde{\eta}_\alpha(\vec{u})$ is defined as:

$$\tilde{\eta}_\alpha(\vec{u}) = \sum_{l=1}^{L} \tilde{m}^l(\vec{u}) \tilde{c}_\alpha^l(\vec{u}) \tilde{v}^l(\vec{u}). \qquad (5.12)$$

This result shows that in encoding space the intensity of a voxel is a weighted sum of at most L different values. Unfolding can be performed voxel-wise in PatLoc encoding space, and therefore only very small matrices must be inverted. Unfolding can be described as a matrix equation upon assembling $\tilde{\eta}_\alpha(\vec{u})$, $\alpha = 1, \ldots, N_c$ and $\tilde{m}^l(\vec{u})$, $l = 1, \ldots, L$ to vectors $\tilde{\boldsymbol{\eta}}(\vec{u})$ and $\tilde{\mathbf{m}}(\vec{u})$ and upon combining $\tilde{c}_\alpha^l(\vec{u})$ to matrix $\mathbf{C}^{\vec{u}}$ and the quantities $\tilde{v}^l(\vec{u})$ to a diagonal matrix $\mathbf{V}^{\vec{u}}$. The magnetization can then be calculated as:

$$\tilde{\mathbf{m}}(\vec{u}) = (\mathbf{V}^{\vec{u}})^{-1}(\mathbf{C}^{\vec{u}})^+ \tilde{\boldsymbol{\eta}}(\vec{u}). \qquad (5.13)$$

Discretizing this equation on a Cartesian grid Σ_{cart} in PatLoc encoding space shows that this approach is equivalent to the reconstruction presented in the previous section (cf. Eq. 5.7). It is straightforward to show that the discretized version of Eq. 5.13 reduces to the Cartesian SENSE equation [135] by defining $\vec{\psi}(x_j, y_j, z_0) := \mathrm{id}(x_j, y_j \bmod N/L, z_0) = (x_j, y_j \bmod N/L, z_0)$, where N is the number of elements of Σ_{cart} along the second dimension, L is the acceleration and $z = z_0$ is the slice position. For arbitrary SEMs the discretized version of Eq. 5.13 is more general than Cartesian SENSE, but becomes formally equivalent by defining $\bar{\mathbf{m}}(\vec{u}_\rho) := \mathbf{V}(\vec{u}_\rho)\hat{\mathbf{m}}(\vec{u}_\rho)$, $\vec{u}_\rho \in \Sigma_{cart}$:

$$\bar{\mathbf{m}}(\vec{u}_\rho) = (\mathbf{C}^\rho)^+ \tilde{\eta}(\vec{u}_\rho). \tag{5.14}$$

In this abstract formulation there is no inherent difference between PatLoc and SENSE reconstruction and so intensity-modulated PatLoc-reconstructed images should have similar properties to SENSE-reconstructed images as long as they are represented in encoding space. If nonlinear, yet bijective, fields were also considered with SENSE imaging, both reconstructions would even be exactly equivalent. Interestingly, in PatLoc, the non-bijectiveness of the SEMs has the same effect that undersampling has in conventional SENSE imaging.

d) Reconstruction with Multipolar Encoding Fields

The Cartesian reconstruction algorithm presented above shows that the Fourier transform of the PatLoc k-space has a precise meaning that is expressed by Eq. 5.12. The meaning of this mathematical expression is demonstrated here under the assumption that the standard x- and y-gradient fields are generalized to orthogonal multipolar SEMs; these fields have already been introduced with further detail in chapter 3.3.1, page 122ff. The SEM-vector field generated by the two multipolar SEMs with sensitivities b_f and b_p together with the linear z-gradient with sensitivity b_z is three-dimensional; however, according to the assumptions presented above on page 156 in section 5.1.1, the z-gradient is only used for slice selection and therefore the vector field can formally be reduced to 2D:

$$\vec{\psi}(\vec{x}) = \frac{\gamma}{\beta} \begin{pmatrix} b_f(\vec{x}) \\ b_p(\vec{x}) \\ b_s(\vec{x}) \end{pmatrix} = \frac{\gamma}{\beta} \begin{pmatrix} h_L r^L \cos(L\varphi) \\ h_L r^L \sin(L\varphi) \\ g_z z \end{pmatrix} \xrightarrow[\beta := \gamma h_L]{\text{2D imaging}} \vec{\psi}(r, \varphi) = \begin{pmatrix} r^L \cos(L\varphi) \\ r^L \sin(L\varphi) \end{pmatrix}.$$

$$\tag{5.15}$$

The quantity g_z is the gradient strength per unit current and h_L describes the corresponding characteristic property of the multipolar fields. The encoding fields are shown in Fig. 5.4a, c for the case $L = 2$.

The transformation $\vec{\psi}$ induced by the multipolar SEMs is illustrated in Fig. 5.5 for the case $L = 2$. It consists of L "pie-shaped" bijective regions. Two independent distortions occur via this mapping: In the azimuthal

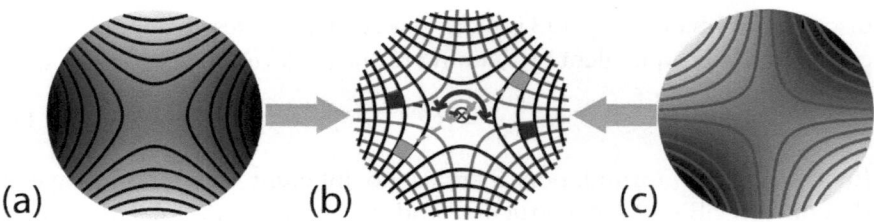

Figure 5.4: (a) and (c) Ideal quadrupolar encoding fields rotated by $45°$. (b) The superimposed contour lines of the encoding fields represent the reconstructed voxel volume in image space. Voxels, rotated by $180°$ around a common center, are equally encoded by the two SEMs.

direction, an Lth fraction of a full circle is mapped onto a complete closed circle; in the radial direction, the inner regions are contracted, whereas the periphery is expanded. Fig. 5.4b illustrates (for quadrupolar SEMs) that voxels, which are rotated in image space by $360°/L$ around the center of the SEMs, are mapped onto the same voxel in encoding space. Interestingly, an analogy to the Riemann surface [37] of the complex valued root function can be established. Orthogonal ideal multipolar fields with $2L$ poles can be described as real and imaginary parts of the complex-valued holomorphic function $f(s) = s^L$ (cf. Appendix A.4, Eq. A.16 on page 302). This function is ambiguous on the complex plane. However, by introducing L leaves of the complex plane, i.e., the Riemann surface of the L-th complex root function, the function can be made unambiguous. More encoding fields, which can (and cannot) be described using this complex-valued formalism can be found in [[159]].

For orthogonal multipolar fields the volumetric correction $\tilde{v}^j(\vec{u})$ does not depend on the subregion V_j and depends only on the modulus of $\vec{u}$; it can be calculated explicitly using Eq. 5.8:

$$\tilde{v}^j(\vec{u}) = (L^{-2}r^{2-2L})|_{u=r^L} = L^{-2}u^{2/L-2}. \tag{5.16}$$

Remark: For central voxels, especially where $\vec{\psi}(\vec{x}) = 0$, the local deformation at the voxel center overestimates the nominal voxel volume (cf. chapter 4.2.2b, page 148ff). According to Eq. 5.7, the nominal voxel volume affects the intensity correction, and therefore, it is to be expected that a signal dropout should occur at the center if the nominal voxel volume is approximated with the local deformation. This behavior is indeed observed

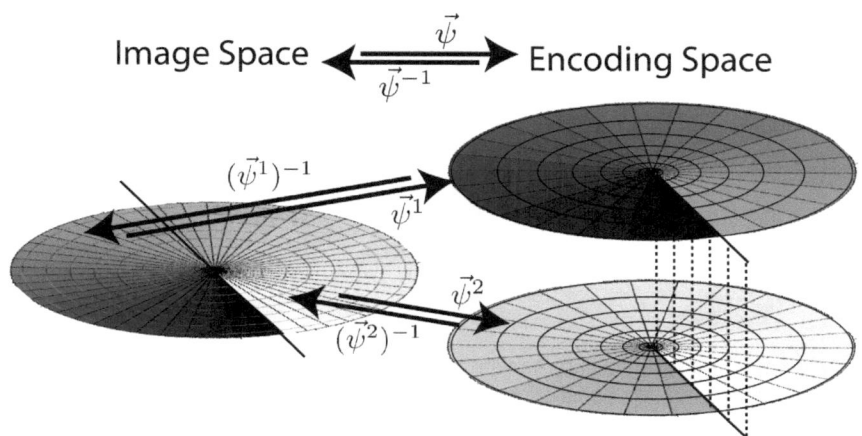

Figure 5.5: Visualization of the induced mapping generated by two orthogonal quadrupolar encoding fields. The circular contour lines indicate that the center is shrunk whereas the periphery is expanded by this transformation. The distance of the radial contour lines and the grayscale in between indicate how the encoding fields act in the circumferential direction: After a half circle, encoding becomes ambiguous. This is indicated by the two leaves in encoding space, which are mapped bijectively onto a half plane in image space.

(see e.g. Fig. 5.13, top left). The dropout is, however, not relevant because at the center, almost no image information is encoded (see next section). With multipolar encoding fields, it is therefore acceptable to use the local deformation to estimate the nominal voxel volume; more precise, however, are the other approaches of chapter 4.2.2b, such as the Voronoi method.

The singularity in Eq. 5.16 at $\vec{u} = 0$ is not problematic because the integral in Eq. 5.10 does not change when this single point is neglected. Equation 5.12 then becomes:

$$\tilde{\eta}^{\alpha}(\vec{u}) = L^{-2} u^{2/L-2} \sum_{j=1}^{L} \tilde{m}^{j}(\vec{u}) \tilde{c}^{j,\alpha}(\vec{u}). \tag{5.17}$$

This equation describes how the magnetization is deformed by multipolar SEMs; In Fig. 5.6 the original magnetization weighted with the sensitivity of one receiver channel of an RF-coil array is compared to its deformed analogue for the case $L = 2$.

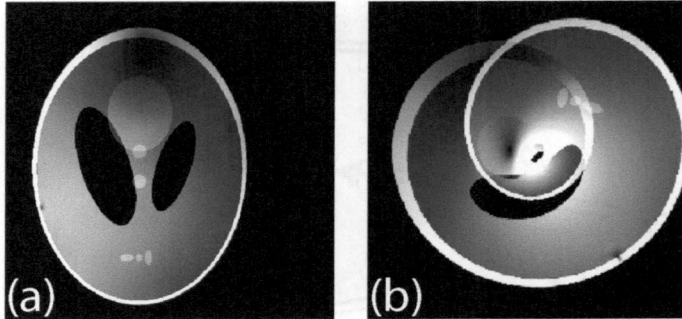

Figure 5.6: Deformed coil image with quadrupolar encoding. (a) Original magneti-zation weighted with the sensitivity of an RF-surface coil element. (b) Corresponding deformed image. The nonlinearities of the SEMs cause intensity modulation (in-crease toward the center) and severe image distortions. The non-bijectiveness of the encoding function is responsible for the fold-over. The effects - increasing information at the periphery and fold-over along the azimuthal direction correspond to the transformation induced by the encoding function, presented in Fig. 5.5.

e) Basic Image Properties

A detailed analysis of image resolution, Gibbs ringing, aliasing and image noise is presented in this section. Image resolution and Gibbs ringing are investigated with two different approaches. The first approach is related to the traditional method of using the FT of the sampling window. The second approach is directly based on the computation and evaluation of the SRF. This second approach is also used to analyze the aliasing artifact. Finally, it is shown that image noise can be determined either using general matrix theory (see chapter 2.1.4, page 52ff) or by referring to the analogy of Cartesian PatLoc reconstruction and SENSE.

Resolution   In general, the nominal voxel volume and image resolution – measured by the width of the main peak – are different. Here, it is shown that image resolution and nominal voxel volume are closely linked to each other in Cartesian PatLoc reconstruction.

Sampling Window Approach   The problem of defining image resolution can be tackled by investigating Eq. 5.11. It states that the coil signal s_α and the distorted magnetization $\tilde{\eta}_\alpha$ form a Fourier transform pair. Sampling PatLoc k-space on a finite grid is equivalent to a convolution of $\tilde{\eta}_\alpha$ with a truncation window consisting of a sinc-function h_s and a comb-function h_c. Although the following calculations are performed in 2D it should be noted that the same reasoning also applies to the 3D case. The value of $\tilde{\eta}_\alpha$ at voxel location (q, q') is given by:

$$(\tilde{\eta}_\alpha)_{q,q'} = (\tilde{\eta}_\alpha * h_s * h_c)(q\Delta u, q'\Delta u). \tag{5.18}$$

According to Eq. 5.4, the value Δu depends on the sampling distance Δk between adjacent k-space locations:

$$\Delta u = 1/(N\Delta k), \tag{5.19}$$

where N is the number of measured k-space values in each dimension. The convolution of $\tilde{\eta}_\alpha$ with h_s leads to a finite resolution of magnitude Δu in the image after performing the FFT-operation. According to Eqs. 5.13, 5.14, the same applies to the reconstructed image as long as it is represented in encoding space under the assumption of smoothly varying coil sensitivity profiles and smoothly varying intensity correction in encoding space. Image resolution is therefore homogeneous in PatLoc encoding space with a FWHM of ≈ 1.21 voxels in units of $\Delta u = 1/(N\Delta k)$. For a more detailed analysis see paragraph *Resolution* in chapter 2.2.1c, page 61f. However, the rewarping to image space (cf. Fig. 5.3e) has two important effects.

The first effect is an increase of the average image resolution compared to standard gradient encoding, caused by the non-bijectiveness of the SEMs (also cf. paragraph *Encoding with Two SEMs* in chapter 3.2.2, page 108ff). To be more precise, depending on the shape of the object, the average voxel volume is approximately by a factor L smaller than in conventional imaging, when the same number of k-space lines are acquired. In other words, the acquisition can be accelerated by a factor of L with respect to conventional imaging to achieve the same average resolution. In situations where the ROI is restricted to the periphery of the imaged region, the effective acceleration factor can be very high.

The second effect is a non-homogeneous image resolution, caused by the nonlinearities of the SEMs. The transformation to image space coordinates locally deforms the voxels according to the derivatives of $\vec{\psi}$ in the corresponding voxel. Image resolution is therefore approximately described by Eq. 5.8, page 162, which has already proven useful in estimating the nominal voxel volume (also cf. chapter 4.2.2b, page 148ff). Size and shape of the deformed voxels can be visualized by plotting $N + 1$ contour lines of both encoding fields in a single image; this is shown in Fig. 3.4, page 109.[5] These voxels define image resolution even more accurately than the local deformation. It is remarkable that for the Cartesian PatLoc method, nominal voxel volume (property of the reconstruction grid) and effective voxel volume (image resolution) are the same. The reason for this equality is that the FFT automatically leads to a reconstruction grid that is rectilinear not in image space, but in PatLoc encoding space.

Analysis of the SRF   With the reconstruction matrix for Cartesian PatLoc imaging, defined in Eq. 5.7, calculations equivalent to those performed for SENSE reconstruction in Eq. 2.43 lead to an SRF of:

$$f_{(l,q,q')}(\vec{x}) = c_{q,q',l}^{virt}(\vec{x}) \cdot f_{q,q',l}^{Fourier}(\vec{x}). \tag{5.20}$$

The individual terms are given by:

$$f_{q,q',l}^{Fourier}(\vec{x}) \quad = \quad v_{l,q,q'}^{-1} \cdot g_N\left(q - \frac{\psi_1(\vec{x})}{\Delta u}\right) g_N\left(q' - \frac{\psi_2(\vec{x})}{\Delta u}\right),$$

$$c_{q,q',l}^{virt}(\vec{x}) \quad = \quad \sum_\alpha \widetilde{C}_{(q,q',l),(\alpha,q,q')}^{+} c_\alpha(\vec{x}),$$

$$\text{with} \quad \widetilde{C}_{(\alpha,q,q'),(q,q',l)} \quad = c_\alpha(\vec{x}_{q,q',l}) = \tilde{c}_\alpha^l(q\Delta u, q'\Delta u).$$

As for conventional PI, the SRF is therefore a combination of the aliased Fourier SRF and a weighting function due to sensitivity encoding.

Recall that image resolution is mainly determined by the width of the main peak of the SRF (see chapter 2.1.3, page 50ff). As coil sensitivities and intensity correction only represent a weighting, the width of the main peak is determined almost uniquely by the Fourier SRF. Image resolution is better analyzed in PatLoc encoding space variables $\vec{u} = \vec{\psi}(\vec{x})$, where it is, according to Eqs. 2.6, 5.8, given by:

$$f_{q,q',l}^{Fourier}(\vec{u}) = \frac{1}{(\Delta u)^2} \cdot g_N\left(q - \frac{u_1}{\Delta u}\right) g_N\left(q' - \frac{u_2}{\Delta u}\right). \tag{5.21}$$

---

[5]Note the similarity to Fig. 4.2f, page 149, where the nominal voxel volume is visualized with the help of contour lines.

In the PatLoc space representation, the Fourier SRF is equivalent to the SRF of standard Cartesian Fourier imaging (cf. Eq. 2.33). Image resolution is therefore homogeneous in PatLoc encoding space with a FWHM of $\approx$ 1.21 voxels in units of Δu. Note that this is exactly the result that has been obtained with the sampling window approach above. The above explanations regarding image resolution therefore apply accordingly.

Gibbs Ringing It is presented here how the Gibbs ringing artifact can be determined. It is shown that the nonlinearities of the SEMs are typically not troublesome; problems in this regard occur, however, when signal is encoded in regions with very low or even vanishing local field gradients.

Sampling Window Approach The Gibbs ringing artifact results from the convolution of the distorted magnetization with the $sinc$-truncation window h_s in PatLoc encoding space. After the FFT, the ringing therefore falls off with $\mathcal{O}(1/u)$ along the main axes in PatLoc encoding space (see paragraph *Resolution* in chapter 2.2.1c, page 61f). This fall-off behavior is typically not heavily influenced by the unfolding operation; however, there is one problem which does not occur in standard imaging: The nonlinearities of the encoding fields may lead to signal accumulation in regions where the SEMs are very flat. The Gibbs ringing originating from those regions can extend over the complete image and mask the true magnetization at locations far away from the source. From a different perspective, the nonlinearities have the consequence that the image must be intensity-corrected; this correction can have a significant influence on the $\mathcal{O}(1/u)$ Gibbs ringing behavior.

For example, with multipolar SEMs, where $u = r^L$, intensity correction is given by r^{2L-2} (see Eq. 5.16). The Gibbs ringing originating from the central voxel at $r = 0$ therefore behaves like $\mathcal{O}(r^{L-2})$. Observe that for $L > 2$ the Gibbs ringing does not diminish with increasing distance from the center; it is even increased toward the periphery! Fortunately, these cases are very rare and can be circumvented with an appropriate encoding scheme, for example by just avoiding regions with vanishing SEM encoding. Note that the final back-transformation to image space coordinates has a predictable effect for Cartesian trajectories: In PatLoc encoding space, the Gibbs ringing primarily occurs along the main axes u_1 and u_2 in encoding space. Correspondingly, the Gibbs ringing artifact occurs along isocontour lines of the SEMs in image space because $\vec{u} = \vec{\psi}(\vec{x})$.

Analysis of the SRF   The SRF presented in Eq. 5.20 also describes the Gibbs ringing artifact. As stated in the previous paragraph, the sensitivity weighting $c_{q,q',l}^{virt}(\vec{x})$ has some influence on the ringing, it is, however, typically not decisive. Therefore, this factor is ignored here. The factor $v_{l,q,q'}^{-1}$ is constant and can therefore also be neglected for the analysis of relative variations of the SRF. Relevant for the Gibbs ringing artifact is therefore again only the Fourier SRF term:

$$f_{q,q',l}^{Fourier}(\vec{x}) = v_{l,q,q'}^{-1} \cdot g_N \left(q - \frac{\psi_1(\vec{x})}{\Delta u} \right) g_N \left(q' - \frac{\psi_2(\vec{x})}{\Delta u} \right). \qquad (5.22)$$

From this equation it can be deduced immediately that the Gibbs ringing artifact occurs mainly along the isocontours of the SEMs. It can also be followed from this equation that the ringing oscillates faster where the field variations are high; on the other hand, extended sidelobes occur in flat SEM regions. In the previous paragraph, it has been argued that Gibbs ringing might extend from regions with flat field geometries. Analysis of the SRF reveals that such a pronounced Gibbs ringing artifact can indeed occur. Recall that the SRF describes the spatial distribution of relative signal contributions to a particular voxel of interest (Eq. 2.6):

$$m_\rho = \int_V m(\vec{x}) f_\rho(\vec{x}) \, d\vec{x}. \qquad (5.23)$$

A problem might therefore occur if (a) $f_\rho(\vec{x})$ is large for some $\vec{x}$ apart from the location of the main peak, and if (b) $f_\rho(\vec{x})$ may have a moderate value, but over a large volume. The Fourier SRF indeed has peaks of equal height with the main lobe; this effect is, however, not responsible for Gibbs ringing, but for aliasing (see below). Therefore, only effect (b) can be responsible for significant signal contributions from distant regions. As stated above, extended sidelobes occur, where the SEMs are flat. If such a region lies along one of the two isocontours passing through the voxel, significant signal contamination might result from that region. Such situations should therefore be avoided when setting up an encoding scheme. The 1D example shown in Fig. 5.7 illustrates the signal contamination issue.

Aliasing   In conventional imaging the sampling window approach can be used to analyze the aliasing artifact because aliasing is related to the violation of the Nyquist criterion (cf. paragraph *Field-of-View* in chapter 2.2.1c, page 62ff). Also in PatLoc, k-space subsampling results in aliasing;

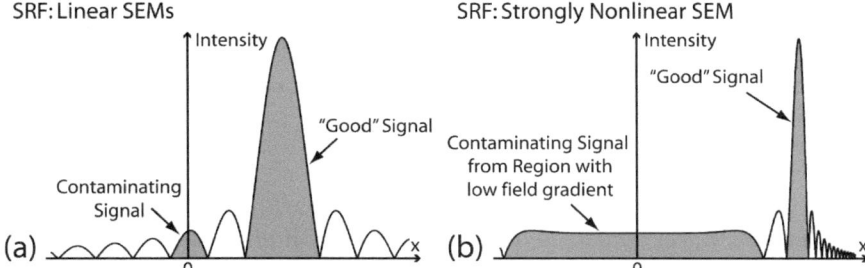

Figure 5.7: Signal contamination from regions with low field gradients. (a) Shown is the absolute value of the sinc-function, the (shift-invariant) SRF belonging to linear gradient encoding. It is shown that the sidelobes contribute some signal to the voxel of interest without overly contaminating the signal. The signal contamination leads to the well-known Gibbs ringing artifact. (b) Shown is the absolute value of the SRF for a strongly nonlinear SEM that is proportional to x^6. At $x = 0$, the gradient of the SEM is zero. The gradient increases toward the edges. It is shown that the nonlinearity of the SEM causes sidelobes to be broader where the field gradients are low (center); on the other hand, sidelobes are narrower where the field gradients are high (right). The main lobe and one broad sidelobe are shaded in gray. In this (extreme) example, the area covered by the sidelobe is larger than the area covered by the main peak of the SRF. This indicates that the signal at the location of interest is strongly contaminated by unwanted signal from the central region. As a consequence, it is to be expected that the Gibbs ringing artifact emanating from the central voxel appears heavily increased in the reconstructed data.

however, also field ambiguities cause multiple locations to be identically encoded. This effect cannot be captured with the sampling window approach; consequently, aliasing is investigated here solely via evaluation of the SRF.

Aliasing Caused by the Non-Bijectiveness of the SEMs Consider first only the Fourier SRF factor in Eq. 5.20, $f_{q,q',l}^{Fourier}(\vec{x})$. It is striking that this factor is the same for all (up to L) locations $\vec{x}$, which are mapped onto the same location u in PatLoc encoding space via $\vec{\psi}(\cdot)$. The SRF therefore has up to L main peaks, one for each subregion V_l, with the property that the aliased locations do not have the regular spacing of conventional PI, but a spatial distribution that depends on the geometries of the SEM subregions.

Also in PatLoc, parallel reception offers a possibility to suppress these multiple peaks. According to the condition of weak reconstruction (Eq. 4.20, page 147), the sensitivity weighting has the important property that

$$c_{q,q',l}^{virt}(\vec{x}_{q,q',l'}) = \delta_{l,l'}. \qquad (5.24)$$

The weak reconstruction therefore demands that the central locations of the aliased Fourier peaks are fully suppressed. Differences to SENSE occur because the locations where the sensitivity weighting is defined are not equidistant, but have a varying distance from one another. Problems may occur in regions where the aliased locations are close to each other, because it is not possible to generate high spatial frequencies, required to differentiate between two close-by locations, by RF-coil sensitivities, which always have smooth spatial variations. This has especially consequences for SNR (see the paragraph *Image Noise* on the next page), but also for not well-suppressed sidelobes that are distant to the aliased locations.

Aliasing Caused by Subsampling   Parallel reception is not only useful in suppressing aliasing that results from the non-bijectiveness of the encoding fields as shown in the previous section, but also in suppressing aliasing that results from k-space subsampling. This approach corresponds to the typical approach in accelerated conventional PI. Again, consider the Fourier SRF represented in PatLoc coordinates:

$$f_{q,q',l}^{Fourier}(\vec{u}) = \frac{1}{(\Delta u)^2} \cdot g_N\left(q - \frac{u_1}{\Delta u}\right) g_N\left(q' - \frac{u_2}{\Delta u}\right). \qquad (5.25)$$

As already stated above, this function has exactly the same dependency on the PatLoc space variable $\vec{u}$ as the Fourier SRF has on the image space variable $\vec{x}$. Therefore, the results from the analysis of the Fourier SRF (see paragraph *Field-of-View* in chapter 2.2.1c, page 62ff) can be translated directly to PatLoc: It is useful to introduce the concept of FOV also in PatLoc. Suppose the object covers the region W in image space. In PatLoc space, the region $\vec{\psi}(W)$ is then covered by the object. Aliasing is avoided as long as $\vec{\psi}(W)$ lies within the region $\square_{FOV}^{PatLoc}$, where the superscript $PatLoc$ indicates that the FOV is measured in PatLoc space coordinates. $\square_{FOV}^{PatLoc}$ is rectangularly shaped with an edge length of $N\Delta u$. If the object is larger than the FOV, fold-over occurs as known from conventional imaging. More important for the actual experiment is, however, the Nyquist relation expressed in image space coordinates. Assume that $\vec{\psi}^{-1}(U)$ describes the set of locations, which are mapped onto U by $\vec{\psi}$. Then the "PatLoc Nyquist criterion" has two alternative descriptions:

$$\vec{\psi}(W) \subset \Box_{FOV}^{PatLoc} \quad \text{or} \quad W \subset \vec{\psi}^{-1}(\Box_{FOV}^{PatLoc}). \tag{5.26}$$

This equation generalizes the corresponding equation of Fourier imaging (cf. Eq. 2.35, page 63).

PatLoc-SENSE Consider now the case where a FOV is chosen smaller than the object in order to accelerate image acquisition. In this case, aliasing occurs. This aliasing can, however, also be suppressed by combining SENSE reconstruction with PatLoc reconstruction. Assume a PatLoc ambiguity of L and a SENSE acceleration of R. Then there are up to $L \cdot R$ aliased locations in the Fourier SRF. These locations must be suppressed by ensuring that $c_{q,q',l}^{virt}(\vec{x}_{q,q',l'}) = \delta_{l,l'}$, where l, l' run over all $L \cdot R$ aliased locations. To this end, the aliased locations must be determined, for example, by calculating the multiple locations by evaluating $\vec{\psi}^{-1}[\vec{\psi}(\vec{x}) + \vec{d}]$, where $\vec{d}$ is zero or a shift of one (PatLoc) FOV along the phase encoding direction.

Remark concerning ultimate SNR in Cartesian PatLoc: The condition represented by Eq. 5.24, i.e. $c_{q,q',l}^{virt}(\vec{x}_{q,q',l'}) = \delta_{l,l'}$, imposed on the virtual coil sensitivity, is formally equivalent to the corresponding condition in PI (see Eq. 2.47, page 79). Recall from chapter 2.3.1d, page 82ff, that this condition is also required to formulate the constraints for the calculation of ultimate SNR or ultimate g-factor. It can therefore be concluded that, once the locations of aliased voxels are determined, exactly the same algorithm which is used to determine ultimate quantities in PI can be applied to find the corresponding quantities for Cartesian PatLoc reconstruction.

Image Noise It is crucial to determine the error propagation properties of the applied reconstruction algorithm to calculate the SNR in the reconstructed images. In chapter 2.1.4, page 52ff, it is shown that the diagonal matrix elements of $\mathbf{X} = \mathbf{F}\tilde{\mathbf{\Psi}}\mathbf{F}^H$ represent the variance of the noise in the reconstructed image. When more receiver coils are available for signal acquisition than strictly necessary to uniquely solve the reconstruction problem represented by Eq. 4.19 this additional information can be used to optimize the SNR. Following the arguments of chapter 2.1.5, page 56f, where a rectilinear reconstruction grid is assumed, it is straightforward to show that the SNR-optimized reconstruction matrix for non-rectilinear reconstruction grids is given by:

$$\mathbf{F} = \mathbf{V}^{-1}(\mathbf{E}^H \tilde{\mathbf{\Psi}}^{-1} \mathbf{E})^{-1} \mathbf{E}^H \tilde{\mathbf{\Psi}}^{-1}. \tag{5.27}$$

With this reconstruction matrix, the image noise matrix $\mathbf{X}$ can immediately be determined. Then, using the formula of Eq. 2.22 on page 55, it is possible to calculate the SNR, and a "g-factor" for PatLoc imaging can be defined in analogy to SENSE. (cf. chapter 2.3.1c, page 80ff).

In the Cartesian case, another approach serves the same purpose: Compared to SENSE, image reconstruction only differs by the necessity to perform intensity correction. The final back-transformation to image space coordinates should not have a significant impact on SNR. Therefore, the g-factor calculations performed above for SENSE reconstruction (cf. Eq. 2.49, page 82) are also valid for Cartesian PatLoc with the exception that the SNR must be divided by the intensity correction v_ρ^{-1}:

$$SNR_\rho^{PatLoc} = SNR_\rho^{linear} \frac{v_\rho}{\sqrt{L} g_\rho}. \tag{5.28}$$

In this formula, the g-factor is defined exactly as for SENSE reconstruction:

$$g_\rho = \sqrt{\left[(\mathbf{C}^{(q,q')})^H \mathbf{\Psi}^{-1} \mathbf{C}^{(q,q')}\right]_{l,l}^{-1} \left[(\mathbf{C}^{(q,q')})^H \mathbf{\Psi}^{-1} \mathbf{C}^{(q,q')}\right]_{l,l}} \geq 1. \tag{5.29}$$

SNR^{linear} is the optimized SNR when linear gradient fields are used for encoding. L, the number of bijective regions of $\vec{\psi}$, describes the intrinsic acceleration of PatLoc over conventional imaging. Similar to the conventional case, the g-factor is calculated from groups of voxels which are mapped onto the same point by $\vec{\psi}$. Contrary to parallel encoding with linear fields, where these groups are formed by equidistant positions in image space, ambiguously encoded voxels are distributed depending on the shapes of the bijective sub-regions (see previous section). In analogy to SENSE, the g-factor describes the spatial variations of loss of SNR caused by subsampling and/or the non-bijectiveness of the SEMs. As shown above, the correction factor v_ρ describes an intensity correction to account for the nonlinear nature of the SEMs; it is proportional to the nominal voxel volume. Note that by this nonlinear correction, the SNR can be improved compared to conventional imaging in regions of low resolution and it degrades in regions where the resolution is very high. As usual, SNR is traded for resolution.

5.1.2 Methods

a) Simulations

Simulations were performed with Matlab (The Mathworks Inc., Natick, MA, USA). A high-resolution Shepp-Logan head phantom as spin density was used to simulate the signal on a Cartesian k-space trajectory. Ideal orthogonal quadrupolar fields ($L = 2$ in Eq. 5.15) were chosen as SEMs, and, to suppress the Gibbs ringing artifact, the k-space data were multiplied with a Kaiser-Bessel window with appropriately chosen parameters. The sensitivity profiles were based on measured sensitivity data of an eight channel receiver coil array. They were determined as explained in chapter 2.1.2b, page 48f. The images were reconstructed with the presented Cartesian algorithm; intensity-correction was approximated by the local deformation at the voxel centers (cf. chapter 4.2.2b, page 148ff). Interpolation is involved at several steps in the reconstruction process, so the choice of an adequate interpolation method should be made carefully. For the performed simulations and experiments, it was sufficient to use a standard bicubic interpolation method to interpolate the sensitivity data and the derivative information of the SEMs on the image space reconstruction grid. For the final interpolation of the image values onto a high-resolution (typically 512×512) Cartesian grid, the multilevel b-spline method [94] was implemented.

b) Experiments

Experimental data of a kiwi fruit and a phantom consisting of several tubes filled with doped water were acquired on a 9.4 T BioSpec system (Bruker BioSpin MRI GmbH, Ettlingen, Germany) using the PatLoc prototype coil, which generated nearly-orthogonal quadrupolar SEMs. Details about the coil and its integration into the scanner hardware environment are presented in chapter 3.3.2, page 124ff. A standard spin echo and a gradient echo sequence (see chapter 1.2.4, page 33f) with Cartesian trajectories were applied to the modified PatLoc hardware.

According to Eq. 4.5, the applied currents through the PatLoc coils must be known for correct determination of the k-space variables. In the measurements, the current strengths could be controlled, and they were set as high as the coils could safely tolerate. The dwell time Δt was chosen such that the object was completely covered by the field-of-view. This is the case when the condition of Eq. 5.26 holds. According to that equation and Eq. 5.19, as well as Eqs. 4.5, 4.6, and considering that adjacent k-space locations have the distance $2\pi \cdot \Delta k$, the condition is met for the readout SEM if $\Delta\omega_f|_W < 2\pi/I_f\Delta t$. Here I_f denotes the current through the readout coil and $\Delta\omega_f|_W$ is the (angular) frequency dispersion per unit current generated by the readout coil. It is measured over the region W, covered by the object. With an estimate of object size and position, it can be calculated from measured SEM sensitivity profiles. The maximum SEM sensitivity of the coil was $23.5\,\mu T/A$ at $3\,cm$ from the center (also cf. table 3.1, page 131). Recall from chapter 3.3, page 121ff, that highly-resolved images could not be acquired with the PatLoc prototype coil because of SNR restrictions and large dwell times. With $I_f = 8.25\,A$, the dwell time was set to $100\,\mu s$ for the measurement of the kiwi fruit. As the sensitivity of the amplifiers was actually not calibrated in the controlling software, dummy values for the FOV needed to be specified to realize the above settings. Such issues and other problems associated with the first PatLoc prototype coil could be solved with subsequent coil designs, resulting in a superior image quality (cf. the last paragraph in chapter 3.3.3 on page 132).

For the determination of the sensitivity profiles of the eight-channel Tx/Rx coil array and for the acquisition of the SEM field maps the standard linear gradient coil setup was used. In order to assess the quality of the PatLoc-encoded images, reference images with the conventional linear gradient system were obtained. All relevant imaging parameters could then be calculated based on the above experimental settings.

c) Determination of the Encoding Fields

For PatLoc imaging, it is crucial to correctly determine the SEMs. In the Cartesian algorithm the following issues have to be considered:

- PatLoc reconstruction involves an intensity correction step. This correction is determined here approximately by calculating derivatives of

$\vec{\psi}$. The calculation of derivatives is in general very sensitive to noise, so the SNR needs to be high in the numerical representation of $\vec{\psi}$.

- In the final reconstruction step, the image has to be transformed to image space coordinates. Errors in $\vec{\psi}$ result in distortions of the reconstructed image, similar to nonlinearities of conventional gradient fields.

- As the RF-coil sensitivity maps are known in image space variables, but have to be calculated for values in encoding space, erroneous $\vec{\psi}$ results in erroneous coil sensitivity information. The robustness of the reconstruction against errors in the sensitivity maps is similar to SENSE reconstruction (cf. Eq. 5.14). Fortunately, SENSE has proven to be robust against moderate errors in the sensitivity profiles of the receiver coil array.

An adequate estimate of $\vec{\psi}$ was found based on raw field maps of the encoding fields. Raw field maps of the SEMs were acquired using two standard single-echo gradient echo measurements with identical T_E for each SEM with the PatLoc coil placed inside the magnet bore and connected to a DC current source. One measurement was performed without current through the PatLoc coil and a second one with a positive DC current I_{DC}. The purpose of the second measurement was to create an additional inhomogeneity indicating the field strength $B_{1,2}^{raw}$ of the magnetic field generated by PatLoc coil $1, 2$. The field strength $B_{1,2}^{raw}$ was calculated by taking the phase difference map of both measurements:

$$B_{1,2}^{raw}(\vec{x}) = \frac{\Delta\phi_{1,2}(\vec{x})}{\gamma T_E}. \tag{5.30}$$

The current I_{DC} was set sufficiently low to avoid voxel shifts in the readout direction. Noise-free field maps $B_{1,2}^{SEM}(\vec{x})$ were modeled by fitting a low number N_b of solid harmonics $B_j(\vec{x})$, $j = 1, \ldots, N_b$ evaluated at the polar angle $\theta = 90°$ to the raw field maps:

$$B_{1,2}^{SEM}(\vec{x}) = \sum_{j=1}^{N_b} a_{ij} B_j(\vec{x}), \quad \text{with} \quad i = 1, 2. \tag{5.31}$$

This model allows gridding to arbitrary positions and the calculation of reliable derivatives. The coefficients a_{ij} were determined by a standard least-squares fitting approach. According to the discussion following Eq. 4.5 on page 137, $\vec{\psi}$ is then given by $\psi_{1,2}(\vec{x}) = (\gamma/\beta I_{DC})\, B_{1,2}^{SEM}(\vec{x})$.

In principle, the inverse of $\vec{\psi}$ has to be determined in order to calculate the positions in image space corresponding to the grid points in each leaf of multiple encoding space. This is simple for ideal quadrupolar fields, especially when the encoding fields are derived using complex-valued algebra (see discussion of Fig. 5.5 on page 165). However, measured sensitivity maps deviate from exact quadrupolar fields, and the problem becomes more intricate. Therefore, a different approach was taken. In fact, the problem can be simplified because the Cartesian algorithm makes use of the fact that the same grid in each leaf of encoding space is chosen. In this case, it is sufficient to determine the multiple points $\vec{x}_{l,\rho}$ in image space corresponding to a single grid location $\vec{u}_\rho$ in encoding space (cf. Fig. 5.1, page 159). Newton's method was used to determine those ambiguous locations by solving the nonlinear equation $\vec{\psi}(\vec{x}_{l,\rho}) = \vec{u}_\rho$ for each location $\vec{u}_\rho$. This approach also avoids the problem of defining cutting lines through each encoding space leaf joining the neighboring leaves (cf. Fig. 5.5, page 167). In order to ensure correct convergence to the two different solutions, the method was initialized twice with points in the vicinity of the true solutions. This was possible because of the similarity of the experimental SEMs to ideal quadrupolar fields, where the two solutions can be determined analytically.

It should be recalled here that unlike receiver coil sensitivities, SEMs do not depend on coil loading. It is therefore sufficient to determine $\vec{\psi}$ only once after coil installation (also compare with last paragraph of chapter 2.1.2b on page 49).

5.1.3   Results

The topics discussed in the theory section (reconstruction algorithm and resulting image properties like resolution, Gibbs ringing, aliasing and SNR) are verified here for quadrupolar PatLoc SEMs with numerical simulations and experimental data.

a)   Simulations

Simulation results based on a numerical phantom are schematically shown in Fig. 5.3. The workflow in this figure confirms, in accordance with Eqs.

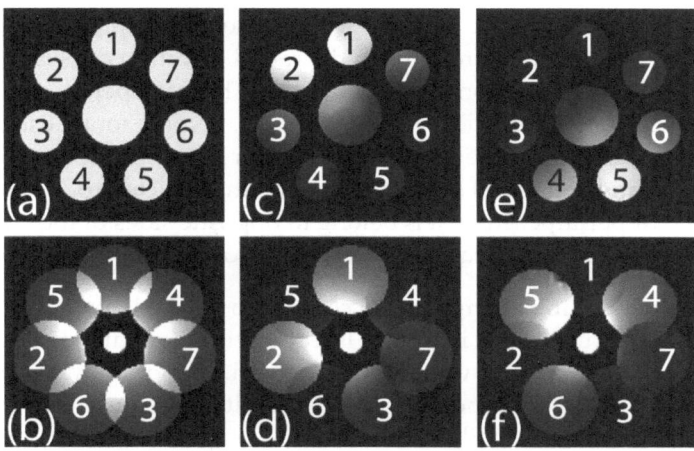

Figure 5.8: Simulated images of a numerical phantom for conventional gradient encoding (top) and for PatLoc encoding using quadrupolar fields (bottom). (a) and (b): Uniform receiver coil sensitivity. (c) and (d): Non-uniform receiver coil sensitivity of a surface coil placed at the top left of the object. (e) and (f): Similar surface coil placed at the bottom right. A deformation is visible in the radial direction. The circles at the periphery are numbered in order to indicate that, for the quadrupolar fields, the object appears aliased because the azimuthal angle is doubled compared to conventional encoding. The intensity of neighboring circles in (d) and (f) is very different such that very weak aliasing occurs when multiple, circumferentially-distributed surface coils are used.

5.12, 5.17, and Fig. 5.6, that a coil-wise FFT of the signal data leads to aliased, intensity-modulated and highly distorted coil images. It is depicted that the matrix inversion step resolves aliasing, the subsequent intensity correction removes the intensity modulation and the final visualization step unwarps the severe distortions.

Fig. 5.8 illustrates the transformation described by Eq. 5.17 for an example test object in detail. In this figure, simulated coil images are shown for a numerical phantom using conventional gradient encoding and PatLoc encoding with quadrupolar fields. Reconstructed images are compared both assuming a single homogeneous sensitivity as well as a set of real-world surface coil sensitivity maps. Fig. 5.8 clarifies in particular two properties of encoding with quadrupolar fields: First, aliasing occurs because the multipolarity of the encoding fields causes a doubling of the angle in the azimuthal direction in the coil images. At the same time, the quadratic dependency of the field strengths in the radial direction causes shrinking at the center and expansion at the periphery. These properties are a direct consequence of the properties of $\vec{\psi}$ (see Fig. 5.5). Second, for realistic surface coils aliasing is weak at the periphery. This can be understood by realizing that the sensitive region of surface coils is often restricted to only a part of the object. Superimposed voxels belong to opposite sides of the object and therefore the surface coil basically only "sees" one of the two voxels.

Resolution and Gibbs Ringing   According to Fig. 3.4b, page 109, the resolution in each dimension increases linearly with the radial distance from the center. This result is verified by simulating and analyzing the PSF at different locations in the image. The results are shown in Fig. 5.9a-c. Figure 5.9a,b shows the PSF at two example locations. One can clearly appreciate that the resolution is higher for the voxel which is farther off-center. In Fig. 5.9c, this result is quantified for a large set of voxel locations. The double logarithmic plot of Fig. 5.9c was generated in the following way: The PSF was calculated for locations belonging to a regular grid in image space. An area was selected, where the PSF's intensity was higher than half the maximum value. The resolution was than defined as the square root of this area. Some scattering of the data is introduced with this method because the resolution only takes discrete values and because gridding the data to image space coordinates introduces some deviations from the theoretical value. A linear least-squares fit of the data points resulted in the slope $m = 0.99 \approx 1$ thus confirming a proportionality of resolution and radial distance from the center.

Before applying the 2D-FFT, the signals in Fig. 5.3 and Fig. 5.9a-c were actually multiplied by a Kaiser-Bessel filter with window parameter $\alpha = 1.5$ and $\alpha = 2.0$ respectively, as defined in Eq. 2.37, page 71. This filtering operation was used to suppress the Gibbs ringing artifact. Fig. 5.9d,e indicate what happens if the reconstruction is performed without this filtering operation. According to Fig. 5.9d, for a source voxel located close to the center, a pronounced Gibbs ringing artifact appears as streaks going from the center to the edges of the images. The images were simulated on a low-resolution 64×64 grid to emphasize the effect. At higher resolution, these artifacts are much less prominent. Fig. 5.9d also indicates that the PSF is aliased outside its central position. The reason for this artifact is that the reconstruction algorithm assumes a coil sensitivity depending on the

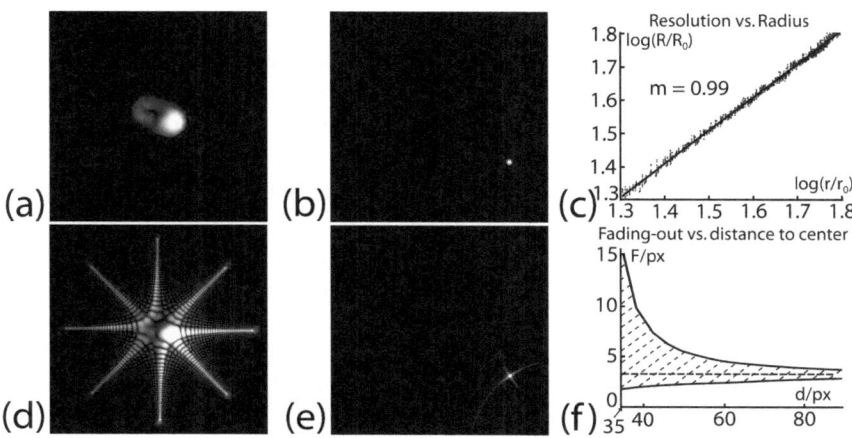

Figure 5.9: Resolution and Gibbs ringing for quadrupolar fields by point spread function (PSF) analysis. The top row shows results with filtered data, the bottom row without filtering. (a) and (b): The resolution is lower toward the center than at the periphery. (c) A quantitative analysis based on a simple numerical evaluation of the width of the PSF at different locations shows that the resolution is proportional to the radius. (d) Without filtering the PSF has long-reaching Gibbs ringing tails which even show some aliasing. (e) Both artifacts are less prominent farther away from the center. The Gibbs ringing behavior is quantified in (f). For each voxel location, the main tails fall off differently. In this plot, F indicates the distance in voxels in encoding space, until which the ringing has fallen off to 10%. These values are plotted against the radial image space distance from the center. All values remain between an upper and a lower bound, which converge at the periphery toward the fall-off behavior for conventional imaging, represented by the dotted line. The convergence expresses the fact that at the periphery the imaging properties are similar to conventional imaging.

corresponding position in the image. The weighting is therefore only correct for the central position of the PSF. The more distant the ringing extends from the central position, the more the weighting deteriorates.

For voxels at the periphery like the one chosen in Fig. 5.9e, aliasing is much weaker because the interplay of more distant aliased points along with less extended ringing leads to a close-to-exact reconstruction also outside the central lobe of the PSF. The ringing toward the edge of the image is less extended in image space for voxels at the periphery because of two reasons. First, in image space the voxel volume is smaller and therefore the same fall-off behavior per voxel has smaller extent. Second, this fall-off behavior varies with distance from the center and with its direction because the reconstructed image is not adequately intensity corrected outside the PSF's center. This behavior is sketched in Fig. 5.9f. The number of voxels F in encoding space, where the intensity of one of the main tails of the PSF has fallen off to less than 10%, varies throughout the image. However, all values are restricted to an upper and a lower bound. At the periphery, these bounds converge toward a common value. This value is the same as in Fourier imaging, which can be found by analyzing the properties of the sinc-function. At the periphery, the ringing artifact is similar to the conventional artifact because locally the gradient fields are constant and so the signal distribution is locally well-behaved. Toward the center the nonlinearity of the fields must be taken into account, the intensity of the signal distribution becomes strongly non-uniform and therefore deviations to the conventional case occur. In the limit $r \rightarrow 0$, where r is defined as the distance to the center, the tails toward the edges remain constant in intensity, whereas the tails toward the center fall off faster, proportional to r^{-2} instead of r^{-1} compared to conventional imaging. This result is in conformity with the theoretical considerations performed on page 171 in the paragraph *Gibbs Ringing* of section 5.1.1e.

Spatially Undersampled Datasets   Fig. 5.10 illustrates the undersampling artifact and presents reconstruction results of a combined PatLoc-SENSE reconstruction. In Fig. 5.10a the acquisition space is fully sampled; the object lies within the rectangular FOV in encoding space. The image can be reconstructed correctly as shown in Fig. 5.10b. The shape of the FOV in image space is given by the inverse mapping $\vec{\psi}^{-1}$ of the SEMs applied to the rectangular FOV in encoding space. In Fig. 5.10c the acquisition is accelerated by a factor of 2 by undersampling the PatLoc k-space. In encoding space, a similar fold-over artifact as in conventional imaging is produced. In the PatLoc-reconstructed image, shown in Fig. 5.10d, the aliasing appears at several locations depending on the number of bijective subregions of the SEMs. The mapping to image space yields a reduced intensity of the artifact in regions where the encoding fields are flat because the back-folded artifact is spread out. If the readout SEM and the accelerated phase encoding SEM were swapped, the artifacts would occur at 45° with respect to the aliasing shown. Fig. 5.10e demonstrates that aliasing can be removed by combining PatLoc reconstruction with SENSE reconstruction. The combination of the

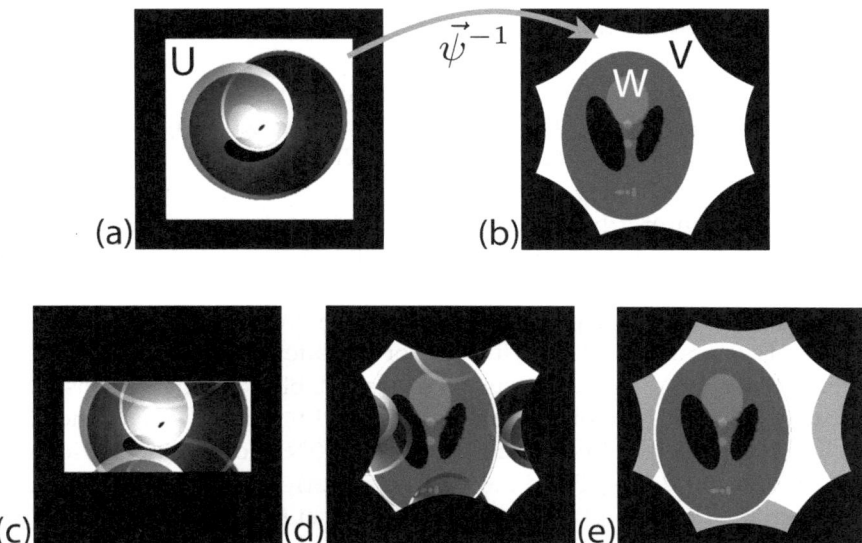

Figure 5.10: Illustration of the concept of FOV in PatLoc imaging, the aliasing artifact and combined PatLoc-SENSE reconstruction. (a) The area U of the FOV is a rectangle in encoding space. (b) In image space, the area V of the FOV is given by the inverse mapping of the SEM vector field applied to this rectangular region; i.e., $V = \vec{\psi}^{-1}(U)$. No aliasing occurs because the covered area of the object W lies within the borders of V. (c) In encoding space undersampling leads to the conventional fold-over artifact. (d) The non-unique mapping to image space leads to a fourfold appearance of the aliasing artifact in image space. (e) This aliasing can be resolved by combining PatLoc and SENSE reconstruction. This combination effectively leads to an extension of the reduced FOV (white) to the full FOV (gray).

two methods is possible because both rely on the fact that spins at different, yet known, positions are identically encoded by the SEMs, but differently weighted by the sensitivity profiles of the receiver coils. Once the aliased positions are determined,[6] an adequate matrix inversion leads to the desired recovery of the original spin density, provided that the sensitivity matrix is well-conditioned.

SNR The simulation results shown in Fig. 5.11a represent a validation of theoretical predictions for the SNR as given by Eq. 5.28. The images

---

[6] A method is described in the paragraph *Aliasing – PatLoc-SENSE* in chapter 5.1.1e on page 175.

of Fig. 5.11 show results along a line, which crosses the common center of the quadrupolar fields. According to Eq. 5.28, it is useful to separate the SNR into three contributions apart from the factor $\sqrt{L}$ describing the intrinsic acceleration. These contributions are depicted in Fig. 5.11b-d. As a reference, Fig. 5.11b depicts the optimal SNR when linear gradient fields are applied. The SNR is calculated according to Eq. 2.48, page 81, under the assumption of a homogeneous magnetization. The SNR should be given by the root-sum-of-squares of the coil sensitivities. Recall that these were estimated with a method that results in sensitivities that are weighted with the root-sum-of-squares of those. Therefore, the plot shown in Fig. Fig. 5.11b is nearly constant, with a minor deviation from unity at the center, where not enough signal intensity was available for reliable sensitivity estimation. The g-factor is shown in Fig. 5.11c. It is inverse to the SNR divided by voxel size because the reference SNR for linear gradients is nearly constant. In Fig. 5.11d the volumetric correction factor is visualized. The combination of Fig. 5.11b-d indicates that at the periphery, the SNR is mainly determined by the volumetric correction factor and therefore the SNR almost exclusively depends on the voxel volume at the corresponding location. At the center, the SNR-benefit resulting from the large voxel size outweighs any SNR-degradation toward the center resulting from an ill-condition of the sensitivity matrix.

Fig. 5.12 shows a comparison of g-factor maps for SENSE imaging, PatLoc imaging using quadrupolar fields and a combination of both. In addition, ultimate g-factor maps are depicted. Fig. 5.12a-d show the results for a circular receiver coil arrangement with eight channels. As depicted in Fig. 5.12a,b, the g-factor for such a circular arrangement is much lower at the periphery ($g < 1.01$) compared to SENSE with acceleration 2 (Fig. 5.12b), which has a peak value of more than 1.25 at the periphery. At the center, where image resolution is low, the g-factor is higher than that for SENSE imaging. Combining PatLoc imaging using quadrupolar fields with a SENSE acceleration of 2 results in up to fourfold aliasing. In Fig. 5.12c the resulting g-factor map is shown. Although the SENSE acceleration introduces non-circular aliasing, the overall g-factor is still considerably lower than the g-factor for a SENSE acceleration of 4 with the conventional gradient system, which is depicted in Fig. 5.12d.

Whereas in Fig. 5.12a-d one particular receiver coil geometry was used, which might be non-optimal in either case, Fig. 5.12e,f show results of the

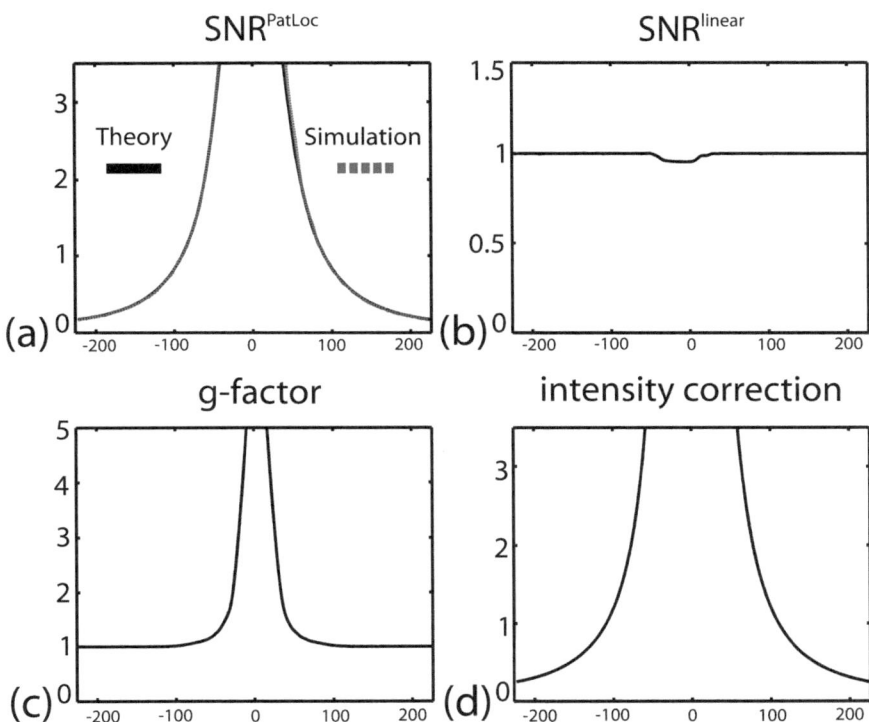

Figure 5.11: Example SNR and its components (cf. Eq. 5.28) for quadrupolar fields and an eight-channel receiver coil array. Shown is a profile through the center of the 2D imaging data. (a) Calculated (solid line) and simulated (discontinuous line) SNR. The lines lie on top of each other, a difference is barely visible. Numbers on the y-axis above unity indicate higher SNR compared to the SNR for fully-encoded Fourier images. Spatial variations in SNR are in this case not dominated by the g-factor, but rather by the correction due to varying voxel size. (b) Optimal SNR for Fourier imaging. The SNR has been normalized to unity at the edges. It is nearly constant for the method that was used to estimate the coil sensitivities. (c) Calculated g-factor. The g-factor is very near to unity except at the center. It is proportional to noise amplification and SNR degradation. (d) Calculated correction factor. For quadrupolar fields, it has an adverse effect on SNR as a consequence to the enhanced resolution toward the periphery.

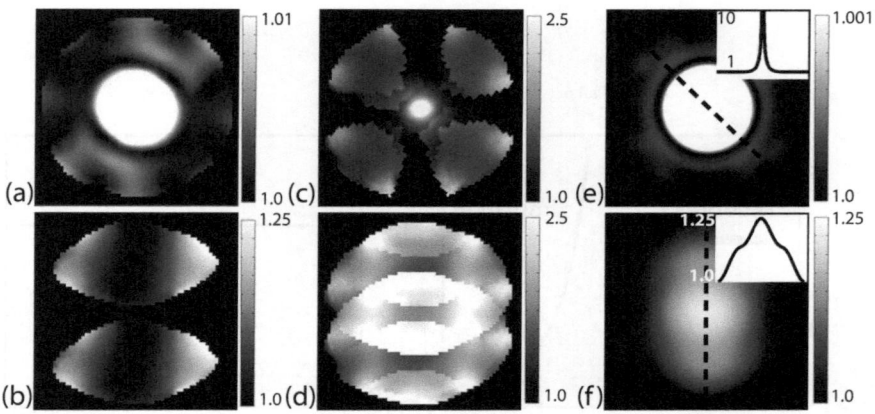

Figure 5.12: g-factor maps for PatLoc imaging using quadrupolar fields (top) and pure SENSE imaging (bottom). An eight-coil receiver array with circular arrangement has been used in (a)-(d). (e) and (f) show ultimate g-factor maps. (a) For a fully acquired dataset the g-factor is very near to unity (lower than 1.01) at the periphery. Only at the center, the g-factor is unfavorable (also cf. Fig. 5.11c). (b) For the same coil arrangement the g-factor for SENSE, accelerated in the vertical direction ($2x$) has peak values of more than 1.25. (c) Apart from the central region, the g-factor of the accelerated ($2x$) PatLoc-encoded image is below 2 almost in the whole image. (d) For pure SENSE ($4x$) the g-factor reaches values of more than 2.5. (e) The ultimate g-factor for accelerated PatLoc imaging ($2x$) reveals that the noise enhancement at the center cannot be overcome for purely quadrupolar SEMs. However, an optimal coil array might be capable of reducing the g-factor close to unity in the major part of the object. (f) For conventional imaging with SENSE ($4x$) the ultimate g-factor is limited to a certain range, but it remains significant farther away from the center of the object. Note the different scaling in (a) and (b) as well as in (e) and (f).

ultimate geometry factor. The ultimate geometry factor is derived from the ultimate SNR in each position, i.e., the highest possible SNR compatible with Maxwell's equations. It depends on the frequency of the RF field, material properties, object size and its shape and also on the imaging method and the applied reconstruction algorithm. The concept of ultimate SNR has been introduced in [117] with an extension to parallel imaging in [119]. In this investigation, the ultimate SNR was calculated in analogy to [200] using a multipole expansion of the electromagnetic field to create an approximately complete basis of the solution space to Laplace's equation involving $2 \cdot 71^2$ basis functions of lowest order. The theoretical background of ultimate SNR is reviewed in chapter 2.3.1d, page 82ff. The *Remark* on page 175 clarifies that the concept of ultimate SNR can immediately be used in Cartesian PatLoc imaging. As the presented PatLoc design is particularly relevant to brain imaging, a homogeneous sphere with diameter of 12 cm was chosen and material properties of average brain tissue at 3 T were taken from Table 1 in [200], i.e., relative dielectric constant $\epsilon_r = 63.1$ and conductivity $\sigma = 0.46/\Omega m$. The relative magnetic permeability μ_r was assumed to be unity.

In addition to the 2D images, Fig. 5.12e,f also sketches profiles along the dotted lines. The same imaging setup was used as in Fig. 5.12c,d. The profile in Fig. 5.12e indicates that the ultimate g-factor diverges toward the center of the quadrupolar fields. The disadvantage toward the center is compensated by a reduced ultimate g-factor toward the periphery. For the largest part of the object, the ultimate g-factor is very close to unity. Fig. 5.12f shows that for conventional imaging with SENSE-acceleration of 4, the ultimate g-factor is bound to the interval $[1.0, 1.23]$ in the complete object. In contrast to quadrupolar SEMs however, the ultimate g-factor remains above unity also farther away from the center of the object. It is to be noted, however, that ultimate g-factors are rarely achieved experimentally (cf. for example Fig. 5.12c,d with Fig. 5.12e,f).

b) Experiments

Measurement of a phantom consisting of several tubes filled with doped water and a kiwi fruit are shown on the left in Fig. 5.13;[7] these measurements were performed with the PatLoc prototype coil. PatLoc images are compared to reference measurements using the conventional gradient system with comparable sequence parameters. The tube phantom data were acquired using a spoiled gradient echo sequence. For the PatLoc experiment, $T_E = 11.2$ ms and $T_R = 0.5$ s were chosen. For the reference measurement, $T_E = 7.2$ ms and $T_R = 0.1$ s were used. The kiwi fruit data were acquired using a spin echo sequence. For both, the PatLoc experiment and the reference measurement, $T_E = 50$ ms and $T_R = 2$ s were used. The PatLoc and the reference measurement results show a fairly good agreement.

The PatLoc images clearly have a resolution gradient toward the periphery. Aliasing is barely visible in the reconstructed images and intensity is

---

[7]The images of the kiwi fruit are also depicted in Fig. 3.16a, page 127.

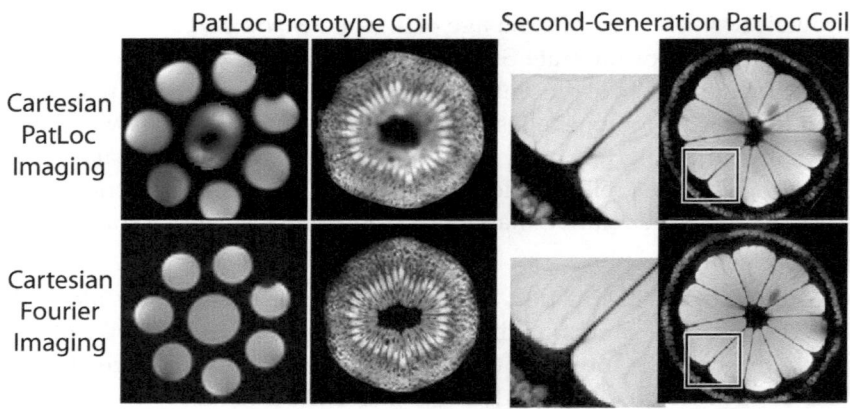

Figure 5.13: Experimental results. Top left: Reconstructed images of a 64×64 spoiled gradient echo PatLoc-experiment with a phantom consisting of several tubes filled with doped water and of a 128×128 spin echo experiment with a kiwi fruit. The data were acquired with the first PatLoc prototype coil. Bottom left: Corresponding reference images acquired using the conventional gradient system. Right: PatLoc image and reference of a lemon acquired with a 256×256 RARE sequence using a second-generation high-performance PatLoc coil developed at Bruker BioSpin MRI GmbH, Ettlingen, Germany. The images on the right were presented at the Annual Meeting of the ISMRM 2010 in Stockholm (cf. [120]) and are courtesy of Stéphanie Ohrel from Bruker BioSpin MRI GmbH.

correctly represented - apart from the central region, where signal dropout occurs caused by having used an approximate continuous method to esti-mate the intensity correction (cf. the *Remark* on page 166f). Some geometric distortions are visible in the images; these can be attributed to inaccurate calibration data (cf. section 5.1.2c, page 178ff). Overall, a robustness of the reconstruction algorithm with imperfect input can be appreciated.

On the right-hand side of Fig. 5.13, an image of a lemon is shown that has been acquired using a 256×256 RARE sequence [60] with $T_R = 5$ s, $T_E = 14$ ms and RARE factor of 8. The image has been acquired with an improved second-generation small-bore PatLoc coil developed at Bruker BioSpin MRI GmbH, Ettlingen, Germany. No geometric distortions are visible in the reconstructed image. It can also be seen that, at the periphery, image resolution is improved compared to the reference image. The image of the lemon verifies that fast, accurate and robust reconstruction is possible with the Cartesian image space reconstruction method presented in this chapter also under realistic experimental conditions.

5.1.4 Discussion

The results presented in the previous section show that the Cartesian reconstruction algorithm is suitable for performing the reconstruction of 2D images using orthogonal non-bijective quadrupolar encoding fields. Aliased voxels are unfolded and the intensity is correctly determined, despite the strong nonlinearities of the involved encoding fields. With the first PatLoc prototype coil, some image deformations were visible; this problem could be eliminated with an optimized second-generation coil design. Similar high-quality results could be achieved with the larger human system (see e.g. Fig. 7.7, page 258). The quality of the reconstructed images presented here is remarkable considering the simplicity of the used signal model, where only the influence of the SEMs onto the phase factor is considered. It was therefore not a priority to enhance the image quality of the reconstructed images by refining the model; for example, by also considering field inhomogeneities of the main magnetic field, as has been done in [121]. Also, typical measurement errors of RF and SEM sensitivities affect the reconstructed images only moderately.

The Cartesian PatLoc reconstruction algorithm is similar to Cartesian SENSE reconstruction [135]. However, the strong nonlinearities of the SEMs require some modifications of this method and cause alterations of image properties. In contrast to conventional SENSE imaging, where the g-factor has only moderate variations, the g-factor for PatLoc imaging using quadrupolar fields is very high at the center, whereas it is close to unity at the periphery (Fig. 5.12). This behavior can be understood qualitatively by investigating the relative distance of aliased voxels with respect to each other. In conventional SENSE imaging the distance of aliased voxels is constant, whereas for quadrupolar fields, the distance is high at the periphery and low toward the center. The variations in the coil sensitivity profiles therefore allow discrimination of voxels with almost no SNR decrease at the periphery, whereas at the center the variations are low and so discrimination is only possible with a high g-factor penalty, which is, however, negligible compared to the SNR enhancement due to the large voxels at the center (Fig. 5.11).

The benign behavior of SNR at the periphery remains partly preserved when the PatLoc dataset is accelerated by a factor of two. In SENSE imaging aliased points lie equidistantly along one single line, whereas in accelerated PatLoc imaging, the points are distributed over the image. This is similar to 3D SENSE imaging with acceleration in two directions. PatLoc imaging might therefore be used with possibly higher acceleration factors than conventional imaging. A circular receiver coil arrangement naturally seems to exploit the inherently radially symmetric aliasing pattern of images fully encoded with quadrupolar fields (Fig. 5.12a), whereas much effort was required to optimize RF-coil arrangements for SENSE imaging (e.g. [194]). However, when PatLoc-encoded data are accelerated, some room for RF-coil optimization remains: The ultimate g-factor indicates that acceleration by a factor of two does not necessarily lead to a significant decrease in SNR (cp. Fig. 5.12a,c,e.) An optimal RF-coil arrangement depends on many parameters, such as object size, acceleration factor and application. In PatLoc, an optimal arrangement also depends on the SEMs. Therefore, it can be expected that PatLoc imaging will profit from the current trend of continually increasing the number of receiver coil elements.

In PatLoc, image resolution is a local property depending on the spatial variations of the gradient fields of the SEMs. In this chapter, quantitative results have been derived based on the choice of a regular grid in encoding space rather than in image space, the natural choice for conventional imaging. This is almost optimal in terms of resolution because it allows direct application of the FFT at the first step of the reconstruction and no information is lost using the FFT operation. The image resolution is in principle defined by the corresponding pattern given by the local gradient strength. Deviations might result because local variations in the RF-sensitivity maps include information, which can be used to locally improve resolution ([170], [125], also cf. chapter 2.3.1e, page 86ff). This effect is often negligible; it should be considered, however, when the RF variations are considerable compared to the intra-voxel variations produced by the SEM system. Such a situation occurs in low-resolution imaging such as spectroscopic imaging ([170], [125]). In the context of PatLoc imaging, RF-sensitivity variations gain considerable value in regions, where the SEMs become very flat. An example is shown later, in Fig. 7.7, page 258, where PSFs are depicted that indicate improved resolution at the center of a quadrupolar SEM-combination if an iterative method is used for image reconstruction.

In terms of the computation time, it is a crucial advantage of the direct Cartesian PatLoc reconstruction algorithm that an FFT is performed because it results in a numerical complexity of only $\mathcal{O}(N \log N)$ for each coil and each dimension. With the FFT the aliased image is represented in encoding space. It is also possible to reconstruct directly onto a regular grid in image space with a non-uniform FFT of type 2 (an explanation of this operation is found in the paragraph *Non-Uniform FFT* in chapter 7.1.3, page 248f). This has the advantage that the RF-coil sensitivities do not need to be interpolated on the PatLoc encoding space grid, and it is no longer required to finally rewarp the image back to image space. As shown later, in chapter 7, page 235ff, the main advantage of choosing a regular grid in image space rather than in encoding space is that the pronounced Gibbs ringing artifact is suppressed - if iterative reconstruction algorithms are applied. However, for the direct reconstruction, that is the topic of the present chapter, this benefit is not observed; the artifact can even be intensified by the non-uniform FFT.

The PatLoc image properties are similar to those found in conventional imaging except for regions where no field gradients are generated during the entire measurement. In such regions, a pronounced Gibbs ringing artifact results that lacks symmetry and aliasing is observed. This problem can be addressed in several ways:

- Via image reconstruction: At the expense of image resolution, the artifact is diminished by data filtering. There are also some limited possibilities to use intra-voxel RF-receiver variations to improve the localization of the signal, for example with the iterative CG reconstruction, see chapter 7, page 235ff.

- Via excitation: Additional object information can be encoded with multiple tailored RF-excitation profiles. Alternatively, the problem can simply be circumvented by only selectively exciting those regions where the gradients are sufficiently strong. Prolonged pulses can be shortened by parallel excitation [81, 215, 185]; however, additional energy deposition in tissue has to be taken into consideration.

- Via modification of the sampling trajectory: In the next chapter, it is shown that radial instead of Cartesian sampling can have beneficial properties. Also other sampling strategies combined with an adequate reconstruction technique may be useful [190].

- Via additional SEM Encoding: To avoid a priori that regions of vanishing gradient fields occur. This may be achieved by phase preparation (for example, signal contamination from low gradient regions would be reduced by adding a linear field prior to signal acquisition) or by appropriately varying the effective gradient field during the encoding process (an example is the 4D trajectory described in [[42]]). Such approaches require that the linear gradient fields are not merely replaced by NB-SEMs, but that a multi-channel system is available that combines a multitude of linear and nonlinear SEMs.

Such extensions, that add flexibility to the encoding process, have been subject to recent research activities. A theoretical approach is presented in [[100, 101]], where different field modes of a PatLoc gradient coil array are determined based on the SVD of the fields that are generated by the individual array elements. A technological improvement is the multi-channel PatLoc hardware configuration for head imaging, described in chapter 3.3.3, page 126ff. A very interesting approach is the "O-Space" parallel imaging technique, where a quadratic SEM is applied in addition to the linear gradient fields [177]. With the signal equation of Eq. 4.9, this imaging modality uses $\psi(\vec{x}) := \gamma\beta^{-1}(b_0, g_x x, g_y y, 1/2(x^2 + y^2))^T$ and m projections $\mathbf{k}_m(t) := -2\pi G t \beta \gamma^{-1}(b_0^{-1}(x_m^2 + y_m^2), -2g_x^{-1}x_m, -2g_y^{-1}y_m, 2h^{-1})^T$, where G is a common "gradient strength" and t the time. The quantities b_0, g_x, g_y and h describe the characteristic properties of the constant linear and quadratic fields, and $(x_m, y_m)^T$ are different center placements. Several center placement patterns are described in [22]. Important is the work presented in [204], where linear and high-order field gradients are generated with a common matrix gradient coil design.

Such multi-channel designs introduce new options for MRI signal encoding; however, images cannot be reconstructed with an FFT as described in this chapter because the number of SEMs exceeds the number of encoded spatial dimensions. Reconstruction methods suitable for such multi-dimensional encoding strategies are explained in detail in chapter 7.1.1 and 7.1.2, page 237ff.

5.1.5 Conclusions

It has been shown that the image space PatLoc reconstruction algorithm presented above is an efficient and robust implementation of the general weak matrix approach (see chapter 4.2.2, page 144ff.); it is applicable to Cartesian sampling trajectories for an experimental setup where the gradient coils are replaced by coils capable of producing nonlinear and non-bijective magnetic encoding fields. By solving the reconstruction problem in encoding space, the reconstruction becomes a generalized version of SENSE reconstruction. This formal relationship is exploited to quantitatively analyze basic image properties by adapting established techniques to the usage of nonlinear and non-bijective encoding fields. The theoretical investigations were verified in numerical simulations and experiments for orthogonal quadrupolar SEMs only; however, note that the presented algorithm is not restricted to quadrupolar SEMs. Images generated with arbitrary field geometries can be reconstructed and the resulting image properties can be described quantitatively.

A k-space based reconstruction method also suitable for Cartesian trajectories is briefly presented in the following section. The two subsequent chapters deal with image reconstruction beyond Cartesian encoding.

5.2 Direct k-Space Reconstruction

The analysis of the previous section has shown that a modified version of SENSE can be used to reconstruct PatLoc images that have been encoded with a Cartesian trajectory. Here, it is discussed to what extent it is also possible to apply GRAPPA for image reconstruction in PatLoc. It seems natural to assume that GRAPPA is a feasible method regarding the close relationship of GRAPPA and SENSE (cf. chapter 2.3.2b, page 99ff). However, it is demonstrated here that it is not valid to draw this conclusion. In PatLoc, partial unfolding is possible with GRAPPA, but it is problematic to acquire sufficient calibration data needed for complete GRAPPA image reconstruction. Different reconstruction strategies are compared to each other and the results are discussed to gain further insight into k-space based image reconstruction from Cartesian PatLoc measurement data.

5.2.1 Physical Limitation: Calibration Data

Why does a SENSE-variant work, but not a GRAPPA-variant? First, examine Fig. 5.14. The figure depicts the analogy of SENSE and the Cartesian PatLoc algorithm presented in the previous section (also cf. Eq. 5.14, page 165). The figure also illustrates that the perfect image space analogy is not perfect in k-space: In conventional imaging, the fold-over artifact does not occur, if k-space is not undersampled; in PatLoc, however, voxels are aliased even for a densely sampled PatLoc k-space (cf. Fig. 5.14h).

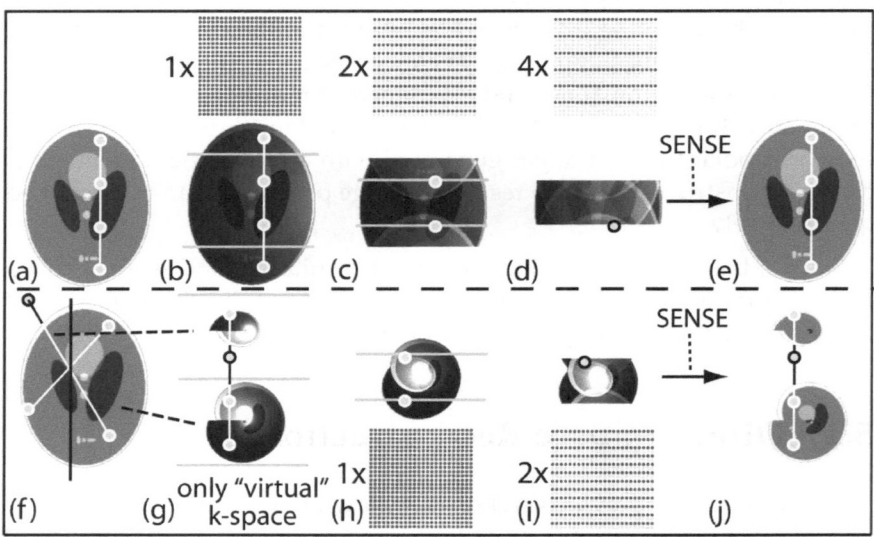

Figure 5.14: Analogy of image space Cartesian PatLoc reconstruction and SENSE and limited analogy for pure k-space based approaches. Depicted are examples encoded with linear SEMs (top) and quadrupolar SEMs (bottom). Top row: Increasing acceleration leads to increased aliasing. The image can be unfolded using SENSE. Bottom row: The situation is similar in PatLoc. If the image is represented in PatLoc encoding space (see subfigures (g - j)), the analogy becomes perfect: In this case, aliased image locations are also equidistantly distributed as in SENSE. This analogy is not perfect in k-space: Whereas an R-fold aliased image corresponds to an R-fold subsampled k-space in conventional imaging, PatLoc k-space is only $R/2$-fold subsampled, if R voxels are aliased. No physical, but rather a "virtual" k-space corresponds to the unfolded image in PatLoc.

Recall that GRAPPA uses calibration data to fill unsampled regions of k-space. If, however, k-space is densely sampled, there are no unsampled regions in k-space to be filled. Therefore, GRAPPA can (generally) not be applied to resolve all ambiguities in PatLoc imaging. One solution would be to introduce a "virtual" k-space that corresponds to the unfolded image displayed for example in Fig. 5.14g. This space is, however, only "virtual" in that sense that it is not a physical space, and therefore it is not (immediately) possible to acquire adequate calibration lines (more on this issue in the discussion section below, page 203ff).

But why does a SENSE-variant work properly? In SENSE, calibration data are not acquired; instead, a separate scan is performed to explicitly measure RF-sensitivity data, and this scan is done with the conventional gradient system also in PatLoc. Therefore, full information about the RF data required for voxel unfolding is available. On the other hand, from the calibration data in GRAPPA, only aliased RF-sensitivity maps can be retrieved (as also shown in the following two paragraphs), and voxel unfolding is not completely possible with GRAPPA.

In chapter 2.3.2b, page 99ff, a relationship of SENSE and GRAPPA is established by directly analyzing the corresponding encoding matrices. It was found that the "GRAPPA encoding matrix" $\hat{\mathbf{E}}_s$ is basically a truncated version of the SENSE encoding matrix $\mathbf{E}$, where the pure RF-sensitivity maps are replaced by the signal data, or, equivalently, by in vivo RF-sensitivity data. Both differences - truncation and in vivo version of the sensitivity data - were proven to merely modify the reconstruction without introducing a profound difference: SENSE and GRAPPA are very similar in conventional imaging.

This seems to be different in PatLoc, and therefore a fundamental difference should also be found by analyzing the corresponding encoding matrices. For the image space reconstruction, the encoding matrix still contains pure RF-sensitivity data (see Eq. 5.5, page 160). The k-space reconstruction matrix, does, however, not contain in vivo sensitivity data any more. Recall that the encoding GRAPPA matrix actually contains signal data. According to Eqs. 5.11, 5.12, the signal data in PatLoc is the k-space version of the aliased and distorted magnetization, and not of the magnetization simply weighted with the RF sensitivities. It can be concluded that the image space encoding matrix contains unaliased sensitivity information, whereas the k-space encoding matrix does not. It has been demonstrated above, that this is exactly the reason, why a SENSE-variant can be applied in PatLoc, but (generally) not a GRAPPA-variant.

In the remainder of this chapter, it is shown that, despite the general problem associated with GRAPPA in PatLoc, k-space based reconstruction can still be a powerful tool for image reconstruction also in the context of non-bijective encoding.

5.2.2   Applicability to Subsampled PatLoc k-Space Data

It may not be possible to acquire calibration data for the reconstruction of a completely unfolded image in PatLoc; however, if the PatLoc data are subsampled, a densely sampled set of calibration data can be acquired - and it is possible to use this calibration data to fill missing lines of PatLoc k-space using GRAPPA *without modification* to the original algorithm. But is this a valid method?

Theory   Reconsider Fig. 5.14. This figure illustrates the fact that an $R\times$ subsampled PI dataset is fully equivalent to an $R/2$-fold subsampled PatLoc dataset (acquired with quadrupolar SEMs). This analogy allows one to replace the problem whether densely sampled calibration data can be used to reconstruct an image from $R/2$-fold subsampled PatLoc data by the following problem: In the context of conventional imaging, is it possible to use $2\times$ subsampled calibration data to reconstruct a $2\times$ subsampled image from an $R\times$ subsampled dataset? This unusual situation, of using subsampled calibration data for image reconstruction, is depicted in Fig. 5.15, and it is compared to the equivalent situation in PatLoc in the same figure.

Consider the more general situation of an $(R{\cdot}L)$-times subsampled Cartesian trajectory, encoded with linear SEMs, and L-times subsampled calibration data. It is shown here that it is possible to calculate appropriate GRAPPA weights $\mathbf{w}_\alpha^{(m)}$ that can be used to fill in each L-th k-space line, thus leading to an L-fold aliased image.

Recall that the GRAPPA weights $\mathbf{w}_\alpha^{(m)}$ are determined by minimizing the l_2-norm of the following expression (cf. Eq. 2.57, page 98):

$$
\left\| \mathbf{w}_\alpha^{(m)} \hat{\mathbf{E}}_s^{(m,ACS)} - \mathbf{s}_\alpha^{ACS} \right\|^2
$$
$$
= \sum_\kappa \left| \sum_{\alpha',\beta} (w_\alpha^{(m)})_{\alpha',\beta}\, s_{\alpha'}^{ACS}(\vec{k}_\kappa - \vec{k}_\beta^{(m)}) - s_\alpha^{ACS}(\vec{k}_\kappa) \right|^2 . \quad (5.32)
$$

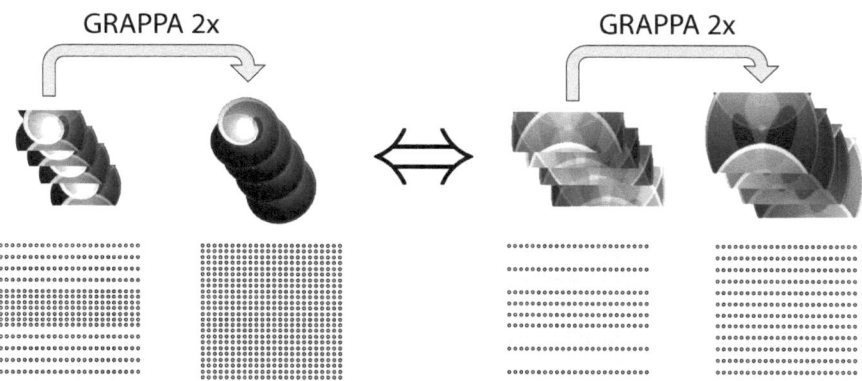

Figure 5.15: Equivalent GRAPPA reconstruction problems for subsampled PatLoc imaging and its linear analogue: It is valid to apply GRAPPA to $2\times$ subsampled Pat-Loc data if and only if GRAPPA can be used in conventional imaging to reconstruct $2\times$ aliased images from $4\times$ subsampled data using $2\times$ subsampled calibration data. It can be shown that this is indeed possible, and therefore the GRAPPA algorithm can be applied without any modification to the subsampled PatLoc dataset.

This equation implies that the weights are found by approximating the signal of each coil at k-space locations $\vec{k}_\kappa$ by a weighted sum of all signals at different k-space locations, defined by the GRAPPA kernel $\mathcal{L}$: For $\beta = (\beta_x, \beta_y) \in \mathcal{L}$ the relative k-space shifts are given by $\vec{k}_\beta^{(m)} = 2\pi\Delta k \cdot (\beta_x \vec{e}_x + (\beta_y R \cdot L - m)\vec{e}_y)$, where $R \cdot L$ is the assumed acceleration factor (cf. chapter 2.3.2a, page 97ff).

In Fig. 5.16 it is illustrated that for a subsampled set of calibration data, it is not possible to determine the GRAPPA weights for each m. To be precise, only each L-th set of GRAPPA weights (i.e., $m = \{L, 2L, (R-1)L\}$) can be determined with an $L\times$ subsampled set of ACS-data. Fig. 5.16 also illustrates that the fitting for each possible $m = \{L, 2L, (R-1)L\}$ is the same, whether the ACS-data are subsampled or not. Observe that the GRAPPA weights are determined independently for each m. Therefore, it is not problematic to determine a reduced set of valid GRAPPA weights from the subsampled ACS-data.

This shows that it is indeed possible to calculate appropriate GRAPPA weights $\mathbf{w}_\alpha^{(m)}$ that can be used to reconstruct each L-th k-space line, thus leading to an L-fold aliased image after performing an inverse 2D-FFT to

Densely Sampled ACS-lines

2x Subsampled ACS-lines

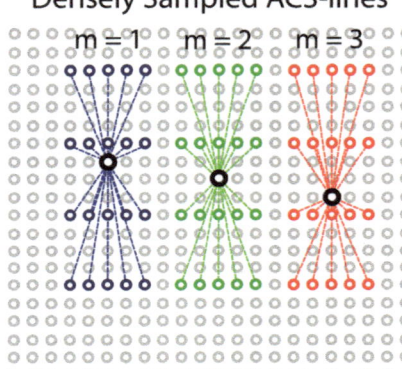 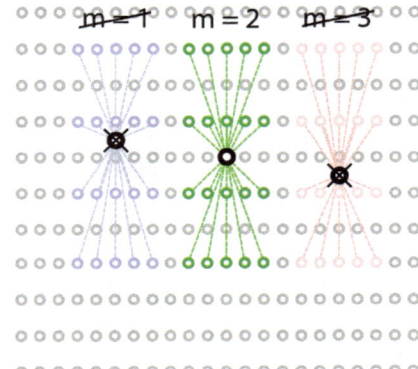

Figure 5.16: Determination of GRAPPA weights from densely sampled (left) and $2\times$ subsampled (right) calibration data. The k-space locations of the ACS-data are in gray. Weights are determined for a $4\times$ subsampled trajectory using a 5×4-GRAPPA kernel. Left: It is illustrated that the relative k-space locations (colored circles) used to fit for a particular k-space location (black circle) are different for each $m = 1, 2, 3$. Right: If only a subsampled set of ACS-data is available, fitting for $m = 1, 3$ is not possible. However, for $m = 2$, fitting is not affected by subsampling of the ACS-data.

the reconstructed k-space data. Because of the analogy to PatLoc imaging, this result can be applied correspondingly to non-bijective encoding with the important consequence that the original GRAPPA algorithm can be used in conjunction with a subsampled PatLoc dataset, as long as a sufficient amount of densely sampled calibration data are acquired. The PatLoc image, reconstructed with GRAPPA, will still exhibit aliasing that is caused by the non-bijectiveness of the SEMs. The Cartesian PatLoc reconstruction method presented above can then be used to finalize image reconstruction.

Methods   Several algorithms for the reconstruction of subsampled imaging data were tested with numerical simulations and experiments. The reconstruction algorithms are presented in Fig. 5.17; the algorithms depicted in Fig. 5.17a-d are applicable to data encoded with linear SEMs, and Fig. 5.17e,f illustrates reconstruction from PatLoc data encoded with quadrupolar SEMs. A detailed description of the methods is found in the figure caption. The involved image space reconstruction was performed as explained in chapter 2.3.1a, page 74ff, and section 5.1.1b, page 160ff.

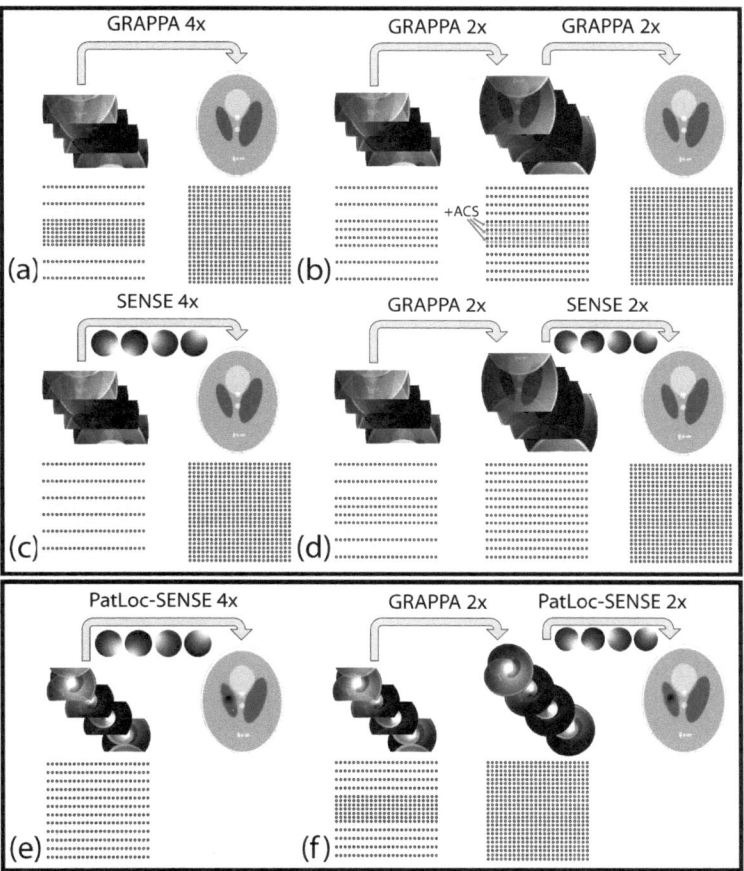

Figure 5.17: Different reconstruction methods for undersampled Cartesian imaging data. (a-d) Encoded with linear SEMs. (e,f) Encoded with quadrupolar SEMs. (a) All calibration lines are used to calculate the GRAPPA weights required to reconstruct the individual missing lines. (b) In a first step, only each second calibration line is used to calculate half of the missing lines. Then, ACS-lines are added and the remaining aliasing is unfolded using GRAPPA again. (c) SENSE is used to reconstruct the image from a $4\times$ subsampled dataset. (d) First, GRAPPA is used as in method (b), but the remaining aliasing is resolved with SENSE and not with GRAPPA. (e) A $2\times$ subsampled PatLoc dataset is reconstructed using the Cartesian PatLoc image space method. (f) First, standard GRAPPA is applied to the subsampled PatLoc dataset using additional calibration lines. In a second step, the remaining aliasing is reconstructed using the Cartesian PatLoc image space method. Observe the similarity of approaches (c,e) as well as (d,f).

GRAPPA image reconstruction was done according to chapter 2.3.2a, page 97f.

Matlab (The Mathworks Inc., Natick, MA, USA) was used to program the algorithms and to perform simulations. Two densely sampled 256×256 datasets, one for linear SEM encoding, the other for quadrupolar SEM encoding, were generated using a Shepp-Logan head phantom and RF-coil sensitivities mimicking an eight-channel real world coil array. White noise was added to the coil data. Subsampled data were simulated by extracting every fourth k-space line of the linear data and every second line of the PatLoc data. For the linear dataset, 32 densely sampled, and 16 subsampled calibration lines were taken for $2\times$ and $4\times$ GRAPPA reconstruction. For the PatLoc dataset, 16 calibration lines were used. GRAPPA was based on a 7×2-kernel to reduce subsampling by a factor of 2 as well as 4. The data were reconstructed with the algorithms illustrated in Fig. 5.17.

In vivo imaging data from the head of a volunteer were acquired with the human system presented in detail in chapter 3.3.3, page 126ff. A fourfold subsampled 256×64 dataset with 32 ACS-lines was measured with the linear gradients, and a twofold undersampled 256×128 dataset with 16 ACS-lines was acquired with the PatLoc coil. The data were then reconstructed using the algorithms shown in Fig. 5.17.

Results   Fig. 5.18 shows simulation results as well as experimental data; depicted are reconstructed images that were encoded with the standard linear SEMs. Two $4\times$ subsampled k-space datasets served as input data for the four algorithms illustrated in Fig. 5.17a-d. The presented images verify that it is indeed possible to use subsampled calibration data to partially unfold the image in a first step. In a second step, the remaining aliasing is well resolved using SENSE, or, with additional ACS-lines, using GRAPPA a second time. Comparison with the images reconstructed using SENSE and standard GRAPPA demonstrates that the two algorithms which assume subsampled calibration data lead to very similar results. Close inspection shows that the two-step approaches seem to yield images with less artifacts, especially compared to pure SENSE reconstruction (see figure caption for more details). It is a counterintuitive result that, at least for the simulated data, the two-step GRAPPA reconstruction yields images with less noise than the one-step GRAPPA reconstruction. This aspect should be further explored in the future.

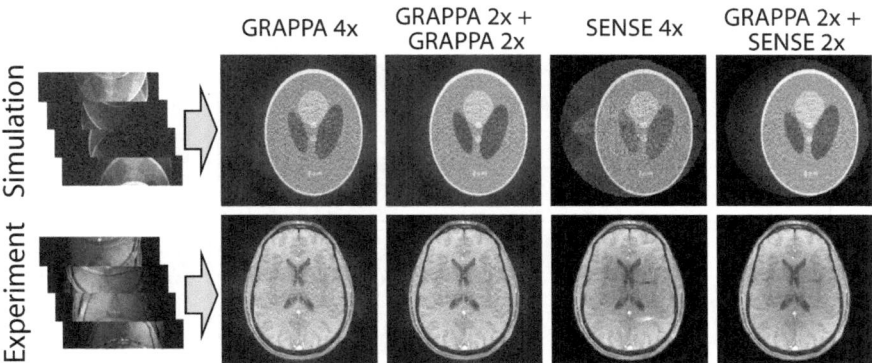

Figure 5.18: Reconstruction results for conventional PI. One simulated, and one measured, subsampled dataset is reconstructed with the four algorithms that are illustrated in Fig. 5.17a-d. All algorithms lead to similar results. Some differences are visible concerning residual aliasing and SNR. The worst result concerning both artifacts yields $4\times$ SENSE reconstruction, where the artifacts have sharp boundaries (also cf. Fig. 2.14b, page 85). In the numerical simulations, the one-step GRAPPA reconstruction seems to be a little bit worse concerning SNR with respect to the two-step reconstructions. Such a difference is not visible in the measured data. No significant differences are to be seen between both two-step reconstructions.

Based on this result and the analogy to PatLoc imaging, established above, it is to be expected that GRAPPA effectively resolves the fold-over artifact also for a subsampled PatLoc dataset. This is confirmed by Fig. 5.19. The reconstruction is then finalized using the PatLoc image space method. The reconstruction results are compared to pure image space reconstruction in Fig. 5.19. Differences can hardly be seen. Though less prominent, but in conformity with linear encoding (Fig. 5.18), image quality seems to be slightly improved with the two-step approach.

5.2.3 Discussion

It has been shown above that aliasing cannot be removed completely in Pat-Loc by applying GRAPPA without any modification. However, it has been demonstrated that it is possible to use GRAPPA for partial unfolding. Theoretically, this has been proven by referring to an analogy to conventional PI.

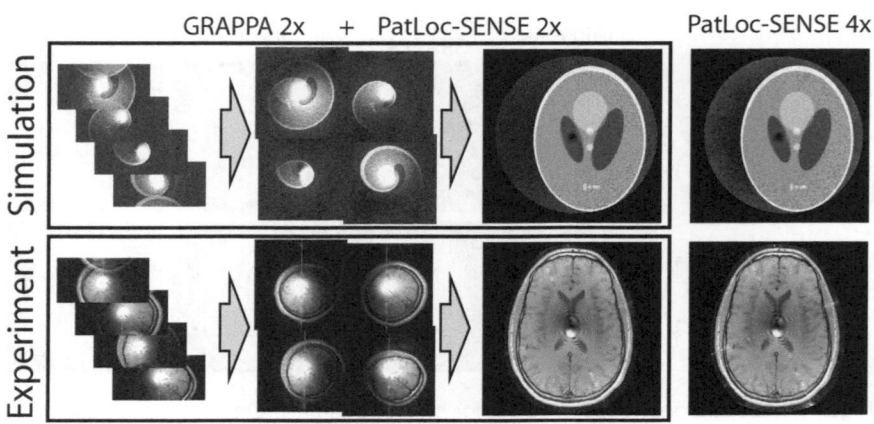

Figure 5.19: Reconstruction results for PatLoc-encoded images. For a simulated and a measured dataset, pure image space reconstruction is compared to partial GRAPPA reconstruction in combination with finalizing image space reconstruction (cf. Fig. 5.17e,f). The two-step reconstruction seems to yields slightly better results than the one-step approach. The data were not filtered; therefore, a pronounced streaking artifact is visible (cf. Fig. 5.9, page 183).

The k-space analysis has clarified that, physically, there is a fundamental difference, whether aliasing is caused by field ambiguities or by subsampling. The two artifacts can be separated from each other with GRAPPA, and it has been demonstrated that this property is essential for k-space based PatLoc image reconstruction because only the latter can actually be unfolded with GRAPPA. Interestingly, this is different with SENSE. For SENSE, both aliasing artifacts are equivalent and cannot be differentiated. Interestingly, with SENSE, partial unfolding is not possible at all: The two different kinds of aliasing artifacts must be unfolded simultaneously involving the inversion of a single combined sensitivity matrix.

The theoretical analysis of k-space based PatLoc reconstruction could also be verified with numerical simulations and in vivo measurement results. The findings have shown that the reconstructions are very similar, be they purely image space based or k-space/image-space hybrids. The hybrid k-space/image-space reconstruction seems to slightly outperform pure image space reconstruction, mainly because the partial usage of GRAPPA avoids sharp artifact boundaries that are a typical feature of pure image space reconstructions like SENSE or PatLoc-SENSE (cf. for example Fig.

5.12a-d). However, also the overall artifact power seems to be reduced in conformity with GRAPPA theory (see chapter 2.3.2, page 96ff). Overall, it can be concluded that a hybrid GRAPPA-SENSE-like reconstruction can compete with, if not even excel, pure image space reconstruction in terms of image quality.

Especially interesting is such a hybrid k-space/image-space method for accelerated non-Cartesian acquisition trajectories, where direct image space reconstruction is often problematic (dense encoding matrix, cf. e.g. chapter 2.2.2a, page 67f; artifacts, cf. e.g. Fig. 6.9b, page 227); therefore, iterative reconstruction is often used instead (see chapter 7, page 235ff). In k-space, a GRAPPA-variant, pseudo-Cartesian GRAPPA [165], has shown to be useful in the context of conventional PI. This method or variations thereof should also be applicable to subsampled non-Cartesian PatLoc trajectories and would allow non-iterative image reconstruction in combination with the Cartesian PatLoc image space method. Assessment of such a reconstruction is still work in progress.

A hybrid k-space/image-space method still requires a separate scan for the acquisition of RF-sensitivity profiles. It can be useful to purely rely on calibration data (cf. chapter 2.3.2, page 96ff.). Calibration data can, however, only be acquired in PatLoc k-space, and are therefore not available to unfold the aliasing resulting from the non-bijectiveness of the SEMs. Complete unfolding would require "virtual" k-space calibration data belonging to the completely unfolded image; such a k-space has been found to exist not physically, but only "virtually" (cf. Fig. 5.14g), thus preventing acquisition of adequate calibration data.

However, if it would be possible to give the virtual k-space a physical background, purely k-space based reconstruction should be feasible. One possibility is to use a separate low-resolution scan with the standard gradient system to synthesize adequate calibration data. However, such a scan would be similar to the additional RF-sensitivity scan required for the hybrid method, and not much would be gained. It is probably more useful to supplement non-bijective SEM encoding with RF-transmit encoding such that acquisition of calibration lines in the virtual k-space becomes possible. The feasibility of such an approach is also part of ongoing research.

5.2.4   Conclusions

In the second part of this chapter, it could be shown that a k-space oriented reconstruction of PatLoc imaging data forms a valuable alternative to the Cartesian image space method, which has been the topic of the first part. The above analysis has revealed fundamental differences between the image space SENSE-like reconstruction and the k-space based reconstruction involving GRAPPA. Whereas in image space, the nonlinearities of the PatLoc-SEMs necessitate modifications to SENSE reconstruction, in k-space, no modifications are required to the GRAPPA algorithm. This is different with respect to the non-bijectiveness of the SEMs. Image-space reconstruction can cope with subsampling as well as non-bijective encoding alike; on the other hand, pure k-space reconstruction can only handle subsampling and must be supplemented with the Cartesian PatLoc image-space method to resolve the remaining aliasing. Non-bijective PatLoc encoding is problematic in k-space because calibration data cannot readily be acquired. Initial ideas were presented how this problem can be circumvented in k-space; however, more research has to be performed to substantiate those ideas and algorithms have to be implemented to verify the effectiveness of the proposed methods.

Chapter 6

Direct Reconstruction for Radial PatLoc Imaging

THE previous chapter has shown that the fundamental character of Cartesian acquisition trajectories is preserved when moving from linear to nonlinear and non-bijective encoding. Also non-Cartesian trajectories play an important role in standard MRI; of particular interest is radial imaging (cf. chapter 2.2.2, page 66ff). In the present chapter, such radial acquisitions are analyzed in the context of PatLoc imaging. This chapter is based on work published in [[157, 158]].

The examination is facilitated by the fact that PatLoc imaging with two SEMs and standard accelerated PI were found to be analogous in the last chapter. Therefore, most principles that govern PI are also valid in PatLoc imaging. Recall, however, that the analogy requires that the magnetization is represented in PatLoc encoding space. This space is interesting because it allows separation of trajectory-dependent effects from those that are caused by the nonlinearities of the SEMs: First, consider that the PatLoc encoding space is the Fourier space of the PatLoc k-space; such a Fourier relation also exists in standard imaging, and therefore many similarities and differences between conventional radial and Cartesian imaging have an analogous counterpart in PatLoc imaging. Second, consider that in PatLoc encoding space the magnetization is intensity-modulated and distorted, and these effects are caused solely by the nonlinearities of the SEMs. It is clear that these arguments are not, by themselves, sufficient to derive exact quantitative results; however, some interesting aspects can already be noted:

- Radial sequences can show a high tolerance to undersampling in situations with high imaging contrast and have inherent self-navigating properties, resulting from oversampling of the k-space center (cf. e.g. [10], page 899). These advantages are primarily related to the manner of how k-space is traversed; these and other trajectory-related properties make radial imaging useful for medical imaging also in the context of PatLoc imaging.

- In conventional MRI, image contrast is the same for Cartesian and radial trajectories as long as equal sequence parameters like T_E, T_R or flip angle are used. With these parameters, the same image contrast also results in PatLoc imaging, whether PatLoc k-space is traversed on a Cartesian grid or following a radial pattern.

- In standard PI, image resolution is mainly determined by the extent of k-space. The particular type of k-space traversal only has secondary effects like deviations in Gibbs ringing or aliasing behavior. Thus, the particular sampling pattern of PatLoc k-space should not have a significant effect on image resolution. Spatial variations of image resolution from radially encoded PatLoc data should be similar to Cartesian data and are therefore mainly defined by the gradients of the SEMs; problems can be expected in regions, where the gradients vanish.

These aspects are in principle valid for any reconstruction method from radial acquisitions. However, an exact quantitative analysis of image properties is possible only for a concrete image reconstruction algorithm. A fast and easy-to-interpret direct reconstruction method for radial acquisition schemes is developed and investigated in this chapter.

The basic observation is that, whereas in conventional imaging a projection is taken along one straight line, in PatLoc imaging projections are also taken along two or more curved lines. Standard back-projection of the data can therefore not directly result in a reconstructed image, but this observation is useful for the development of efficient reconstruction algorithms. The iterative reconstruction methods presented later in chapter 7.1.1 to 7.1.3, page 237ff, may be used to solve the problem. Under certain circumstances, for example for undersampled datasets, iterative methods are indeed the methods of choice. Iterative methods can be used to significantly reduce a prominent star-shaped artifact that is a particular feature of radial PatLoc imaging with quadrupolar SEMs. However, such iterative approaches are more computation-intensive and other problems are associated with them (more details are found in the next chapter, page 235ff). These problems are avoided here with a direct reconstruction method.

It is shown that the direct Cartesian algorithm, presented and thoroughly analyzed above, can be incorporated into the reconstruction from radially acquired data by first performing standard reconstruction from projection data before applying the Cartesian PatLoc reconstruction algorithm. In view of the special designs of the realized PatLoc hardware (cf. chapter 3.3, page 121ff), the present chapter focuses again on a set of two orthogonal multipolar SEMs. It is demonstrated that for such fields, the reconstruction is simpler and more elegant in a polar coordinate representation. The resulting image properties are compared to Cartesian PatLoc acquisitions. Then, the polar algorithm and its properties are verified and evaluated with simulated and in vivo imaging data. One interesting result is that the isotropy of the radial PSF leads to a significantly reduced Gibbs ringing artifact at the imaging center compared to Cartesian encoding. At the end of this chapter a few remarks are given concerning generalizations of radial PatLoc imaging including arbitrary non-Cartesian trajectories and generalized projections.

6.1 Presentation of Image Reconstruction Methods

The reconstruction methods presented in this chapter are applicable to an imaging modality with the following two assumptions:

1. Two nonlinear and non-bijective SEMs for 2D imaging are applied.
2. Radial sampling trajectories are used.

The encoding strategy treated in this chapter is therefore similar to the imaging situation that is discussed in the previous chapter. However, not a Cartesian trajectory, but a radial trajectory is assumed for image acquisition.

The Cartesian image space method turned out to be an efficient implementation of the general weak matrix approach, which is presented in chapter 4.2.2, page 144ff. Both, the strong as well as the weak matrix approach can in principle be used for image reconstruction also when the image is encoded with a radial trajectory. In radial Fourier imaging, it was shown that the matrix approaches were not practical because the encoding matrix is dense in that case (see chapter 2.2.2a, page 67f); it can be shown that the same problem hinders direct application of the general matrix approaches also in the context of radial PatLoc imaging. An alternative represents radial GRAPPA [48] in combination with the Cartesian image space reconstruction method (see chapter 5.2,page 195ff).

In this chapter, a different approach is taken that has been shown to be effective also for Cartesian trajectories (cf. chapter 5.1.1c, page 163ff). An efficient image reconstruction method is developed by directly analyzing the signal equation. Based on this signal equation, a reconstruction is formulated that can be applied to arbitrary SEMs. Then, an efficient algorithm for multipolar SEMs is developed and analyzed in detail.

Recall that for Cartesian trajectories, this approach, based on the analysis of the signal equation, has turned out to yield the same reconstruction as the weak matrix approach. For non-Cartesian trajectories, this is different. It was demonstrated in paragraph *Relationship to Direct Matrix Inversion* in chapter 2.2.3, page 71f, that gridding reconstruction in conventional non-Cartesian imaging is a useful and efficient approximation of the strong matrix approach. It is left to the interested reader to show that the reconstructions presented below for radial PatLoc imaging are also closely related to the general matrix approaches.

6.1.1 Signal Equation in Radial PatLoc Imaging

In compliance with the previous chapter, also here, 2D imaging with two NB-SEMs is assumed. Therefore, the PatLoc signal equation has the same continuous form (cf. Eq. 5.9, page 163):

$$s_\alpha(\vec{k}) = \int_V m(\vec{x}) c_\alpha(\vec{x}) e^{-i\vec{k}\vec{\psi}(\vec{x})} \, d\vec{x}. \tag{6.1}$$

The explicit form of the phase factor $\vec{k}\vec{\psi}(\vec{x})$ is given by $k_1\psi_1(\vec{x}) + k_2\psi_2(\vec{x})$. Recall that, except for a scaling factor, the two components of $\vec{\psi}$ are equivalent to the SEM sensitivities (cf. Eq. 4.6, page 138). The PatLoc signal equation as described by Eq. 6.1 generalizes the signal equation known from standard radial imaging. In conventional radial imaging, $\psi_1(\vec{x}) \propto x$ and $\psi_2(\vec{x}) \propto y$. In PatLoc, $\psi_{1,2}$ take different shapes, depending on the architecture of the SEM system.

6.1.2 Interpretation of PatLoc Projection Data

In conventional radial acquisition, the inverse one-dimensional Fourier transform of the signal projections (= readouts) are projections of the magnetization taken at different angles (also cf. Fig. 2.7, page 68). This is a direct consequence of the projection-slice theorem. However, with arbitrary encoding fields, the situation is more complicated and the question arises how the signal projections can then be interpreted. This question can be answered by looking at the effective encoding field ψ_{res} during readout:

$$\psi_{res}(\vec{x}; \Theta_j) = \cos(\Theta_j)\psi_1(\vec{x}) + \sin(\Theta_j)\psi_2(\vec{x}). \tag{6.2}$$

It consists of a superposition of the two individual SEMs (Fig. 6.1). These SEMs are differently mixed for each projection angle Θ_j, $j = 1, \ldots, N_p$. Signal projections $s_\alpha(k, \Theta_j)$ are typically acquired with the N_p projection angles equidistantly distributed in the interval $[0°, 180°]$.

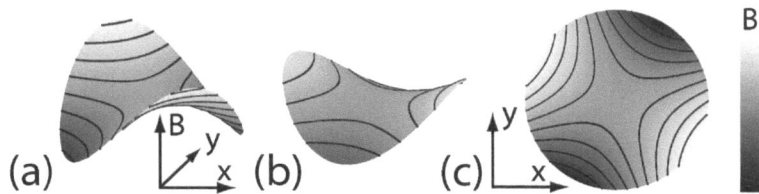

Figure 6.1: Radial encoding with orthogonal quadrupolar SEMs. (a) and (b) The two orthogonal encoding fields are rotated against each other by $45°$. The field strength of the individual SEMs depends on the projection angle. Higher magnetic field strength is indicated by brighter grayscale and extension along the vertical axis. (c) The effective encoding field is a superposition of the SEMs. The resulting field shares the quadrupolar geometry of the two individual SEMs.

If linear gradient fields are used for encoding, the effective encoding field is also linear. This linear field rotates incrementally from one projection to the next. This geometrical similarity property of the effective encoding field does not hold for the general case of arbitrary SEMs. However, it is preserved if quadrupolar (or multipolar) encoding fields are used (cf. Fig. 6.1c) with the property that a field rotation of $90°$ - instead of $180°$ for the standard case - is sufficient to cover all necessary projection angles. From Eq. 6.1

it can be deduced that the projections $P_\alpha(p, \Theta_j) = \mathcal{FT}_k^{-1}\{s_\alpha(k, \Theta_j)\}(p, \Theta_j)$ are given by:

$$P_\alpha(p, \Theta_j) = \int_V m(\vec{x}) c_\alpha(\vec{x}) \delta\left(p - \psi_{res}(\vec{x}; \Theta_j)\right) d\vec{x}. \tag{6.3}$$

As ψ_{res} is proportional to the magnetic field strength, the projections are taken along isocontour lines of the encoding field applied during the acquisition.

The presentation of the previous chapter has shown that the variable transformation $\vec{u} := \vec{\psi}(\vec{x})$ simplifies the mathematical treatment of the *Cartesian* reconstruction problem. The reason for this fact is that, with $U := \vec{\psi}(V)$, the signal data

$$s_\alpha(\vec{k}) = \int_U \eta_\alpha(\vec{u}) e^{-i\vec{k}\vec{u}} d\vec{u} \tag{6.4}$$

and $\eta_\alpha(\vec{u})$ form a Fourier transform pair. As shown in the previous chapter, the coil images $\eta_\alpha(\vec{u})$ represent highly distorted, intensity modulated and aliased versions of the true image. Because of the Fourier pair property the coil images are given by:

$$\eta_\alpha(\vec{u}) = \int_U s_\alpha(\vec{k}) e^{i\vec{u}\vec{k}} d\vec{k}. \tag{6.5}$$

According to Eqs. 6.4, 6.5, the variable transformation $\vec{u} := \vec{\psi}(\vec{x})$ also leads to a different interpretation of the PatLoc projection data: In the distorted coordinate system, represented by $\vec{u}$, projections are formed by just taking ordinary projections of $\eta_\alpha(\vec{u})$ in the same way as image projections are taken in conventional imaging. The theoretical justification lies in the application of the projection-slice theorem, which is equivalent to formulating Eq. 6.3 in $\vec{u}$-coordinates:

$$P_\alpha(p, \Theta_j) = \int_U \eta_\alpha(\vec{u}) \delta\left(p - \cos(\Theta_j) u_1 + \sin(\Theta_j) u_2\right) d\vec{u}. \tag{6.6}$$

The practical justification, however, lies in the fact that in the distorted coordinate system, the encoding fields are linear fields - like the gradient fields in conventional imaging - as can be seen from the latter equation. In this space representation not the geometry of the encoding field, but rather the object itself is distorted. Moreover, the effective linear field shows exactly the same behavior as the encoding field in standard radial imaging.

In this regard, PatLoc imaging and standard imaging are equivalent. The meaning of "image" projections in the context of PatLoc SEMs is illustrated in Fig. 6.2a-c.

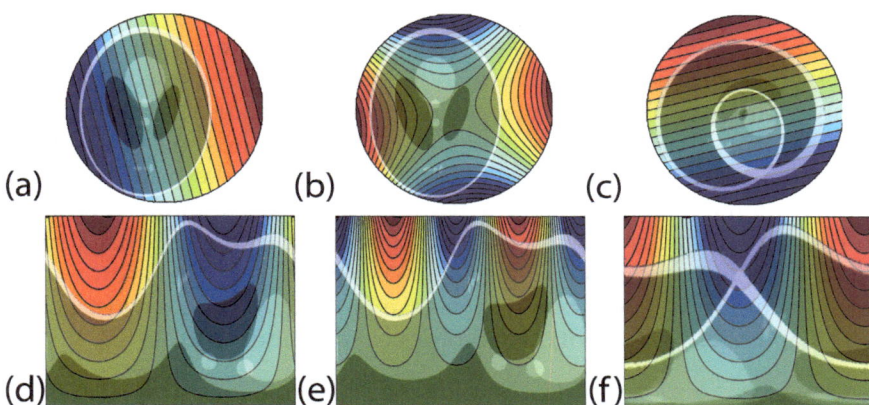

Figure 6.2: Analysis of a single projection with linear and quadrupolar encoding. (a) For linear gradient fields a projection is found by integrating along straight isocontour lines parallel to each other. (b) For quadrupolar encoding fields, the isocontour lines along which the projections are taken are bent and occur on two distinct positions on opposite sides of the image. (c) In PatLoc encoding space, the magnetization overlaps with itself and is heavily distorted. The magnetic field, however, forms equidistant and straight isocontour lines equivalent to linear gradient fields. (d) The linear gradient field is represented in polar coordinates along with the encoded object. (e) In polar coordinates, the quadrupolar encoding field has a similar shape, however, distorted in the radial direction and with four sign changes along the azimuthal direction. (f) The transformation to PatLoc encoding space is simpler than in the Cartesian representation. Quadratic stretching along the radial direction and linear stretching along the azimuthal direction can be observed.

6.1.3   Reconstruction from Projection Data with Arbitrary Encoding Fields

The variable transformation $\vec{u} := \vec{\psi}(\vec{x})$ also offers a profound basis for formulating adequate direct reconstruction methods in radial PatLoc imaging. For Cartesian acquisitions, $\eta_\alpha(\vec{u})$ is found by the inverse 2D-FFT of the acquired signal data. For radial acquisitions, as a result of the variable transformation to $\vec{u}$, the reconstruction can be realized equivalently to conventional reconstruction from projection data using linear gradient fields: According to Eq. 6.6, conventional reconstruction from radial data results in $\eta_\alpha(\vec{u})$ on a Cartesian grid. Thus, the image can be reconstructed by applying the Cartesian PatLoc Reconstruction algorithm to $\eta_\alpha(\vec{u})$.

Filtered back-projection (FBP) (cf. chapter 2.2.2b, page 68f) may be used to determine $\eta_\alpha(\vec{u})$. With multipolar SEMs it is recommended to use the more accurate cubic spline interpolation method because the faster linear interpolation can result in small intensity variations across the image. Even better image quality might be achieved by using more elaborate back-projection methods [122, 180], which typically require more computing time. The FBP approach along with subsequent Cartesian image space PatLoc reconstruction corresponds to the reconstruction steps shown at the top part of Fig. 6.3. Alternatively, instead of FBP, gridding reconstruction (cf. chapter 2.2.3, page 69ff) may be employed to find $\eta_\alpha(\vec{u})$.

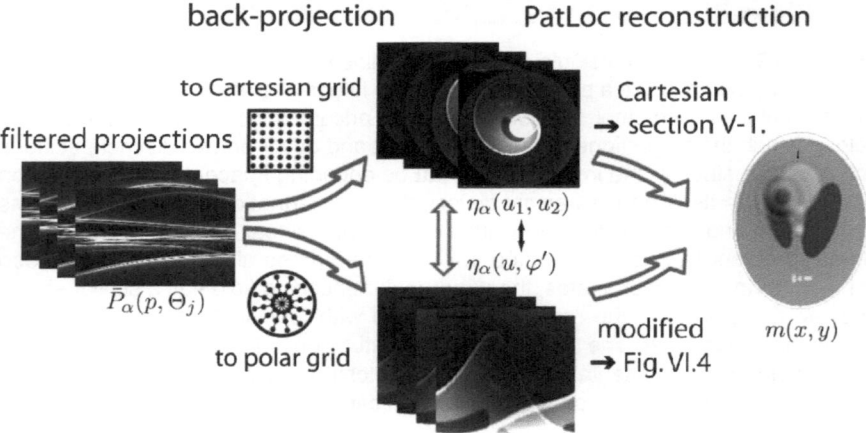

Figure 6.3: Reconstruction algorithms for 2D PatLoc with radial acquisition schemes. Upper path: Standard FBP can be combined with the Cartesian PatLoc reconstruction algorithm. Lower path: If the back-projection is not performed onto a Cartesian grid, but onto a polar grid, the Cartesian reconstruction algorithm must be modified (cf. Fig. 6.4). The images back-projected onto different grids are linked to each other by a simple coordinate transformation from Cartesian to polar coordinates. The images shown are based on simulations. The images are accompanied with nomenclature as used in the text body.

6.1.4 Reconstruction from Projection Data with Multipolar Encoding Fields

The situation is particularly interesting when orthogonal multipolar SEMs are used for encoding because this allows one to simplify image reconstruction. An efficient algorithm is discussed in this section.

a) Reconstruction Algorithm

Multipolar SEMs are best described in polar coordinates. With adequate scaling, they are represented by $\psi_1(r, \varphi) = r^L \cos(L\varphi)$ and $\psi_2(r, \varphi) = r^L \sin(L\varphi)$, see Eq. 5.15, page 165. Consider quadrupolar fields with $L = 2$; the calculations shown in this section can be generalized to SEMs with different multipolarity L in a straightforward manner. The polar coordinate representation of the combined encoding function is given by:

$$\vec{\psi}_0(r, \varphi) = \begin{pmatrix} \psi_1(r, \varphi) \\ \psi_2(r, \varphi) \end{pmatrix} = r^2 \begin{pmatrix} \cos(2\varphi) \\ \sin(2\varphi) \end{pmatrix}. \tag{6.7}$$

This representation better reveals the symmetry of the fields than the Cartesian analogue, where

$$\vec{\psi}_0(x, y) = \begin{pmatrix} \psi_1(x, y) \\ \psi_2(x, y) \end{pmatrix} = \begin{pmatrix} x^2 - y^2 \\ 2xy \end{pmatrix}. \tag{6.8}$$

Note the multiplicative separability of the two variables r and φ. In the polar representation, linear and quadrupolar fields are very similar (Fig. 6.2d-f). This is different for Cartesian coordinates, where the transformation from image space coordinates to PatLoc encoding space coordinates is not obvious (Fig. 6.2a-c). Expressed in polar coordinates, the signal projections for quadrupolar fields take the following concrete form:

$$s_\alpha(k, \Theta_j) = \int_{r=0}^{\infty} \int_{\varphi=0}^{2\pi} r m(r, \varphi) c_\alpha(r, \varphi) e^{-ikr^2 \cos(\Theta_j - 2\varphi)} \, dr \, d\varphi. \tag{6.9}$$

The expression can be derived from Eq. 6.1 using addition theorems for trigonometric functions. Substituting $u = r^2$ and $\varphi' = 2\varphi$ gives:

$$s_\alpha(k, \Theta_j) = \int_{u=0}^{\infty} \int_{\varphi'=0}^{4\pi} m(u, \varphi'/2) c_\alpha(u, \varphi'/2) e^{-iku \cos(\Theta_j - \varphi')} \, du \, d\varphi'. \tag{6.10}$$

In the variable φ' two rotations must be evaluated; it is, however, possible to evaluate both rotations at the same time:

$$s_\alpha(k, \Theta_j) = \int_{u=0}^{\infty} \int_{\varphi'=0}^{2\pi} u\eta_\alpha(u, \varphi')e^{-iku\cos(\Theta_j - \varphi')} \, \mathrm{d}u \, \mathrm{d}\varphi', \qquad (6.11)$$

with

$$\eta_\alpha(u, \varphi') = \frac{1}{u}\left[m(u, \varphi'/2)c_\alpha(u, \varphi'/2) + m(u, \varphi'/2 + \pi)c_\alpha(u, \varphi'/2 + \pi)\right]. \qquad (6.12)$$

Equation 6.11 is equivalent to the standard formula, expressed in polar coordinates, known from conventional radial imaging. η_α is the same as presented in Eq. 6.5, where (u_1, u_2) has been replaced by its polar coordinate representation (u, φ'). In this case, it is advantageous to alter the back-projection step. Normally, the projections are back-projected onto a Cartesian grid Σ_{cart} (cf. chapter 2.2.2b, page 68f). Instead of using this Cartesian grid, a polar back-projection grid $(u, \varphi') \in \Sigma_{polar}$ can be chosen. If the same number of grid points is chosen, there is no influence on the reconstruction time and the implementation of the back-projection is done equivalently to back-projecting onto a Cartesian grid. The only difference is that the back-projected data are directly represented in a different coordinate system. According to Eq. 6.12, and using the fact that $\varphi = \varphi'/2$, $\varphi \in [0, \pi]$, one therefore finds:

$$m(u, \varphi)c_\alpha(u, \varphi) + m(u, \varphi + \pi)c_\alpha(u, \varphi + \pi) = u\sum_{j=1}^{N_p} B(\bar{P}_\alpha(\cdot, \Theta_j))(u, \varphi)\Delta\Theta. \qquad (6.13)$$

In this polar representation, PatLoc reconstruction is particularly simple. The left hand side of the latter equation is just the Cartesian SENSE equation (cf. Ref. [135] or Eq. 5.14, page 165) with acceleration along the φ-direction. Apart from the final transformation from polar coordinates to Cartesian coordinates, image intensity and distortion need to be corrected only along the direction of the u variable. In Fig. 6.3 the two different back-projection methods are shown together with their mutual relationship. Based on Eq. 6.13, Fig. 6.4 presents each step of the algorithm that is termed *direct polar reconstruction* in this chapter.

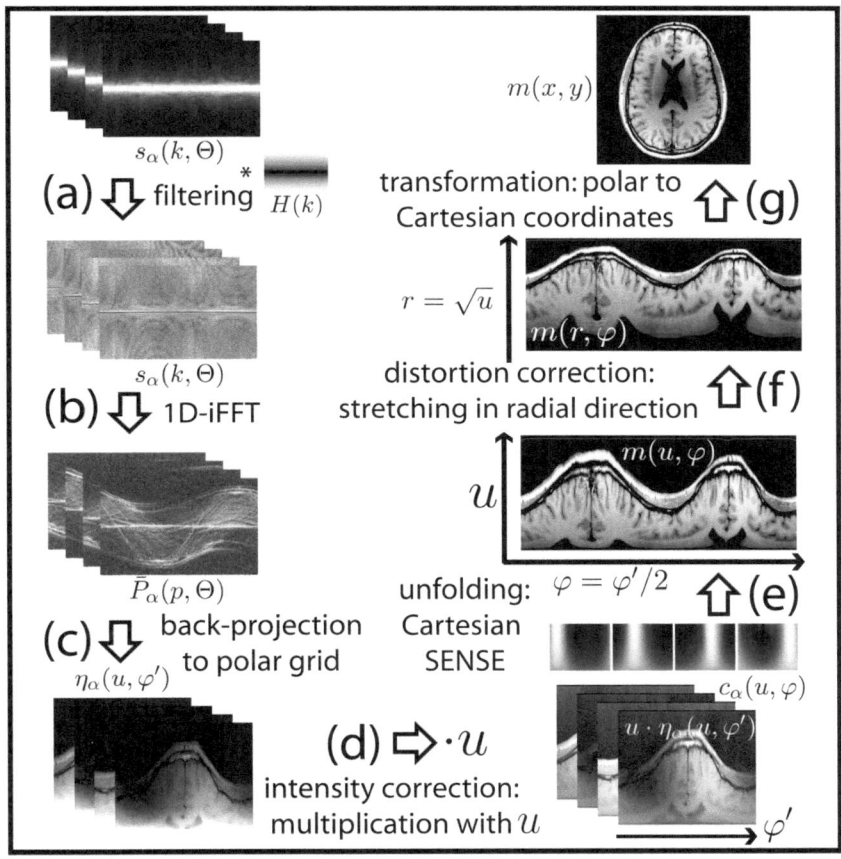

Figure 6.4: Proposed direct reconstruction algorithm for radial PatLoc data encoded with quadrupolar SEMs. (a) First, for each coil, the radially acquired signal projection data are filtered. (b) Then, an inverse 1D-FFT is applied to each signal projection. (c) The resulting filtered projections are back-projected onto a polar grid. (d) The different coil images are intensity-corrected by multiplication with a linear intensity ramp. (e) The Cartesian SENSE algorithm is applied with the azimuthal direction corresponding to the accelerated direction. To this end, the RF-coil sensitivity information is represented in the same space as the coil data by describing the sensitivity profiles in polar coordinates and quadratically stretching them in the radial direction. (f) The distortions are undone by reversing the quadratic stretching of the image in the radial direction. (g) Finally, the image is again represented in Cartesian coordinates. Note the similarity to the algorithm shown in Fig. 5.3, page 163, applicable to Cartesian trajectories.

b) Image Properties

Image resolution and SNR resulting from reconstruction with the algorithm that is described in the previous section are discussed here. More details are found in [[158]].

Image Resolution In the introduction to this chapter it has already been argued that radial PatLoc acquisitions should yield a distribution of spatial resolution similar to Cartesian acquisitions. This claim can be substantiated through a precise analysis of the polar reconstruction algorithm. As shown in Fig. 6.3, the reconstruction can be decomposed into two steps: First, the image is back-projected and second, the aliased images are unfolded. The equivalence of the second step to the Cartesian algorithm of the previous chapter shows that differences may occur only as a result of the first step, where the FBP is applied instead of the DFT. However, both operations lead to homogeneous resolution patterns; the conclusion can be drawn that image resolution is indeed the same for radial and Cartesian sampling with a resolution gradient that is proportional to r^{1-L}, where L is the multipolarity of the encoding fields. Differences occur, however, in the sidelobe behavior of the PSF because the FBP and the DFT have different properties in this regard.

Signal-to-Noise Ratio Also the SNR that results from Cartesian and polar reconstruction is expected to have the same spatial distribution because both, FBP and FFT, lead to a uniform noise distribution which is altered in the same way by the subsequent reconstruction steps. Analogous to Cartesian sampling (cf. Eq. 5.28), the SNR is given by:

$$\mathrm{SNR}^{PatLoc} = \mathrm{SNR}^{linear} r^{2-2L} \Big/ \sqrt{L}g, \tag{6.14}$$

where g describes the g-factor and SNR^{linear} the SNR that results from FBP applied to a standard radial dataset.

6.2 Application to Simulated and Measured Imaging Data

The image reconstruction methods of the previous section were implemented, imaging data were generated and reconstructed. The first part of this section (Methods) gives more details on how these steps were performed and the second part (Results) gives an overview of the most important findings.

6.2.1 Methods

Numerical simulations as well as in vivo measurements were performed to verify the properties of a particular implementation of the polar reconstruction algorithm. Below, a special emphasis is placed on the determination of the SEMs and their approximation by exactly orthogonal quadrupolar fields, the geometry that is assumed by the polar reconstruction algorithm.

a) Simulations

Image resolution and SNR analysis was performed with Matlab (The MathWorks Inc., Natick, MA, USA). The spatial resolution of the reconstructed images was analyzed with PSF-plots. The PSF analysis was performed in three steps: First, the signal (Eq. 6.1) was evaluated at predefined locations. Then, the evaluated signals were reconstructed and finally visualized with a surface plot. In particular, the evaluation of the signal equation requires RF-coil sensitivity profiles, SEMs and the k-space trajectory. The RF-coil sensitivity profiles were designed to mimic an eight-channel receiver coil whose elements were positioned symmetrically around the object. Orthogonal quadrupolar SEMs were chosen according to Eq. 6.8. A Cartesian (64 phase-encodes) and a radial (103 projections) trajectory with 64 readout samples were generated, where the k-space sampling distance Δk was selected such that the (centered) field-of-view (FOV) of the projections coincided with the (centered) FOVs of the coil sensitivity profiles and the SEMs. According to Eqs. 5.19, 5.26, this is ensured when:

$$1/\Delta k = 2 \cdot \|\vec{\psi}_0(\vec{x}_{edge})\| = 2 \cdot \|\vec{x}_{edge}\|^2, \qquad (6.15)$$

where $\vec{x}_{edge}$ is a location at the edge of the FOV. The factor 2 takes into account that the SEMs have positive as well as negative field strengths. The Cartesian dataset was reconstructed with the Cartesian PatLoc method and the radial dataset was reconstructed with the direct polar method.

SNR was investigated by simulating the noise propagation properties of the direct polar reconstruction algorithm. For the analysis, 100 images were reconstructed from assumed white Gaussian noise in the RF channels and then the images were averaged. Further investigations were performed by comparing the resulting noise distribution with the noise generated by standard FBP and the Cartesian method.

b) Experiments

In vivo measurements of a volunteer were performed on a MAGNETOM Trio, A Tim System 3T (Siemens Healthcare, Erlangen, Germany). The scanner was equipped with a modified encoding hardware for head imaging using quadrupolar PatLoc coils. The PatLoc hardware and its integration into the scanner environment is described in detail in chapter 3.3.3, page 126ff.

For reception, a conventional eight-channel head RF-coil array was used and sensitivity data were acquired and processed with standard methods, explained in chapter 2.1.2b, page 48f. The quadrupolar SEM-profiles were mapped with an improved variation of the protocol that was used to determine the SEMs of the smaller PatLoc prototype coil (see chapter 5.1.2c, page 178ff). For the in vivo experiments, a more flexible hardware configuration permitted simultaneous switching of linear and PatLoc SEM gradient pulses (cf. Fig. 3.18c, page 129). In the new SEM-mapping pulse sequence, a spoiled gradient echo was played out with 8 echoes acquired each TR. The first four echoes were used to map the heterogeneity of the static B_0 field. Between each of the last four echoes, a SEM-gradient pulse with predefined current and duration was applied to induce a small phase accumulation between each echo. With the B_0 field determined, the phase accumulation caused by the SEMs was calculated and the SEM profiles were derived.

Spin echo images were acquired with a radial sequence (cf. Fig. 6.5), which was programmed similar to a conventional radial sequence with the obvious difference that instead of the linear gradient coils, the quadrupolar PatLoc coils were switched during the encoding process. The projection angles

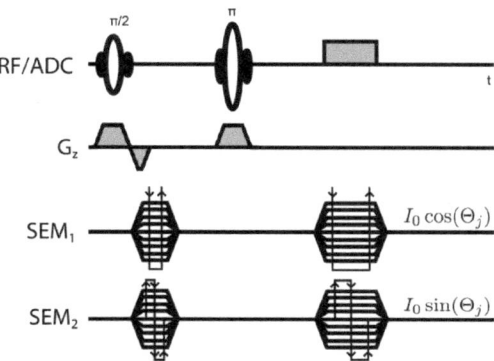

Figure 6.5: Radial measurement protocol. A radial spin echo protocol was used with the standard gradient system for reference measurements (cf. Fig. 2.6, page 66). The protocol was slightly modified for the PatLoc measurements to allow for operation of the PatLoc coils instead of the linear gradient coils. The only difference (apart from a different base current I_0) between reference and PatLoc measurements was that different encoding fields were applied resulting in images of the same contrast. The formulas on the right describe how the applied currents in the corresponding PatLoc coils changed depending on the projection angle.

were determined to cover a full circle. In order to distribute the effects of trajectory inaccuracies like switching delays of the SEMs more evenly in PatLoc k-space, alternating encoding directions were selected from one projection to the next. According to Eq. 6.15, the k-space distance was chosen to match the FOVs of acquired RF-coil profiles and PatLoc measurement data. For comparison, a Cartesian spin echo image was acquired with the same hardware as well as radial spin echo images with the standard hardware. For all measurements, the same imaging parameters of TR $= 500\,\mathrm{ms}$ and TE $= 11\,\mathrm{ms}$ were assumed. 256 phase-encodes were acquired for the Cartesian trajectory and 410 projections for the radial trajectory. Each readout comprised 256 samples. For a separate investigation, fourfold undersampling was mimicked by only retaining 64 phase-encodes and 103 projections. The direct polar algorithm and the image space Cartesian method were used to reconstruct images from the acquired datasets.

c) Reconstruction

The reconstruction algorithms require information about (a) the PatLoc measurement data (b) the RF-coil sensitivity profiles and (c) the SEMs. The data were provided as described in section 6.2.1a and 6.2.1b.

Implementation   The Cartesian PatLoc algorithm was programmed as explained in the previous chapter. The polar reconstruction algorithm is described in detail in the caption of Fig. 6.4. A standard implementation of SENSE reconstruction (cf. Ref. [135]) was used and FBP was implemented with a Ram-Lak filter [96] and cubic spline interpolation for back-projection. The distortion correction was implemented in the following way: The equidistant grid $\mathcal{I}_N = \{0, 1/(N-1), \ldots, 1\}$ was transformed to a new grid $\mathcal{J}_N = f(\mathcal{I}_N)$, where $f(u) = \sqrt{u}$ for all $u \in \mathcal{I}_N$. Then, $\mathcal{J}_N$ was regridded on the regular grid $\mathcal{I}_{2N}$ with cubic interpolation. Cubic interpolation was also used for image transformations between polar and Cartesian coordinates.

SEM Approximation for In Vivo Measurements   In order to simplify the direct polar reconstruction, the acquired SEMs were approximated by two identical ideal orthogonal quadrupolar SEMs. It was assumed that the fields could sufficiently be modeled by the standard form $\vec{\psi}_0(\vec{x})$ (see Eq. 6.7) and only a few additional parameters:

$$\vec{\psi}_m(\vec{x}) = h\vec{\psi}_0(\mathbf{R}(-\varphi_0)(\vec{x} - \vec{x}_0)). \tag{6.16}$$

The parameters describe (a) the magnetic field sensitivity h in $[T/(m^2 A)]$ (b) a field rotation φ_0 and (c) the position of the common field centers $\vec{x}_0$. The parameters were found by a least-squares fit to the measured fields. The modeled fields deviated from the measured fields nowhere more than 1.5% compared to the field strength at the edge of the FOV. The RF-coil sensitivity maps were acquired centered around $\vec{x}_0$. Therefore, $\vec{x}_0 = 0$ could be assumed in the reconstruction. The magnetic field sensitivity was $h = 1.4\,\mathrm{mT/m^2 A}$ (also cf. table 3.1, page 131) and the field rotation was $\varphi_0 = 21.95°$.

The SEMs have the interesting property that it is possible to rotate k-space instead of the SEMs because $\vec{\psi}_0(\mathbf{R}(-\varphi_0)\vec{x}) = \mathbf{R}(-2\varphi_0)\vec{\psi}_0(\vec{x})$. The characterizing properties h, φ_0 can therefore be absorbed in an effective k-space vector $\vec{k} := h\mathbf{R}(2\varphi_0)\vec{k}$ such that the effective encoding function is just the standard form $\vec{\psi}_0(\vec{x})$. The phase factor in Eq. 6.1 is then modeled by two equivalent expressions: $\phi(\vec{k}, \vec{x}) = \vec{k}\vec{\psi}_m(\vec{x}) = \vec{k}\vec{\psi}_0(\vec{x})$.

The advantage of this redefinition for the reconstruction is that images can be reconstructed exactly with the same implementation as used for the simulated datasets without having to introduce additional data rotations. In practice, $2\varphi_0$ is just formally added to the projection angles before starting the reconstruction. With the latter equation, the SEM-sensitivity parameter h can also be interpreted as a k-space scaling factor. It does not influence the back-projection. However, according to Eqs. 4.5, 4.6 and Eq. 6.15, the sensitivity scaling h influences the acquisition. With the two-layer coil structure (cf. Fig. 3.18a, page 129), the SEM sensitivities of the two PatLoc coils differed significantly from each other. This was compensated for by using slightly different coil currents for a unit step in k-space when the sequence was played out.

It is obvious that the model does not fully represent the geometry of the experimental encoding fields. The model does not consider that the individual fields are not just equivalent versions from each other rotated by $45°$. However, for the experimental setup the individual fields resembled each other to a high degree. The measured fields were rotated by $44.2°$ and the centers of the individual fields were less than one millimeter apart from each other. Small asymmetries in the coil design also lead to a finite field strength at the field centers. Compared to the field strength at the edge of the FOV the field offset was far less than 1%. The effect is almost negligible and only visible at the center of the reconstructed images, where small frequency offsets become noticeable. This effect was corrected by considering its linear influence on the phase of the acquired signals.

6.2.2 Results

In vivo reconstruction results are presented here, image resolution and SNR are analyzed, and the consequences are illustrated that are caused by subsampling image acquisitions.

a) Radial Images with Linear and Quadrupolar Fields

For better visualization, a larger version of the reconstructed image of Fig. 6.4, found with the direct polar algorithm, is depicted in Fig. 6.6b. It is

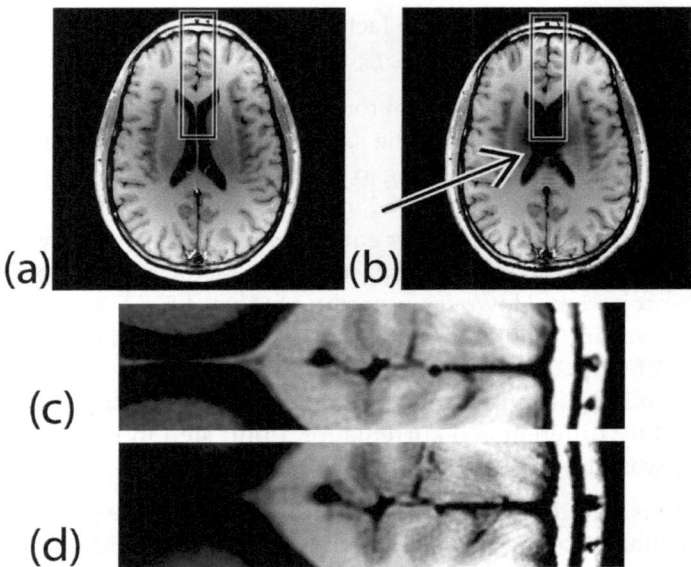

Figure 6.6: Measurement results. (a) Radial acquisition with the standard linear gradient system reconstructed with filtered back-projection. (b) Radial acquisition with the PatLoc SEM system reconstructed with the direct polar method. The images were encoded with a $90° - 180°$-spin echo sequence using TR = 500 ms, TE = 11 ms and a slice thickness of 4 mm. 410 projections were acquired with a 256-readout. (c) The zoomed section corresponds to the rectangle in plot (a). A homogeneous resolution can be appreciated. (d) The corresponding section for the PatLoc image shows a resolution gradient from the center (arrow in plot (b)) toward the periphery. From about half way on toward the periphery, the resolution is higher in the PatLoc image compared to the image acquired with linear gradients.

compared to an equivalent radial image acquired with the standard linear gradient system (Fig. 6.6a). Apart from the obvious resolution gradient toward the periphery (Fig. 6.6d), the images look very similar. In particular, no significant geometric distortions can be noted and the PatLoc reconstructed image shows no visible unfolding artifact. This is similar to the results obtained in the previous chapter with a Cartesian trajectory. Some signal relocalization is visible at the center with a nearly circularly shaped region of low intensity.

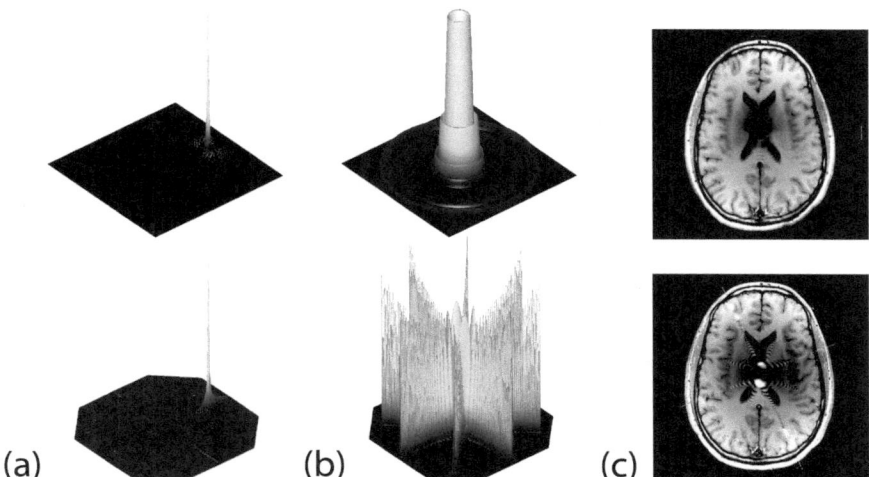

Figure 6.7: PSF analysis and Gibbs ringing. Top: Direct polar reconstruction for a radial trajectory. Bottom: Cartesian PatLoc reconstruction for a Cartesian trajectory. (a) The PSFs for a peripheral source location are well-behaved for both algorithms. (b) The PSFs for a central location are problematic and depend significantly on the chosen reconstruction method. For the Cartesian reconstruction the main peak vanishes because of the intensity correction. The polar reconstruction shows that the resolution is very low at the center compared to the peripheral PSFs. The destructive sidelobe behavior of the Cartesian method cannot be observed with direct polar reconstruction. (c) The dominant PSFs from the central locations are clearly visible in the reconstructed in vivo data as pronounced Gibbs ringing artifacts. The PSFs have lower resolution than the acquired in vivo images to show the ringing effect more clearly.

b) PSF and Noise Analysis

Fig. 6.7 presents PSFs for two different source locations and reconstructed brain images. The PSFs for the polar reconstruction method (Fig. 6.7, top row) are compared to PSFs of the direct image space Cartesian reconstruction method (Fig. 6.7, bottom row). As reported in the previous chapter, for Cartesian trajectories, the signal accumulation at the center leads to pronounced Gibbs ringing appearing as clearly defined streak artifacts (Fig. 6.7c, bottom) with origins at the center of the multipolar encoding fields separated by $45°$. For radial trajectories, the polar reconstruction method shows strongly suppressed Gibbs ringing artifacts (Fig. 6.7c, top). More details are found in the figure caption.

Fig. 6.8 presents simulation results for the noise behavior of the direct polar reconstruction method. In particular, Fig. 6.8b illustrates that Cartesian and radial PatLoc have the same SNR distribution. Fig. 6.8c shows that the theoretical predictions of Eq. 6.14 are accurate. These statements to Fig. 6.8b and c are valid apart from low radii, where differences occur because of the special implementations of the intensity and distortion correction steps. However, this difference can be ignored because of the low image information in this region.

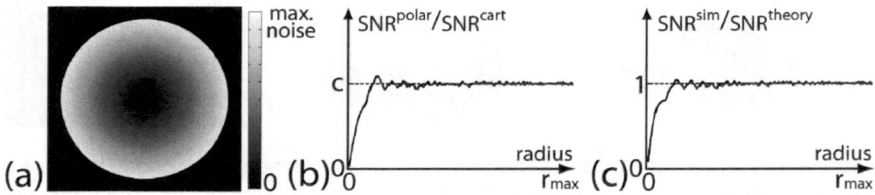

Figure 6.8: Noise propagation of the direct polar reconstruction method. (a) The noise level is very low at the center and increases toward the periphery. The plot shows that the noise distribution has an azimuthal symmetry. (b) The SNR of polar and Cartesian reconstructions are proportional except for very low radii. Shown are simulation results. The presentation of a 1D plot is sufficient because of the radial symmetry. (c) Apart from very low radii, the theoretical predictions for the SNR of the polar reconstruction match the simulated results. The oscillations are due to statistical effects and interpolation errors.

c)   Reconstruction from Undersampled Datasets

Undersampled datasets are shown in Fig. 6.9a-c. For Cartesian trajectories, fourfold undersampling leads to a characteristic fold-over behavior (also cf. Fig. 5.10d, page 185) appearing at four positions in the image (Fig. 6.9a). In contrast to standard radial imaging with linear encoding fields, undersampled PatLoc encoding with quadrupolar fields results in coherent undersampling artifacts: star-shaped stripes, which run from the center toward the edge of the image, starting at some distance from the source (Fig. 6.9b).

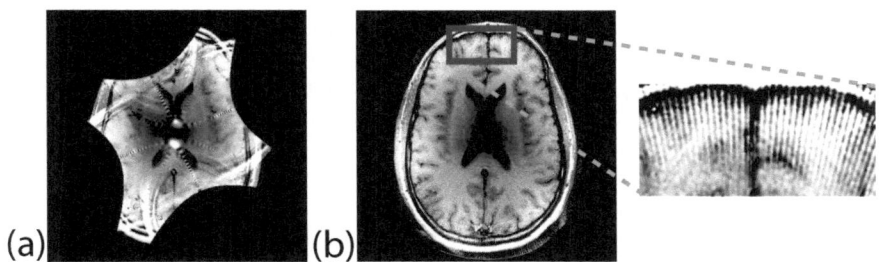

Figure 6.9: Undersampling artifact. (a) For Cartesian trajectories with fourfold undersampling, parts of the image are folded in at four different positions. (b) For radial trajectories, star-shaped stripes appear at some distance from the center when the polar reconstruction method is used.

6.3 Evaluation

In concordance with the developed theory, the results show that an elegant direct reconstruction from PatLoc encoded projection data exists, which produces high-quality images. An unusual star-shaped stripe artifact is caused by undersampling. The algorithms and the resulting image properties are discussed here in detail, and generalizations of the presented algorithms are briefly addressed.

6.3.1 Reconstruction Algorithms

Algorithms for arbitrary field geometries were presented as well as a particular implementation applicable to multipolar SEMs.

a) Arbitrary Encoding Fields

A method for the reconstruction of radial data with arbitrary encoding fields has been presented above: a direct reconstruction, which combines standard projection reconstruction methods with an algorithm originally developed for Cartesian PatLoc trajectories. This approach works because in PatLoc encoding space a combination of two arbitrary magnetic encoding fields appear as a linear field, which rotates from projection to projection. Such field rotations are also known from conventional radial imaging with linear gradients. Therefore, standard projection reconstruction methods can be used. However, they result in the warped encoding space representation of the magnetization (Fig. 6.2c). This representation is also known from Cartesian acquisitions (cf. e.g. Fig. 5.3, page 163) and therefore the image space algorithm, developed for Cartesian trajectories, is also applicable to radial trajectories.

b)   Multipolar Encoding Fields

A simplified version of the Cartesian reconstruction algorithm for multipolar SEM encoding has been derived in this chapter. The crucial point about the Cartesian algorithm is that it transforms the image from PatLoc encoding space back to natural image space coordinates. For multipolar SEMs, this back-transformation can be done more easily when polar coordinates are used. The reason for this simplification is that in polar coordinates the transformation takes a simple form, resulting in a separation of distortion (radial axis) and aliasing (azimuthal axis). Moreover, aliasing is equidistant and therefore Cartesian SENSE is applicable to remove the fold-over artifact that arises from the non-bijectiveness of the SEMs.

These considerations have beneficial consequences in setting up the reconstruction algorithm because, in contrast to a general implementation, presented in chapter 5.1, page 155ff, it allows one to use only very basic or common reconstruction operations. It is a significant advantage that Cartesian SENSE can be applied directly without having to perform the difficult search for image locations, which are aliased. This search must be done with more general encoding fields by performing a detailed analysis of the field geometries.

Besides Cartesian SENSE, intensity correction and image rewarping are very simple operations with quadrupolar encoding fields. Intensity correction corresponds to a linear intensity ramp and rewarping is done by first stretching the images to undo the quadratic distortions in the radial direction and then transforming the images from polar to Cartesian coordinates. The situation does not become much more difficult when arbitrary multipolar fields of order L are considered. The simplicity of these reconstruction operations therefore favors the usage of polar coordinates instead of Cartesian coordinates whenever multipolar fields are used for encoding.

For radial trajectories, standard FBP and subsequent transformation to polar coordinates can be combined by directly choosing a polar back-projection grid. This simplifies the reconstruction, however, a stretching in the radial direction is still necessary. It is, in fact, also possible to perform the distortion correction *within* the back-projection step, by just choosing a back-projection grid, which directly accounts for the distortions, given by $u = r^2$. This advantage comes, however, at the expense of longer reconstruction times: In this case, distortion correction and SENSE are swapped with the consequence that more voxels must be unfolded because of finer discretization (see paragraph *Implementation* in the above section 6.2.1c, page 222).

6.3.2 Influence of Field Approximations

The experimental fields deviated from the exact quadrupolar shape. These deviations have in general well-behaved effects on the resulting image quality for the direct polar reconstruction: Geometric distortion can occur and inaccurate RF-coil sensitivity information might lead to incorrect unfolding. However, the smoothness of the RF-coil sensitivities tolerates minor displacement errors. These errors were small in the measurement data, and therefore the reconstructed images are only slightly affected. This result is supported by Fig. 6.6, where the PatLoc image is compared to an image acquired with the standard system. Note that deviations from the exact multipolar field geometry can be considered with iterative methods (see following chapter) if accurate measurement data of the SEMs are available.

6.3.3 Image Properties and Artifacts

The properties of the images reconstructed with the direct method can generally be predicted by combining experience from standard projection reconstruction and Cartesian PatLoc reconstruction because image reconstruction is basically a concatenation of both methods.

Image Resolution   The r^{1-L}-law of image resolution not only holds for Cartesian, but also for radial trajectories. In fact, this law is independent of the chosen trajectory: Spatial variations of image resolution are primarily caused by spatial variations of the Jacobian of the SEMs. The r^{1-L}-law is exact in the continuous formulation. Deviations occur because of the discreteness of the reconstruction. The effect is negligible except for the center, where resolution is finite and not infinite as suggested by the law. For example, the circularly shaped, low-intensity region in Fig. 6.6b is related

to the size of the central image voxel (also cf. the PSF image on the top of
Fig. 6.7b).

Gibbs Ringing   The chosen trajectory does, however, have a significant influence on the sidelobe behavior of the PSF. In particular, major differences
in the Gibbs ringing artifact resulting from Cartesian and radial trajectories
could be observed. The most obvious differences are observed at the SEM
center, where the fields flatten out (Fig. 6.7b). The Cartesian method suffers
from destructive streaking artifacts, which extend over the complete image.
The artifact can be avoided, however, not without sacrificing image resolution (cf. previous chapter). In contrast to the Cartesian PSF, the radial PSF is
much more localized. The unwanted signal relocalization is restricted to the
center and does therefore not influence the utility of the proposed methods
in applications. The cause for this beneficial property can be understood
with a different k-space coverage of Cartesian and radial acquisitions. The
first has the shape of a square, the latter the shape of a disc. The Fourier
transform (FT) of these shapes have a significant influence on the sidelobe
behavior: The FT of a square is the product of two sinc-functions along the
two spatial dimensions. The PSF is therefore highly anisotropic with a very
slow sidelobe fade-out of $1/r$ along the main axes. On the other hand, the
FT of a disc is proportional to $k/r \cdot J_1(kr)$, where J_1 is the Bessel function of
the first kind of order one. The PSF is therefore isotropic and fades off faster
than $1/r$. The subsequent intensity correction in the reconstruction does
therefore not enhance the sidelobes to a degree, which leads to significant
image deterioration as in the Cartesian method.

Image Noise   In this chapter, the noise propagation properties of the direct
polar algorithm have been investigated. Note that the results also apply
to the SNR because of the linear nature of the direct reconstruction algorithms. The image noise is dominated by the varying voxel size and is
therefore very similar for Cartesian and radial trajectories. It was shown
in this work that the noise variations are actually equivalent for the two
direct reconstruction methods (Fig. 6.8b). Apart from the varying voxel
size, the SENSE reconstruction introduces spatial noise variations. In the
previous chapter (cf. e.g. Fig. 5.12a, page 188), it has been shown that the
g-factor is very low for PatLoc SENSE unfolding. In the polar representation,
this fact can be motivated well with the visual impression of the RF-coil
sensitivity maps sketched in Fig. 6.4e. Apart from the center, the maps

show very sharp intensity bands, which resemble the optimal RF maps needed for Partially-Parallel-Imaging-with-Localized-Sensitivities(PILS)-reconstruction [50]. PILS with optimal RF maps does not result in noise enhancement. This similarity of polar PatLoc reconstruction and optimal PILS reconstruction explains the low g-factor penalty for PatLoc.

Undersampling Artifact It could be observed in this work that, as expected, the undersampling artifact for Cartesian trajectories is not comparable to the artifact resulting from radial undersampling (Fig. 6.9). Similar to conventional imaging the presented projection reconstruction method is not suitable for the reconstruction of undersampled datasets (cf. Fig. 6.9b). In PatLoc, there is an additional problem: For illustration consider the filtered projections in Fig. 6.4 after step (b): Each projection has significant intensity at the zero-frequency. This central intensity can be explained by the fact that a narrow frequency band is generated over an extended region near the SEM center, where the field variations are low. The back-projection results in a coherent star-shaped stripe artifact not known from conventional imaging. This artifact is enhanced toward the periphery by the intensity correction. The stripes appear at a certain distance from the center, where the spatial distance between individual rays exceeds their width.

It has been shown in the literature that iterative reconstruction methods reduce the undersampling artifact in standard radial imaging [186, 13]. In the following chapter, it will be demonstrated that this is also true for undersampled PatLoc data (cf. e.g. Fig. 7.10, page 263). The main reason for this favorable impact on image quality is that iterative methods make full use of the available RF-coil sensitivity information, having positive effects on the point spread function. It remains to be investigated under which conditions k-space based methods like radial GRAPPA [48] or pseudo-Cartesian GRAPPA [165] adapted to PatLoc perform well with undersampled imaging data.

The analysis of the image properties shows that radial acquisitions can be useful in handling the problems which arise from flat encoding regions. Note that these problems do not occur if such flat regions are avoided with additional gradient encoding (see next chapter).

6.3.4 Generalizations Beyond Multipolar Field Encoding and Projection Reconstruction

Two different kinds of generalization are discussed here: acquisition with arbitrary non-Cartesian trajectories and encoding with generalized image projections.

Non-Cartesian Trajectories   In this chapter, reconstruction from a radial imaging sequence has been discussed. Radial acquisition is a special type of non-Cartesian imaging, and the question might arise how arbitrary non-Cartesian imaging sequences can be reconstructed. It has been shown above that a radial PatLoc acquisition cannot only be reconstructed by combining FBP with the Cartesian PatLoc image space reconstruction, but also by using gridding. Recall that gridding reconstruction is feasible with any non-Cartesian trajectory (cf. chapter 2.2.3, page 69ff). It is therefore, in principle, possible to first grid the non-Cartesian PatLoc imaging data onto a Cartesian grid and then apply the Cartesian PatLoc reconstruction algorithm. Keep in mind, however, that, depending on the trajectory, violation of the Nyquist criterion can have a significant impact on the resulting image quality.

Generalized Projections   In this chapter, most of the analysis was based on image projections that were formed by superimposing orthogonal multipolar SEMs. It has been shown that these fields are particularly suited for extended ROIs at the periphery of the object under examination. The resulting resolution gradient is also very well matched with the characteristics of ultrafast imaging techniques like MR-Encephalography [64, 51] and inverse imaging [99]. However, the ROI varies with the application, and other field geometries might be required to maximize the relevant information content. Flexible gradient coil designs [80, 203] seem to be appropriate for the generation of flexible resolution patterns. PatLoc may thus be used to further improve image quality and/or imaging speed with such techniques.

Such a flexible gradient system would allow one to not only superimpose two different SEMs with obvious restrictions on the realizable field geometries during the acquisition of image projections, but to define a nearly arbitrary effective magnetic field geometry $\psi_{res}(\cdot)$ that is different for each projection. For such general projections, image reconstruction, as done in this chapter, is not possible. At least two issues must be considered: First, the effective encoding field $\psi_{res}(\cdot)$ cannot be written as a superposition of two SEMs (cf. Eq. 6.2), a property that has been exploited in this chapter. More subtle is a second issue: For radial trajectories, it is possible to back-project each signal value of a one-dimensional projection along a single ray onto a two-dimensional plane. This operation is sparse and fast implementations exist. However, for general projections, it must be considered that a projection is, to be correct, the projected signal data convolved with a sinc-function [178], and therefore a signal value cannot merely be back-projected along a single ray, but must be mapped onto the complete 2D plane. Image reconstruction is therefore much more challenging. The development of efficient generalized projection reconstruction methods for PatLoc imaging beyond radial encoding with arbitrary SEM designs is a natural generalization of the work presented in this chapter and is a topic of the next chapter, section 7.1.2, page 240ff.

6.3.5 Conclusions

In this chapter, it has been shown that conventional radial imaging methodology is applicable to PatLoc imaging without requiring major modifications to the acquisition protocols. Images can be reconstructed by combining standard projection reconstruction methods with Cartesian PatLoc reconstruction. Also other non-Cartesian trajectories can in principle be reconstructed by concatenating standard gridding with the Cartesian PatLoc algorithm. For multipolar encoding fields, the reconstruction from radial imaging data is simpler and more straightforward when polar coordinate representations of the images are used instead of conventional Cartesian coordinates. The evaluation of simulated data as well as data measured in vivo has illustrated that the k-space isotropy of the radial trajectory significantly reduces the pronounced Gibbs ringing artifact that may occur in PatLoc imaging with Cartesian sampling. A star-shaped artifact, with no direct counterpart in conventional imaging, was found to result from a subsampled set of projections. In the next chapter it will be shown that this artifact is effectively suppressed by iterative image reconstruction.

Chapter 7

Iterative Reconstruction in PatLoc Imaging

TWO specific modalities of PatLoc imaging were analyzed in the previous chapters; Cartesian and radial acquisition with two NB-SEMs, for which highly efficient reconstruction is possible, yielding images with clearly defined properties. In the present chapter, more general imaging modalities are considered, and adequate reconstruction methods are discussed.

Unfortunately, the approaches taken in the previous chapters cannot be used in more general imaging situations. The reconstructions presented above were closely related to the general approaches of chapter 4.2.2, page 144ff, where the encoding matrix is directly inverted. The developed algorithms were efficient either because the encoding matrix was highly structured and could be inverted fast and robustly, or because it was possible to efficiently approximate the inverse with a related method. Such direct solutions to the inverse problem are, in principle, still possible for more general imaging modalities; however, direct inversion can be very inefficient; and it can be problematic because of ill-conditioning of the encoding matrix. One indirect solution – the approach taken here – is to model the imaging process through a linear operation, and to iteratively minimize the error between the measured and the modeled signal data by variation of the unknown spin density. This approach merely involves repetitive evaluation of the forward model, thereby avoiding direct inversion of the encoding matrix.

Typically, the solutions of iterative methods and the properties of the reconstructed images are less well-defined compared to direct solutions because, with noisy data, the algorithms usually do not converge and are often stopped after a relatively small number of iterations; if stopped too late, image quality begins to degrade because artifacts, which result from inaccuracies of the encoding matrix, are enhanced and SNR degradation is observed caused by ill-conditioning of the reconstruction. Nevertheless, iterative methods have proven extremely useful in MR image reconstruction. One reason is that such iterative methods can often be applied to a broad range of encoding strategies. For example, whereas basic SENSE is restricted to Cartesian trajectories, iterative SENSE can be applied to any sort of sampling trajectories. Another advantage of iterative methods is that the reconstruction problem is solved by successive evaluation of the forward operation only. The forward operation directly represents the imaging process. Therefore, it is often easier to appropriately incorporate refined signal models into the reconstruction. Other advantages include the extension of the image reconstruction by constraining the solution to certain prior knowledge [83]. These advantages often come at the expense of a dramatic increase in reconstruction time. Also the possibility to derive image quality measures in a clear manner as for direct reconstruction methods is lost. However, because of their flexible applicability, it is indispensable to develop such iterative methods also in the context of PatLoc imaging.

In this chapter, several iterative reconstruction methods are developed and their properties are compared with each other by evaluating several example datasets. Very relevant is chapter 2.3.1f, page 89ff, where an approach is presented that is applicable whenever the signal is modeled using a linear operation. The approach involves the CG method to update the intermediate quantities for each iteration. The same approach is used in conventional PI [134], and it can also be applied in PatLoc imaging, as done in this chapter; if necessary, an extension to non-equidistant reconstruction grids is considered (cf. chapter 4.2.3, page 152f).

7.1   Presentation of Image Reconstruction Methods

Iterative methods are presented for three different imaging situations. The first situation is the most general, with no restrictions imposed on the encoding strategy; however, the reconstruction is also the slowest of all presented methods. Initial examples of this time-domain reconstruction were presented in [[100]][1]. Much progress in this regard has been achieved by the work published in [[42]]. Other relevant work within the context of this thesis is [[158]] where images, reconstructed with the iterative method

---

[1]This ISMRM abstract has been further elaborated in [[101]].

and with the direct polar method of the previous chapter, are compared to each other.

The second situation involves MRI with generalized projections, where the magnetic field is constant during signal readout, but where the field may change between successive projections by combining an arbitrary number of SEMs without any restrictions imposed. This situation has been the topic of [[153]]. By formulating the problem not in the time domain, but in the frequency domain, it is possible to sparsify the forward operator with positive consequences for reconstruction time.

The last two methods naturally extend the direct reconstruction algorithms of the two previous chapters to arbitrary and subsampled trajectories. Initial steps toward the development of appropriate reconstructions have been presented in [[156]], where it has been observed that the similar structure of the encoding matrix allows one to base reconstruction on previous implementations of the iterative SENSE algorithm. A decisive step forward forms recent work [[86]], where a fast implementation is presented and combined with an adequate regularization term.

7.1.1 Reconstruction in the Time Domain

This section is important because the presented reconstruction method can be applied to any PatLoc encoding strategy (and even beyond PatLoc); no restrictions are demanded. In particular, the imaging situation considered here comprises:

1. An arbitrary number of SEMs.

2. Arbitrary sampling trajectories.

The applicability to any PatLoc encoding scheme makes the time-domain method the most flexible of all reconstruction methods that are discussed in this thesis. The downside of the method is that it is at the same time the slowest with high computational cost and/or memory requirements.

As already stated above, images encoded with a general PatLoc encoding strategy can be reconstructed using the iterative CG method, explained in the context of PI in chapter 2.3.1f, page 89ff, with an extension to non-equidistant reconstruction grids in chapter 4.2.3, page 152f. The main aspects are quickly reviewed here for general PatLoc encoding strategies.

In PatLoc, the signal s (see Eq. 4.9, page 139) is approximately given by s $\approx$ **EVm**, where **m** is the magnetization, **V** is a diagonal matrix that contains the nominal voxel volume of each voxel (cf. chapter 4.2.2b, page 148ff) and **E** is the encoding matrix. According to Eq. 4.18, page 146, the elements of **E** are given by:

$$E_{(\alpha,\kappa),\rho} := c_\alpha(\vec{x}_\rho)e^{-\mathrm{i}\mathbf{k}_\kappa^T\psi(\vec{x}_\rho)}. \tag{7.1}$$

A feasible image **m** is found by minimizing the difference between the measured signal s and the estimated signal **EVm** in the l_2-norm. According to Eq. 4.26, page 152, the minimization leads to the following problem:

$$(\mathbf{E}^H\mathbf{E})\mathbf{V}\mathbf{m} = \mathbf{E}^H\mathbf{s} \tag{7.2}$$

for $N_\rho < N_\kappa N_c$. For $N_\rho > N_\kappa N_c$ as well as for Tikhonov regularization, the modifications presented on page 89f in chapter 2.3.1f apply correspondingly. The latter equation can be solved iteratively with the CG method. A typical algorithm is presented on page 93. Other methods like the algebraic reconstruction technique exist to solve this equation. Here, however, only the CG method is considered, and a reconstruction algorithm, analogous to iterative SENSE (cf. chapter 2.3.1f, page 89ff), is depicted in Fig. 7.1.

Recall from chapter 2.3.1f, on page 93ff, that the bottleneck of the reconstruction is the matrix-vector multiplication of the encoding matrix **E** and its adjoint $\mathbf{E}^H$ with vectors of compatible lengths. It is therefore crucial to perform these matrix-vector multiplications as fast as possible. According to Eq. 7.1, the encoding matrix decomposes into two matrices $\mathbf{E} = \mathbf{GC}$, where **C** describes RF-sensitivity encoding and **G** SEM encoding. The application of the RF-sensitivity encoding matrix **C** can be implemented as a vector-vector multiplication for each RF channel and is therefore very quick. Problematic is the multiplication with the Fourier terms $e^{-\mathrm{i}\mathbf{k}_\kappa^T\psi(\vec{x}_\rho)}$ that form the matrix **G**. Recall that, for iterative SENSE, this multiplication can be accelerated with implementations of the nuFFT. The same is true as long as only two SEMs are used for 2D encoding (cf. section 7.1.3, page 247ff). This possibility to accelerate the reconstruction is not available in the general case with dramatic consequences for reconstruction time.

---

[2]This step is only required if irregular reconstruction grids are used. Alternatively, intensity correction can be performed as part of the matrix-vector multiplication, immediately before the multiplication of the conjugate direction vector with the coil sensitivity data.

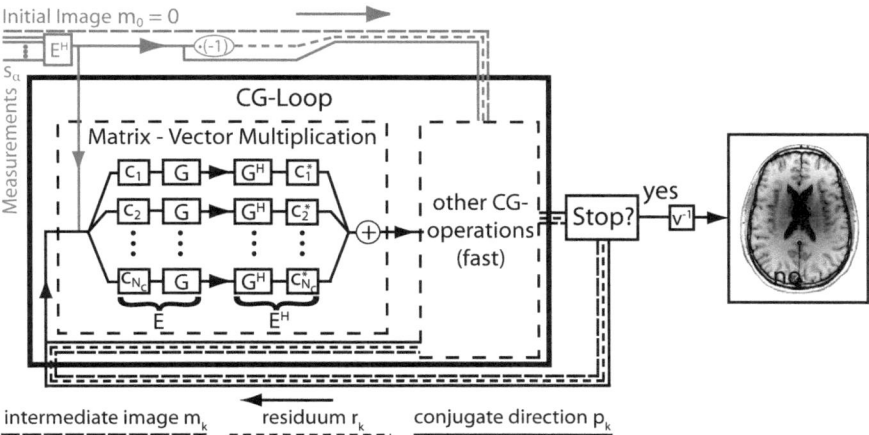

Figure 7.1: General iterative time-domain reconstruction with the CG method. The reconstruction is very similar to iterative SENSE, see Fig. 2.18, page 95. Initialization and termination of the algorithm are the same. A final intensity correction, division by the nominal voxel volume, has been added in this figure.[2] By far the most computation-intensive part of the algorithm is the matrix-vector multiplication. Multiplication with the RF-coil sensitivities $c_j(\cdot)$ and their complex conjugates $c_j^*(\cdot)$ is fast. Very problematic in PatLoc imaging is the multiplication with the matrix $\mathbf{G}$ or its adjoint $\mathbf{G}^H$. These matrices contain the phase terms resulting from SEM encoding. When, in PatLoc imaging, more than two SEMs are applied, these operations cannot be accelerated with fast nuFFT algorithms as is done in iterative SENSE. Note, however, that a matrix-vector multiplication is highly parallelizable, thus offering options to reduce reconstruction time.

To give an example, the first quick-and-dirty Matlab implementation of the iterative time-domain method required about half a week for the reconstruction of a $N_\kappa = 256 \times 256$ acquisition with $N_c = 8$ coils using a reconstruction grid with $N_\rho = 320 \times 320$ lattice points. Simple optimizations like changing the summation order or avoiding repetitive evaluations of expressions that may be reused diminished the computation time almost by a factor of 10. More elaborate multi-core implementations with Matlab reduced the reconstruction time even further by another factor of 10. Initial GPU-implementations resulted in yet another improvement of almost a factor of 20 such that the overall speedup is currently around 1400 for a dataset of the size as assumed above, resulting in a total reconstruction time of a few minutes for 25 iterations. Compared to several days, this is a tremendous acceleration, making 2D reconstructions practical at least for research; however, it will be difficult to achieve high-resolution 2D image reconstructions in the range of seconds in the near future; three-dimensional datasets are currently almost not tractable, even with highly optimized parallelization.

Despite the flexibility of the CG method, its practical usability is limited by the long computation time for the evaluation of the non-optimized matrix-vector multiplication. It is, however, often optimizable. The two previous chapters have already shown that, for Cartesian and radial encoding, fast and robust direct image reconstruction algorithms can be formulated. Similarly, in the following two sections, fast iterative image reconstructions are presented that use optimized matrix-vector multiplications. Their scope of applicability may be more restrictive than that of the general time-domain method; however, the algorithms discussed below offer opportunities to deal with datasets that are too large to be handled with the general time-domain CG method, and are therefore preferable in many situations.

7.1.2   Reconstruction from Generalized Image Projections in the Frequency Domain

The temporal evolution of the MR signal is very complicated because a very large number of spins create time-varying contributions that are all mixed up and received at the same time. It is often much simpler to describe not the temporal, but the frequency content of the MR signal, considering that each spin has a precession frequency that is directly proportional to the applied magnetic field. For a magnetic field that is not time-varying, the precession frequency of each spin does not change over time. Consequently, not all spins contribute to a particular frequency of the MR signal, but only those which lie on the corresponding isosurface of constant magnetic field strength. Thus, the signal is found by simply integrating the spin density over the isocontours of the encoding field.

Such a projection can be regarded as a sparse operation and it is to be expected that also image reconstruction is faster when formulated in the frequency domain. This hypothesis is analyzed in detail in this section under a general imaging condition that involves NB-SEMs and also phase encoding. To be precise, the imaging situation considered in this section has these assumptions:

1. An arbitrary number SEMs is used for encoding.
2. The sampling trajectories are subject to only one restriction: During signal readout, the effective encoding field is assumed to be constant.[3]

On the one hand, the case treated in this section is very general because an arbitrary number of encoding fields is considered. On the other hand, it may appear restrictive because the effective encoding field is required not to change during readout. Note however, that virtually all multi-dimensional trajectories for PatLoc presented in the literature so far (e.g. [178], [[42]]) fall under this category. Some, like the trajectories shown in [[101]] can even be reduced to the 2D case discussed below in section 7.1.3, page 247ff. The case treated here therefore covers a large class of important trajectories. Not covered are trajectories where the encoding field continuously changes during readout; an example from standard imaging are spiral trajectories.

After formulating the signal equation in the frequency domain, it is presented that the frequency-domain signal can be interpreted as a generalized projection. It is shown that the original magnetization can be recovered from the generalized projections using a method that is equivalent to the time-domain algorithm of the previous section. Finally, faster variants of the frequency-domain reconstruction are discussed that make use of an appropriate window function.

Signal Equation in the Frequency Domain First, reconsider the PatLoc signal equation represented in the time-dependent formulation of Eq. 4.7. Assume equitemporal signal recording at time points $t_j \in \Delta t \cdot \mathcal{I}_N$. Then, the signal is given by:

$$s_\alpha(t_j; r) = \int_V m(\vec{x}) c_\alpha(\vec{x}) e^{-\mathrm{i}(\mathbf{k}_r + \mathbf{k}(t_j; r))^T \psi(\vec{x})} \, \mathrm{d}\vec{x}. \tag{7.3}$$

According to the definition of PatLoc k-space and encoding function in Eqs. 4.5, 4.6, the phase contribution from frequency encoding for constant coil currents is given by $\phi(t_j, \vec{x}; r) = \mathbf{k}(t_j; r)^T \psi(\vec{x}) = \omega_r(\vec{x}) t_j$, where $\omega_r(\vec{x}) = \gamma B_r(\vec{x})$ is the frequency offset generated by the effective magnetic encoding field B_r during readout r; i.e., the superposition of the individual SEMs, driven with the currents $I_j(r)$: $B_r(\vec{x}) = \sum_j I_j(r) b_j(\vec{x})$. By abbreviating the

---

[3]Piece-wise constant trajectories like the 4D-RIO trajectory presented in [[42]] are also covered by sub-dividing the readout into several segments, where each of which is treated as a separate readout.

phase resulting from phase encoding with $\phi_r(\vec{x}) = \mathbf{k}_r^T \psi(\vec{x})$, the signal can then be written as:

$$s_\alpha(t_j; r) = \int_V m(\vec{x}) c_\alpha(\vec{x}) e^{-i(\phi_r(\vec{x}) + \omega_r(\vec{x}) t_j)} \, d\vec{x}. \qquad (7.4)$$

In the context of the following derivations, it is useful to formally extend the signal, technically defined only at discrete time points, to a continuous signal, where the time t can take any real number ($t \in \mathbb{R}; s \rightarrow s^{\mathbb{R}}$) by introducing a window function $w(t)$. To a good approximation, this window function can typically be assumed to be unity if data are recorded and zero if no recording occurs. The signal then reads:

$$s_\alpha(t; r) = w(t) s_\alpha^{\mathbb{R}}(t; r) = \int_V m(\vec{x}) c_\alpha(\vec{x}) e^{-i\phi_r(\vec{x})} \left[w(t) e^{-i\omega_r(\vec{x})t} \right] d\vec{x}. \qquad (7.5)$$

In this formulation, the signal has the natural temporal dependency. An equivalent frequency-domain formulation is found by taking the inverse FT (or, in a discrete formulation, the inverse DFT) of the signal along each readout:

$$P_\alpha(\omega; r) = \int_V m(\vec{x}) c_\alpha(\vec{x}) e^{-i\phi_r(\vec{x})} \hat{w}(\omega - \omega_r(\vec{x})) \, d\vec{x}, \qquad (7.6)$$

where $\hat{w}$ denotes the inverse (discrete) FT of the sampling window w. This frequency-domain representation $P_\alpha(\cdot)$ of the signal is termed *generalized projection* in this thesis; this concept is explained in more detail the next section.

Generalized Projections In conventional radial imaging (cf. chapter 2.2.2, page 66ff), a projection is the 1D Fourier transform of the corresponding signal readout and describes the integration of the excited magnetization (weighted with the sensitivity of the receiver coil) along the isocontour lines of the gradient field. The opposite process - back-projection of a 1D signal onto the 2D plane - does not directly represent the inverse operation; it does, however, play an important role in image reconstruction. Both, projection and back-projection in conventional radial imaging, are illustrated in Fig. 7.2a. Also in radial PatLoc imaging, as shown in the previous chapter, the Fourier analogues of the individual readouts can still be interpreted as image projections, where, however, the integration may be performed along multiple, bent isocontour lines of the effective encoding field (see Fig. 6.2, page 213). Observe that radial imaging, with linear SEMs as well as with NB-SEMs, has a special feature: The k-space center is acquired every signal readout. From a theoretical point of view, radial imaging can therefore be regarded as being a pure frequency encoding strategy.[4]

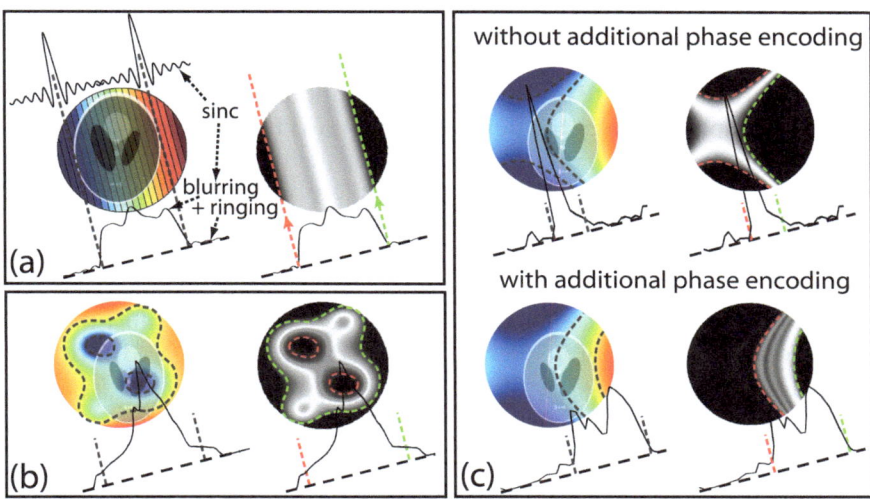

Figure 7.2: Generalized projections: projection and back-projection. (a) In conventional radial imaging, a projection corresponds to the integration of the magnetization along the isocontour lines of the linear gradient field. In practice, the signal is convolved with a sinc-function. The opposite operation, back-projection, cannot directly recover the original magnetization; nevertheless, it often forms a decisive step of image reconstruction. (b) Also for nonlinear field geometries, an image projection is found by integrating along the isocontour lines of the field, and back-projection is still a well-defined mathematical operation. (c) Sometimes, an image projection is defined to result from pure frequency encoding. This concept can be generalized to also include phase encoding performed with a SEM of different geometry prior to frequency encoding. Comparison of the images with and without phase encoding illustrates that the additional phase distribution added by phase encoding has a significant influence on the frequency content of the projected signal. In the depicted example, low-frequency information is strongly suppressed by phase encoding, whereas positive high-frequency information is well displayed in the signal spectrum.

---

[4]Note that, in the actual experiment, pre-phasers are typically involved, cf. Fig. 1.8, page 31.

The notion of image projections is generalized by Eq. 7.6. First, consider pure frequency encoding (i.e., $\phi_r(\vec{x}) = 0$) and assume idealized imaging with a readout of infinite duration and continuous sampling. Then, the frequency-domain window $\hat{w}(\cdot)$ is a delta function, which contributes signal if $\omega = \omega_r(\vec{x}) = \gamma B_r(\vec{x})$. This means that the frequency content of the signal is found by integrating the spin density weighted with the RF sensitivity along the isocontour lines of the effective magnetic field. In other words, $P_\alpha(\cdot)$ describes an image projection as conventionally defined. In contrast to conventional imaging, the field geometry can change nearly unrestrictedly between successive projections. Also for such generalized projections, back-projection is still well-defined. One projection and the corresponding back-projection for an arbitrary field geometry is illustrated in Fig. 7.2b. With additional phase encoding (i.e., $\phi_r(\vec{x}) \neq 0$ for some projection r) the frequency content can be modified even further. Fig. 7.2c,d shows an example for a quadrupolar encoding field, where phase encoding shifts the signal contribution from central frequencies to the edge of the acquired spectrum.

According to the previous paragraph, generalized projections are characterized in that the projections are taken for field geometries of any shape, and in that phase encoding is also considered. Actually, there is a third issue that must be taken into account: Under practical imaging conditions, it is not valid to assume continuous acquisitions of infinite duration. Typically, the data acquisitions are oversampled, such that continuous sampling is a good approximation. However, the finiteness of data sampling is crucial. The window function $w(t)$ has a finite width, and therefore its Fourier representation $\hat{w}(\omega)$ is not a delta function, but a sinc-function. The image projections are therefore blurred with primary contributions from the central contour line, but with signal contamination from other frequencies (cf. Fig. 7.2a). In MRI, the projection is therefore not perfect; this has important consequences for image reconstruction as will be shown in the following sections.

Frequency-Domain Reconstruction   In contrast to the time-domain method, where the data-consistency error between measured signal and modeled signal is minimized, the frequency-domain method minimizes the difference between the projection data and an estimate that is found by discretizing Eq. 7.6:

$$\min_{\mathbf{m}} \left\| \hat{\mathbf{s}} - \hat{\mathbf{E}}_t \mathbf{m} \right\|^2, \quad \text{where} \quad (\hat{E}_t)_{(\alpha,j,r),\rho} := c_\alpha(\vec{x}_\rho) e^{-i\phi_r(\vec{x}_\rho)} \hat{w}(\omega_j - \omega_r(\vec{x}_\rho)),$$
$$(7.7)$$

and where $\hat{s}_{\alpha,j,r} = P_\alpha(\omega_j; r)$, with $\omega_j \in \Delta\omega \cdot \mathcal{I}_N$ and $\Delta\omega = 1/(N\Delta t)$. In the latter equation the hat symbol is used to indicate that reconstruction is based on the frequency-domain formulation of the signal equation. Assuming a regular, normalized, reconstruction grid, i.e., $\mathbf{V} = \mathbb{1}$, the minimization yields the linear system $(\hat{\mathbf{E}}_t^H \hat{\mathbf{E}}_t)\mathbf{m} = \hat{\mathbf{E}}_t^H \hat{\mathbf{s}}$. It is proposed here to solve this system also with the CG method as described above.

The transformed encoding matrix $\hat{\mathbf{E}}_t = \mathbf{iDFT}_t \cdot \mathbf{E}$ (the subscript t indicates taking an inverse 1D-DFT along the temporal dimension) can be interpreted as a projection operator (cf. the latter section *Generalized Projections*), its adjoint operation $\hat{\mathbf{E}}_t^H \hat{\mathbf{s}}$ as the sum of the back-projected projection data. A fast reconstruction would result by simply (back-)projecting along the isocontour lines of the encoding field (cf. Fig. 7.2). This would correspond to a Fourier-domain window $\hat{w}(\cdot)$ of a delta function or a box-shaped function (see Fig. 7.3a,b, top row). However - as already stated above - the correct window is a sinc-function (see Fig. 7.3c, top row) and therefore each point must be projected not only along one line, but the complete image must be taken into consideration for the computation of the projection. This implies a dense encoding matrix $\hat{\mathbf{E}}_t$. Reconstruction is feasible with this method, but there is no improvement in computation time compared to the time-domain reconstruction.

Equivalence to the Time-Domain Method   It is important to note that the frequency-domain reconstruction using a sinc-window gives exactly the same results that are found with the time-domain reconstruction. The reason for this equivalence is that the inverse DFT is unitary. The inverse DFT does not change the norm $\|\hat{\mathbf{s}} - \hat{\mathbf{E}}_t \mathbf{m}\| = \|\mathbf{iDFT}_t(\mathbf{s} - \mathbf{Em})\| = \|\mathbf{s} - \mathbf{Em}\|$. In the frequency-domain method, the term on the left hand side is minimized, whereas the right hand side is the norm which is minimized to solve the corresponding time-domain problem. Both norms are the same, and therefore the reconstruction solves exactly the same problem. Also from a numerical point of view, the inverse DFT has no influence because

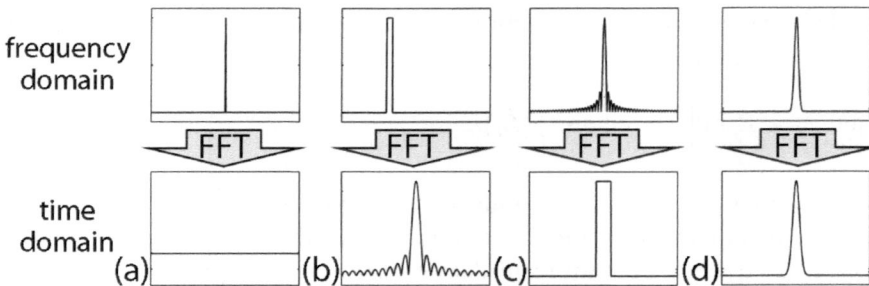

Figure 7.3: Time-domain filter of the signal readout (bottom) and corresponding frequency-domain filter (top). (a) The perfect frequency-domain filter would be a delta function, corresponding to an unrealistic, infinitely long, readout. (b) A fast and simple back-projection algorithm could be implemented assuming a box-shaped frequency-domain support; the corresponding filter in the time domain is a sinc-function that is, however, not useful to be implemented in practice. (c) The natural filter in the time domain is box-shaped with a width that corresponds to the time duration of signal readout. The corresponding frequency-domain filter is a sinc-function with non-local support. (b) With a Kaiser-Bessel filter, both, time-domain and frequency-domain supports, are localized.

it does not change the condition of the reconstruction. Therefore, both, time-domain and frequency-domain reconstruction, yield the same results.

Acceleration of the Frequency-Domain Reconstruction   The computation time can be reduced when the encoding matrix is approximated by a sparser version of it. A straightforward method to achieve sparsity is to simply disregard values of the encoding matrix that fall below a certain threshold [178]. Recently, this method has successfully been demonstrated for 4D-RIO [[43]]; the downside of this approach is that systematic errors are introduced that may lead to severe artifacts. A similar approach is presented here (also cf. [[153]]) that results in a fast, but also much more consistent, reconstruction.

The problems that arise with a threshold can be approached by reconsidering Eq. 7.5; from this equation, it follows immediately that a temporal filter acts on the signal data as well as on the encoding matrix. As implicitly stated above, signal acquisition can be modeled with a rectangular temporal window; correspondingly, the projection data are convolved with a sinc-function. Thresholding the sinc is problematic because it has fairly extended sidelobes, and therefore inconsistencies with the measurement data are generated.

The idea here is to apply, in addition to this natural rectangular filter, a second, artificial filter, in order to suppress the sidelobes, thereby transforming the encoding matrix into a sparser representation, with the consequence that thresholding becomes less problematic. Two methods are described here:

- The encoding matrix is constructed not with the sinc, but with a different filter function. Also the data are filtered in order to ensure consistency. This can be done in the time domain (cf. Eq. 7.5), for example, using a Kaiser-Bessel window. The corresponding window in the frequency domain has significantly suppressed sidelobes (cf. Fig. 7.3d). When these sidelobes are ignored, data consistency is only moderately affected. The consequence is a sparse encoding matrix and significantly accelerated image reconstruction. The downside of this approach is that more CG iterations are required than usual to reach an optimal image resolution.
- In accordance with the first method, the encoding matrix is constructed with an appropriate window function. However, the signal data are not filtered; consistency is guaranteed by applying the inverse of the filter to the filtered encoding matrix instead. It can easily be shown that this method - before thresholding - is equivalent to the unaccelerated time-domain reconstruction.[5] With this method, not more CG iterations are required than usual. The downside is that reconstruction is much more sensitive to data reduction via thresholding compared to the first method.

7.1.3 Fast Reconstruction with Non-Uniform FFT Algorithms

Much faster reconstructions are possible if the number of independent SEMs does not exceed the dimension of the excited imaging volume. In particular, the following assumptions are made in this section:

1. Two nonlinear and non-bijective SEMs for 2D imaging are applied.

---

[5]When the encoding matrix is calculated as $\mathbf{E} = 1/w \cdot \mathbf{DFT}_t \hat{\mathbf{E}}_t^w$, where $\hat{\mathbf{E}}_t^w$ is the filtered frequency-domain representation of the encoding matrix, i.e. $\hat{\mathbf{E}}_t^w := \mathbf{iDFT}_t w \mathbf{E}$.

2. Arbitrary sampling trajectories are used.

The case treated in this section is similar to the imaging situation that has been discussed in the previous chapters in that, again, only two SEMs are applied during acquisition; it is more general because the reconstruction is not restricted to a specific type of sampling trajectory (Cartesian, radial), but the signal can be encoded with any kind of acquisition trajectory. However, it is also more restrictive than the iterative methods presented above because the methods cannot be applied to encoding strategies that involve any number of SEMs.

The previous chapter has revealed that gridding in combination with the Cartesian image space reconstruction method of chapter 5.1 should be useful for densely sampled, arbitrary, trajectories. Gridding is not an appropriate method to fill unsampled portions of PatLoc k-space. However, as discussed in chapter 5.2, pseudo-Cartesian GRAPPA in combination with the Cartesian image space reconstruction might yield useful results.

An alternative, involving the iterative CG method, is presented here. Good results are to be expected because this method makes efficient use of RF-sensitivity encoding. The non-Cartesian nature of the imaging trajectories hinders usage of the FFT. Nevertheless, fast image reconstruction is possible because the nuFFT can be applied instead. The nuFFT is briefly reviewed below before two different reconstruction methods are presented.

Non-Uniform FFT   In conventional MRI there is a Fourier relation between the signal data and the magnetization. Also in PatLoc imaging with two NB-SEMs, the Fourier domain of the signal data is an important space, which has been termed *PatLoc encoding space* in chapter 5 on page 158.

In MRI, only a finite amount of signal data, measured at k-space locations $\vec{k}_\kappa$ is available, and for numerical reasons, also the reconstruction grid must have a finite spacing with locations $\vec{x}_\rho$. For numerical calculations, the continuous Fourier terms must therefore be replaced in practice by a discrete number of terms: $e^{-i\vec{k}\vec{x}} \rightarrow e^{-i\vec{k}_\kappa \vec{x}_\rho}$. In Cartesian Fourier imaging, the discrete version of the FT is termed the *discrete Fourier transform* (DFT), and a fast algorithm to calculate the DFT is the well-known FFT. However, the FFT requires that both, $\vec{k}_\kappa$ and $\vec{x}_\rho$, lie on grids with equidistant spacing. If one or both grids are not equidistantly spaced, the DFT must be replaced by a non-uniform DFT, for which also fast non-uniform FFT implementations exist.

In general, the nuFFT can be subdivided into three different types; these types, together with the FFT, are illustrated in Fig. 7.4 and explained in the figure caption. Note that *gridding* is effectively a realization of a nuFFT of type 1. A typical gridding algorithm is presented on page 70f in chapter 2.2.3. For more information on the nuFFT and fast algorithms for each of the three types, consult the abundant literature on this topic, for example the tutorial [133].

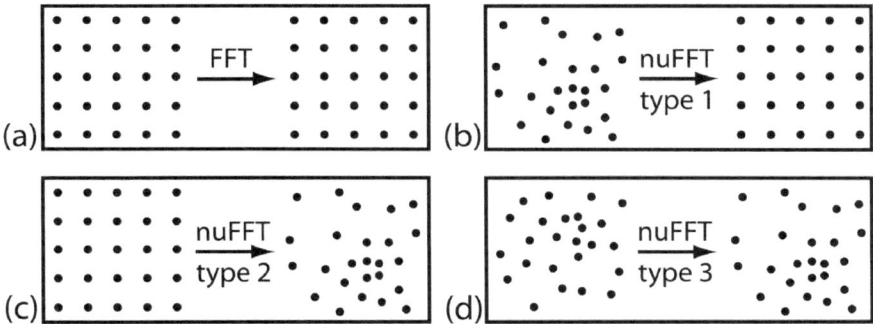

Figure 7.4: FFT and different types of the nuFFT. The FFT and the nuFFT are fast implementations of discrete versions of the continuous FT. Whereas the FFT requires equidistant grids in both Fourier domains, the nuFFT can cope with non-equidistant data samples (the dots represent the distribution of source and target locations). Three different types of the nuFFT can be distinguished with respect to the distribution of the source and target data.

Reconstruction Using the nuFFT of Type 1 and 2 It has been shown above that the matrix-vector multiplication in the CG method is very problematic when more than two SEMs are used. For two SEMs, further acceleration is possible. Recall that, with two SEMs, the general form of the encoding matrix is given by Eq. 5.2, page 157; it is repeated here using a notation which clarifies that the locations $\vec{x}_{l,\rho}$ belong each to a separate bijective region $l = 1, \ldots, L$ of the encoding function $\vec{\psi}$ (cf. Fig. 5.1, page 159):

$$E_{(\alpha,\kappa),(l,\rho)} = \tilde{c}_\alpha^l(\vec{u}_{l,\rho})e^{-i\vec{k}_\kappa\vec{u}_{l,\rho}}, \quad \text{with} \quad \vec{u}_{l,\rho} := \vec{\psi}(\vec{x}_{l,\rho}), \qquad (7.8)$$

where $\tilde{c}_\alpha^l := c_\alpha \circ (\vec{\psi}^l)^{-1}$. The problematic part is the multiplication with the Fourier terms. Recall that the fast reconstruction achieved with the Cartesian PatLoc image space method is a consequence of choosing a rectilinear reconstruction grid not in image space, but in PatLoc encoding space. In this case it is possible to drop the index l from $\vec{u}_{l,\rho}$ because these locations lie on a rectilinear grid with L identical layers (cf. Fig. 5.1, page 159).

This idea of using a rectilinear grid in PatLoc encoding space can also be applied to iterative reconstruction. The Fourier terms $e^{-i\vec{k}_\kappa \vec{u}_\rho}$ then have a form suited for the application of a nuFFT of type 2 because the locations $\vec{u}_\rho$ of the source data are distributed equidistantly, whereas the locations $\vec{k}_\kappa$ of the target data are irregularly sampled (also cf. Fig. 7.4c). The opposite is the case for the adjoint $\mathbf{E}^H$, which maps the irregularly-spaced data at locations $\vec{k}_\kappa$ to the regularly-spaced data at locations $\vec{u}_\rho$. Also this mapping can be performed rapidly, this time with a nuFFT algorithm of type 1 (cf. Fig. 7.4b).

For the design of a particular reconstruction algorithm, it is useful to compare the problem with iterative SENSE. This approach is promising because, as has been shown for Cartesian trajectories already, SENSE and the image space PatLoc method are also closely related to each other. The reason for the similarity is that the encoding matrix has an equivalent structure. This is also true with non-Cartesian trajectories; let $\mathbf{E}_{pat}$ denote the PatLoc encoding matrix and $\mathbf{E}_{lin}$ the corresponding matrix that occurs in iterative SENSE (see Eq. 2.15, page 47). The entries of the encoding matrices are then given by:

$$\underbrace{(E_{pat})_{(\alpha,\kappa),(l,\rho)} = \tilde{c}^l_\alpha(\vec{u}_\rho)e^{-i\vec{k}_\kappa \vec{u}_\rho}}_{\text{PatLoc}} \quad \text{and} \quad \underbrace{(E_{lin})_{(\alpha,\kappa),\rho} = c_\alpha(\vec{x}_\rho)e^{-i\vec{k}_\kappa \vec{x}_\rho}}_{\text{Standard PI}} .$$

$$(7.9)$$

Observe that, regarding the structure of the encoding matrix, the only difference between the two matrices is the additional index $l = 1, \ldots, L$ in the RF-coil sensitivity maps. For convenience of notation, let w. l. o. g. $L := 2$. With the latter equation, $\mathbf{E}_{pat}$ can formally[6] be expressed in terms of $\mathbf{E}_{lin}$ via $\mathbf{E}_{pat} = (\mathbf{E}_{lin,1} \ \mathbf{E}_{lin,2})$. This equation relates the iterative PatLoc reconstruction with iterative SENSE such that it should be possible to perform the matrix-vector multiplication in PatLoc using matrix-vector multiplications of the corresponding PI analogue. To be more concrete, let s be a formal signal space vector and let $\mathbf{m}_{pat} = (\mathbf{m}_{lin,1} \ \mathbf{m}_{lin,2})^T$, where $\mathbf{m}_{pat}$ is a for-

---

[6]*Formal* means here that the expressions are not equal in the usual sense because $\tilde{c}_\alpha \neq c_\alpha$ for nonlinear SEMs, but merely in a formal sense that only relates to the structure of the matrices.

mal PatLoc image space vector and $\mathbf{m}_{lin}$ the corresponding PI vector. The matrix-vector multiplication in PatLoc can then be calculated according to:

$$\mathbf{E}_{pat}\mathbf{m}_{pat} = \mathbf{E}_{lin,1}\mathbf{m}_{lin,1} + \mathbf{E}_{lin,2}\mathbf{m}_{lin,2} \quad \text{and} \quad \mathbf{E}_{pat}^H\mathbf{s} = \begin{pmatrix} \mathbf{E}_{lin,1}^H\mathbf{s} \\ \mathbf{E}_{lin,2}^H\mathbf{s} \end{pmatrix}. \quad (7.10)$$

These equations show explicitly that the matrix-vector multiplications for the iterative PatLoc method can each be performed by applying L-times the matrix-vector multiplications programmed for iterative SENSE reconstruction.

Close inspection of the latter equation shows that there is even room for optimization. Recall from Eq. 2.54, page 94, that the encoding matrix in iterative SENSE can be written as $\mathbf{E}_{lin} = \mathbf{GC}$, where $\mathbf{G}$ contains the time-intensive Fourier terms (which can be implemented as a nuFFT) and where the application of the sensitivity matrix $\mathbf{C}$ can be realized as a quick vector-vector multiplication. Then, $\mathbf{E}_{pat}$ can be written as $\mathbf{E}_{pat} = \begin{pmatrix} \mathbf{E}_{lin,1} & \mathbf{E}_{lin,2} \end{pmatrix} = \begin{pmatrix} \mathbf{GC}_1 & \mathbf{GC}_2 \end{pmatrix} = \mathbf{G}\begin{pmatrix} \mathbf{C}_1 & \mathbf{C}_2 \end{pmatrix}$ and the matrix-vector multiplication evaluates to:

$$\mathbf{E}_{pat}\mathbf{m}_{pat} = \mathbf{G}(\mathbf{C}_1\mathbf{m}_{lin,1} + \mathbf{C}_2\mathbf{m}_{lin,2}) \quad \text{and} \quad \mathbf{E}_{pat}^H\mathbf{s} = \begin{pmatrix} \mathbf{C}_1^H \\ \mathbf{C}_2^H \end{pmatrix} \mathbf{G}^H\mathbf{s}. \quad (7.11)$$

The optimized PatLoc reconstruction therefore requires only a single nuFFT of type 2 to be applied for the forward operation, and a single nuFFT of type 1 for the adjoint operation. This is exactly what needs to be done in iterative SENSE reconstruction. It is to be expected, however, that PatLoc reconstruction is faster than iterative SENSE for a comparable number of image voxels because, in PatLoc, the encoding space grid, which is relevant for the nuFFT, only consists of an L-th fraction ($\vec{u}_\rho$) of all image voxels ($\vec{x}_{l,\rho}$).

Reconstruction Using the nuFFT of Type 3   Instead of reconstructing on a regular grid in PatLoc encoding space, it is also possible to choose equidistant locations $\vec{x}_{l,\rho}$ directly in image space. In this case, however, the locations $\vec{u}_{l,\rho} = \vec{\psi}(\vec{x}_{l,\rho})$ are no longer regularly spaced with the consequence that the Fourier terms $e^{-\mathrm{i}\vec{k}_\kappa \vec{u}_{l,\rho}}$ (see Eq. 7.8) are not suited any more for reconstruction with the nuFFT of type 1 or type 2.[7] However, this situation

---

[7]Only for Cartesian trajectories in PatLoc k-space, the nuFFT of type 1 or type 2 can still be applied. Note however, that, this time, the locations $\vec{k}_\kappa$ lie on a regular grid and $\vec{u}_\rho$ on an irregular grid, whereas in the previous section, it was $\vec{u}_\rho$ that laid on a regular grid, and $\vec{k}_\kappa$

can be tackled with a nuFFT of type 3 when applying $\mathbf{E}$ as well as $\mathbf{E}^H$ (cf. Fig. 7.4d). To be precise, the encoding matrix $\mathbf{E}_{pat}$ can still be written using two components (for $L = 2$) as $\mathbf{E}_{pat} = (\mathbf{E}_1 \ \mathbf{E}_2) = (\mathbf{G}_1\mathbf{C}_1 \ \mathbf{G}_2\mathbf{C}_2)$, where $\mathbf{G}_1$ and $\mathbf{G}_2$ describe the application of the nuFFT of type 3 for $l = 1$ and $l = 2$. Note that in general, $\mathbf{G}_1 \neq \mathbf{G}_2$, even though both operations can be the same, for example when exact quadrupolar SEMs are used. The matrix-vector multiplication then yields:

$$\mathbf{E}_{pat}\mathbf{m}_{pat} = \mathbf{G}_1\mathbf{C}_1\mathbf{m}_1 + \mathbf{G}_2\mathbf{C}_2\mathbf{m}_2 \quad \text{and} \quad \mathbf{E}_{pat}^H\mathbf{s} = \begin{pmatrix} \mathbf{C}_1^H\mathbf{G}_1^H\mathbf{s} \\ \mathbf{C}_2^H\mathbf{G}_2^H\mathbf{s} \end{pmatrix}. \quad (7.12)$$

The matrix-vector multiplication therefore normally requires that the nuFFT of type 3 is applied L-times for the forward as well as for the adjoint operation. Note that further acceleration by applying a single nuFFT on the combined vector $\mathbf{m}_{pat}$ is not always possible; the result might be different to a separate application of the nuFFT on each of the sub-vectors $\mathbf{m}_l$. Also note that a nuFFT algorithm of type 3 is typically not as fast as the nuFFT algorithms of types 1 or 2. However, the difference is often not very high (cf. e.g. [30]).

Considering that iterative PatLoc reconstruction with a nuFFT of type 3 is not much slower than reconstruction with the nuFFT of type 1 and 2, and especially taking into account that a higher image quality can be expected with a nuFFT of type 3 (see discussion below), in many situations, this approach seems to be superior to the approach that uses a rectilinear reconstruction grid in PatLoc encoding space.

7.2   Application to Simulated and Measured Imaging Data

The properties of the reconstruction methods, that were described on a theoretical basis in the previous section, are verified here with simulated as well as experimental data. In this section, it is first explained how the

---

on an irregular grid. As a result, this time, the nuFFT of type 1 can be used in the forward operation and the nuFFT of type 2 for the adjoint operation - which is the opposite of the situation treated in the previous section.

data were generated, reconstructed and analyzed. Then, the corresponding results are presented.

7.2.1   Methods

Further details about the implemented reconstruction algorithms and the generated datasets are given in this section, and it is shown how image resolution and SNR were analyzed.

a)   Reconstruction Algorithms

Several iterative reconstruction methods were implemented in addition to the direct methods that have been presented in the previous chapters.

Time-Domain Reconstruction   The time-domain reconstruction was implemented as shown in Fig. 7.1 and a standard implementation of the CG method similar to the algorithm presented on page 93 was used. The algorithm was stopped after a fixed number of iterations, typically after 25 or 30 iterations. An option was added to enable Tikhonov regularization. The matrix-vector multiplication of the matrix G, which contains the phase terms, or its adjoint with compatible vectors was programmed in two different ways for CPU computations: For small datasets, where the matrix could be stored entirely in the memory, G was precomputed once in order to ensure quick accessibility of the relevant information. For large datasets, the matrix-vector multiplication was performed line by line. This approach reduces the memory requirements drastically, however, as each line has to be recomputed multiple times, this approach is also much slower than if the matrix could be stored completely in the memory. In order to ensure acceptable reconstruction times also for larger datasets, the line-by-line approach was also programmed for GPU-computation using CUDA (Compute Unified Device Architecture; Nvidia, Santa Clara, CA, USA).

Frequency-Domain Reconstruction   The equivalent frequency-domain method was programmed similar to the time-domain method. It differed only in that an FFT was applied to the signal data and that the encoding matrix was not constructed based on Eq. 7.1, but on the frequency-domain analogue, given by Eq. 7.6, with a sinc-filter of appropriate width. For the accelerated reconstructions, a Kaiser-Bessel window with filter parameter $\alpha = 2$ was used, and the encoding matrix was constructed using the corresponding Fourier-domain window. The window was thresholded by setting all values below 0.1% of the maximum value to zero. For comparison, two additional, inconsistent, reconstructions were tested. In the first reconstruction, the encoding matrix was filtered, but no inverse filter was applied, nor were the signal data filtered. In the second example, the signal data were also not filtered and back-projection was implemented according to the box-shaped frequency-domain window shown in Fig. 7.3b.

nuFFT Implementations An iterative method was implemented that was based on the nuFFT of type 1/2. The implemented method used a regular reconstruction grid in PatLoc encoding space, and was applicable to a non-Cartesian PatLoc k-space grid. For the nuFFT of type 1/2, the *image reconstruction toolbox* of Jeffrey A. Fessler was used. The toolbox contains a fast implementation of the min-max interpolation method [36] with a Matlab interface, downloadable for free on Fessler's website [35]. A fast implementation for the PatLoc reconstruction based on the nuFFT of type 3 has recently been developed by Dr. Florian Knoll in a joint project [[86]]. The results shown here, however, have not been accelerated using this method; instead, the accurate, but slow, nuDFT (time-domain reconstruction) was applied without further numerical optimization.[8]

b) Data

The implemented reconstruction algorithms were tested with three different encoding strategies:

1. 2D Cartesian PatLoc trajectory as presented in chapter 5.
2. 2D radial PatLoc trajectory, densely sampled as well as subsampled as presented in chapter 6.
3. 4D PatLoc trajectory as explained below.

Numerical data were generated by discretization of the PatLoc signal equation (cf. Eq. 4.9, page 139). The Shepp-Logan head phantom served as spin density, exact linear and quadrupolar SEMs were assumed and the RF-sensitivity profiles of a real-world eight-channel RF-coil array were taken as input data.

---

[8]The same applies to the Cartesian method described in footnote 7, page 251, that makes use of a nuFFT reconstruction with the types 1 and 2, but with the order reversed compared to the implementation that has actually been applied to generate the results for this chapter.

Measurement data were acquired with the PatLoc hardware, which is described in chapter 3.3.3, page 126ff. Phantom measurements were performed with a cylindrically-shaped object with a diameter of 190 mm. The object contained plexiglass tubes filled with water that had been doped with nickel sulfate and sodium chloride. In vivo head imaging was performed in volunteers. RF-sensitivity profiles and maps of the SEMs were determined as described in the previous chapter (cf. 6.2.1b, page 220f).

The tested 4D PatLoc encoding strategy was the 4-Dimensional Radial In/out vs. radial Out/In (4D-RIO) trajectory developed by Dr. Daniel Gallichan. 4D means here that 4 SEMs, two linear and two quadrupolar fields, are used to encode a 2D slice. For 4D-RIO, the linear and the quadrupolar SEMs both follow a separate radial trajectory. The trajectories are, however, not synchronous, but shifted by half a readout such that when the linear trajectory passes through the center of k-space (in/out), the quadrupolar trajectory approaches the edge of k-space and moves back inward on the next radial spoke (out/in), and vice versa. The temporal delay between the linear and the quadrupolar trajectory leads to complex, but very interesting imaging properties. Here, only a few aspects are presented; for a detailed analysis consult [[44, 42]].

c) Image Quality Analysis

Image resolution and image noise were analyzed based on numerical simulations.

Image Resolution PSF plots were generated for different source locations, different encoding strategies, and different reconstruction algorithms. For quantitative results, the area of the main peak at FWHM was calculated. For the 4D trajectory, image resolution was also estimated from the extent of its local k-space.

Image Noise The noise propagation properties of the algorithms were determined by first reconstructing $100\times$ pure, white Gaussian noise, and then calculating the standard deviation at each location.

7.2.2 Results

Reconstruction results are presented for the Cartesian, the radial and the 4D-RIO trajectory. The 2D datasets were reconstructed with the direct image space methods presented in the two previous chapters as well as with the iterative methods described above. The 4D-RIO trajectory was reconstructed with the (accelerated) frequency-domain and the time-domain method.

a) Cartesian PatLoc Trajectory

Above, it has been shown theoretically that the iterative frequency-domain and time-domain reconstructions are equivalent methods. Also, it has been shown that an artificial filter function can be added to the reconstruction without affecting consistency if appropriately included. These claims are supported by Fig. 7.5.

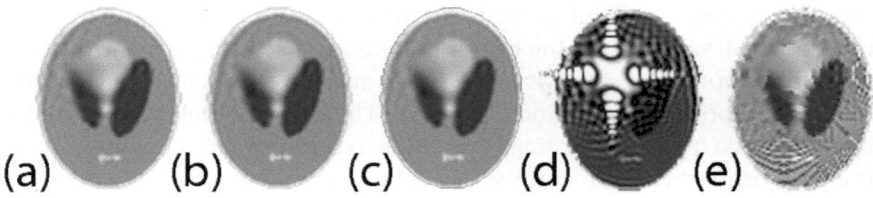

Figure 7.5: Reconstructed images for a Cartesian trajectory with quadrupolar Pat-Loc encoding. All reconstructions were stopped after 30 CG iterations. (a) Unfiltered time-domain and (b) frequency-domain reconstructions give equivalent results. (c) Also the filtered reconstruction yields an identical image. In this example, the encoding matrix was constructed with a Kaiser-Bessel window, Fourier transformed, and divided by the time-domain analogue of the filter to undo the filtering. Thresholding was omitted. (d) Not dividing by the time-domain window leads to an inconsistent reconstruction. (e) Back-projection along box-shaped bands does also not correspond to a consistent reconstruction.

The figure shows images from a simulated 64×64-acquisition reconstructed on a 128×128-grid. It is clearly demonstrated that an appropriate frequency-time-domain filter combination must be chosen to guarantee data consistency (cf. Fig. 7.5c-e). Time-domain, frequency-domain and filtered reconstruction (no threshold) yield identical images, Fig. 7.5a-c.

Fig. 7.6 illustrates that there is a fundamental difference, whether the filtering is undone after application of the filtered encoding matrix or whether the filtering is not undone, but considered by also filtering the signal data. For the depicted very simple unaccelerated PI example, the final image resolution is achieved with the former method right from the start. When the filtering is not undone, however, more than 100 iterations are required to reach the optimal image resolution. Note that only the frequency encoding direction is affected by the intermediate loss of resolution because the encoding matrix is filtered only along the readout direction.

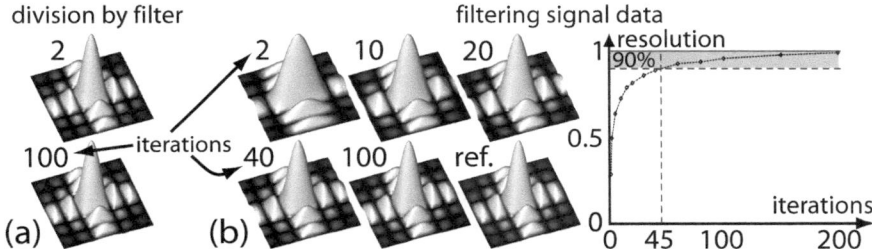

Figure 7.6: Effect of a window function on image resolution. (a) Filtering is undone after application of the encoding matrix. (b) Filtering is not undone, but considered instead by filtering the signal data along the readout direction. Shown are the central parts of a PSF for different numbers of CG iterations reconstructed from unaccelerated Cartesian PI data. Frequency encoding is from left to right. It can be observed in this example that the optimal image resolution is achieved right from the start when filtering is undone. If not, the filtering (here with a Kaiser-Bessel window, filter parameter $\alpha = 2$) reduces the spatial resolution along the frequency encoding direction. The effect becomes smaller with an increasing number of iterations. After about 100 iterations the difference to an optimal reference PSF (obtained from an unfiltered reconstruction) becomes almost negligible. The plot on the right depicts a quantitative evaluation of the resolution loss along the frequency encoding direction. In the presented example, 90% of the optimal resolution is reached after about 45 iterations.

Further details about image resolution and Gibbs ringing for a 2D quadrupolar Cartesian PatLoc trajectory are presented in Fig. 7.7, where these properties are analyzed with the help of PSFs, and where phantom images are shown that were reconstructed with different methods.

The PSFs in Fig. 7.7 were simulated for two different source locations with 64×64 samples. Iterative reconstruction was performed on a grid with 256×256 lattice points. Relaxation effects were ignored. The measurement of the tube phantom, shown in the bottom part of Fig. 7.7, was higher resolved with 128×128 samples and a 256×256-reconstruction grid. The acquisition protocol was a gradient echo with the following sequence parameters:

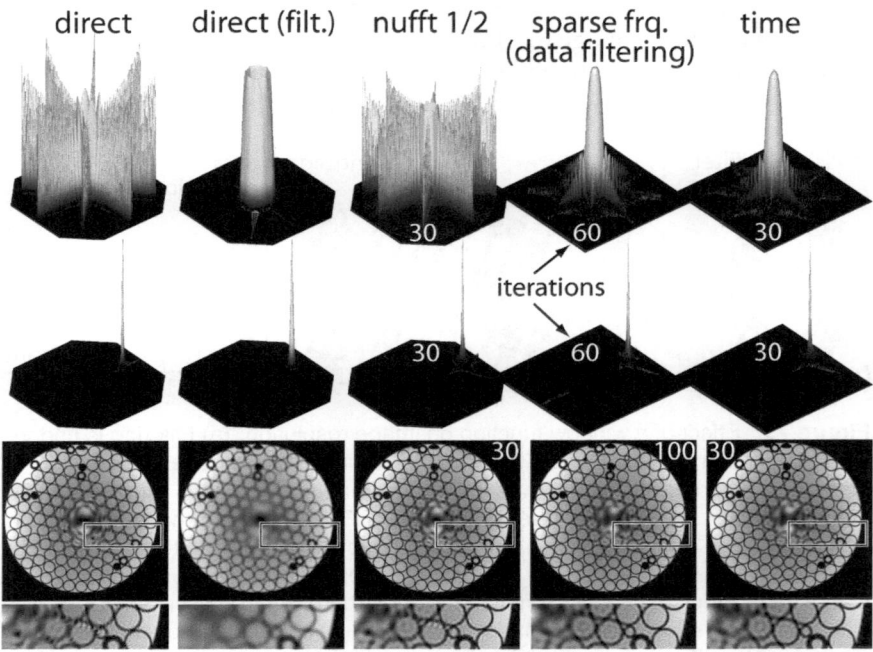

Figure 7.7: PSF analysis and Gibbs ringing of a Cartesian trajectory for quadrupolar PatLoc SEMs. The results for five different reconstruction methods are shown: direct Cartesian; direct Cartesian where the data have been filtered with a Kaiser-Bessel window; iterative nuFFT reconstruction (type 1 and 2); sparse iterative frequency-domain reconstruction, with filtering of the signal data; and iterative time-domain reconstruction. Top row: The PSFs for a central location are problematic and depend significantly on the chosen reconstruction method. Direct Cartesian, but also the nuFFT reconstruction exhibit prominent Gibbs ringing, which is significantly suppressed by a window function at the expense of reduced image resolution. The iterative time-domain (30 iterations), and accelerated frequency-domain reconstruction (60 iterations) give almost exactly the same results, with the highest spatial resolution and no destructive sidelobes. Middle row: The PSFs for a peripheral source location are well-behaved for all algorithms. Some loss of resolution is visible for the filtered direct reconstruction, but not for the filtered iterative frequency-domain method. Bottom rows: The dominant PSFs from the central locations are clearly visible as corresponding pronounced Gibbs ringing artifacts in the reconstructed measurement data. These artifacts are effectively suppressed by the time-domain method and the filtered reconstructions. The PSFs have a lower resolution than the acquired phantom images to show the ringing effect more clearly.

$T_E = 8.7\,\text{ms}$, $T_R = 100\,\text{ms}$, slice thickness $\Delta z = 5\,\text{mm}$, flip angle $\alpha = 20°$. The results shown in Fig. 7.7 are discussed in detail in the figure caption.

In this figure, the results from the iterative methods are compared to those found with the direct image space method of chapter 5.1, page 155ff, whose properties were analyzed in detail above. All images clearly have the expected resolution gradient resulting from the increased SEM variations at the periphery of the FOV. The direct reconstruction from filtered data shows significantly reduced image resolution because a fairly high Kaiser-Bessel window parameter of $\alpha = 2$ was chosen to accentuate the effect. The figure illustrates that the nuFFT implementation reconstructed onto a regular grid in PatLoc encoding space outperforms the direct reconstruction only slightly. Thresholding the frequency-domain reconstruction resulted in a significant improvement in reconstruction time, approximately factor 20 for each CG iteration. Shown in the figure is a result from filtering the signal data. The number of CG iterations was tripled compared to the time-domain reconstruction. This resulted in an image with no increase in noise, and no blurring or PSF anisotropies. Also, the pronounced Gibbs ringing artifact is effectively suppressed by this method.

b) Radial PatLoc Trajectory

In the previous chapter, it has been shown that the main characteristics of PatLoc imaging, for example non-homogeneous image resolution, are very similar for radial trajectories and Cartesian trajectories. Significant differences occur, however, in the sidelobe behavior of the PSFs. Different reconstruction methods also affect the PSF and therefore it is interesting to analyze how iterative methods alter the PSF and thus Gibbs ringing and aliasing. Here, results for a densely sampled and a $4\times$ undersampled radial PatLoc trajectory, encoded with quadrupolar SEMs, are shown. The same dataset has already been analyzed in detail in the previous chapter with the direct reconstruction method. This has the advantage that it is possible to focus here on those aspects, which are caused by choosing iterative reconstruction methods instead of the previously discussed direct reconstruction.

Densely Sampled Trajectory   In Fig. 7.8 image resolution and Gibbs ringing is analyzed. PSFs are shown for two source locations, using 103 simulated projections and 64 samples per readout line. The iterative methods use

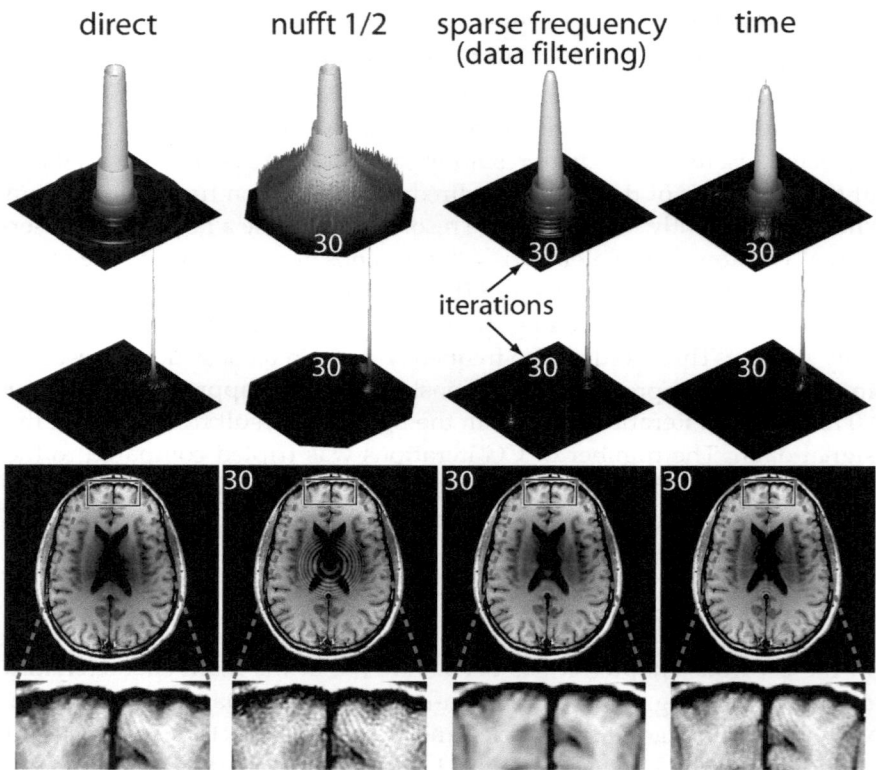

Figure 7.8: PSF analysis and Gibbs ringing; similar to Fig. 7.7, however, with a radial trajectory. Top row: For the central location, direct reconstruction with FBP performs very well. Only the iterative nuFFT algorithm (type 1/2) has significant sidelobes; they quickly vanish with increasing distance from the center - in contrast to the corresponding artifact resulting from Cartesian encoding. Middle row: In this example, the same number of CG iterations (30) was used for all reconstructions. For peripheral locations, the filtered frequency-domain method has a reduced spatial resolution. This shows that more iterations are required to reach optimality when the signal data are filtered prior to iterative reconstruction. Bottom row: The in vivo images support the simulation results: Direct reconstruction gives an excellent image, the nuFFT exhibits prominent Gibbs ringing at the center, and the filtered reconstruction yields reduced resolution when reconstruction is stopped already after 30 iterations.

a 256×256-reconstruction grid and all reconstructions were stopped after 30 iterations. Besides the PSF plots, 2D brain slices are depicted, reconstructed on a 512×512-grid from 410 projections, each consisting of 256 data points.[9]

The figure illustrates that, overall, the image quality with the radial trajectory seems to be higher than the quality that is achieved with the Cartesian PatLoc trajectory. In contrast to Cartesian encoding, the direct reconstruction can, with respect to image quality, compete with the iterative reconstructions. The direct reconstruction exhibits almost no Gibbs ringing, and also image resolution appears to be fairly high. A noisy image with pronounced Gibbs ringing at the center is found with the nuFFT implementation of type $1/2$, where the image is intermediately reconstructed onto a regular grid in PatLoc encoding space. Recent results [[86]] show that significantly better results are found with a nuFFT implementation that reconstructs onto a regular grid in image space, resulting in images that have almost the same quality than those that are reconstructed with the computation-intensive time-domain reconstruction method. Thresholding the frequency-domain reconstruction was more effective than for the lower-resolved Cartesian phantom image, with a speedup factor of approximately 40 instead of 20. Comparison to the time-domain image clearly shows the effect that, after 30 iterations, optimal resolution is almost reached for the unfiltered reconstruction, whereas more iterations are required for the filtered version.

The noise characteristics of the different reconstructions are shown in Fig. 7.9. Again, all iterative methods were stopped after 30 iterations. From the nonlinearities of the SEMs, a quadratic dependency of noise and radius is to be expected. This dependency is less well reproduced with the iterative methods compared to the direct reconstruction. The lowest SNR is found with the nuFFT implementation. With Tikhonov regularization, however, the quadratic dependency can almost be recovered. Interestingly, the time-domain reconstruction shows a slightly increased noise level compared to the direct method, whereas the filtered frequency-domain reconstruction yields images with higher SNR. This behavior is related to the reciprocal property that image resolution is the highest with the time-domain method, and the lowest with the accelerated frequency-domain method, if stopped too early.

---

[9]For details about the acquisition consult the previous chapter, where the same data were used.

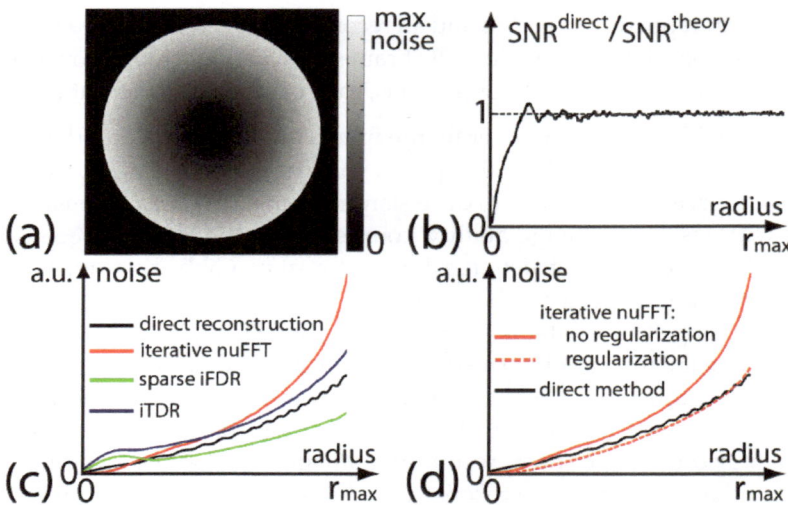

Figure 7.9: Noise propagation for several different reconstruction methods applied to radial PatLoc data. (a, b) repeat Fig. 6.8a,c. (a) With pure quadrupolar encoding, the noise level increases almost quadratically toward the periphery for the direct method. (b) This is in conformity with theoretical calculations. (c) Also the images reconstructed with the different iterative methods (all stopped after 30 iterations) have a higher noise level with increasing radius. There are, however, significant differences, with a more than quadratic increase of noise for the nuFFT implementation. (d) Tikhonov regularization seems to be appropriate to recover the quadratic dependency of the noise also for the nuFFT implementation.

Subsampled Trajectory   The previous chapter has shown that direct reconstruction is problematic if subsampled radial trajectories are used. As iterative methods have the potential to process RF-sensitivity data more effectively, it can be expected that the undersampling artifact is diminished with iterative methods. Fig. 7.10 shows that this is indeed the case for a fourfold subsampled radial trajectory. One aspect of the filtered reconstruction should not be overlooked: In contrast to Fig. 7.8, image resolution is not reduced, even though the reconstruction was stopped earlier than the time-domain method (25 instead of 30 iterations). The reason for this positive effect is that no window function was applied to the signal data, but the filtering was undone after application of the filtered encoding matrix. For this radial trajectory, the slight data inconsistency resulting from thresholding manifests as a prominent Gibbs ringing at the center, similar to

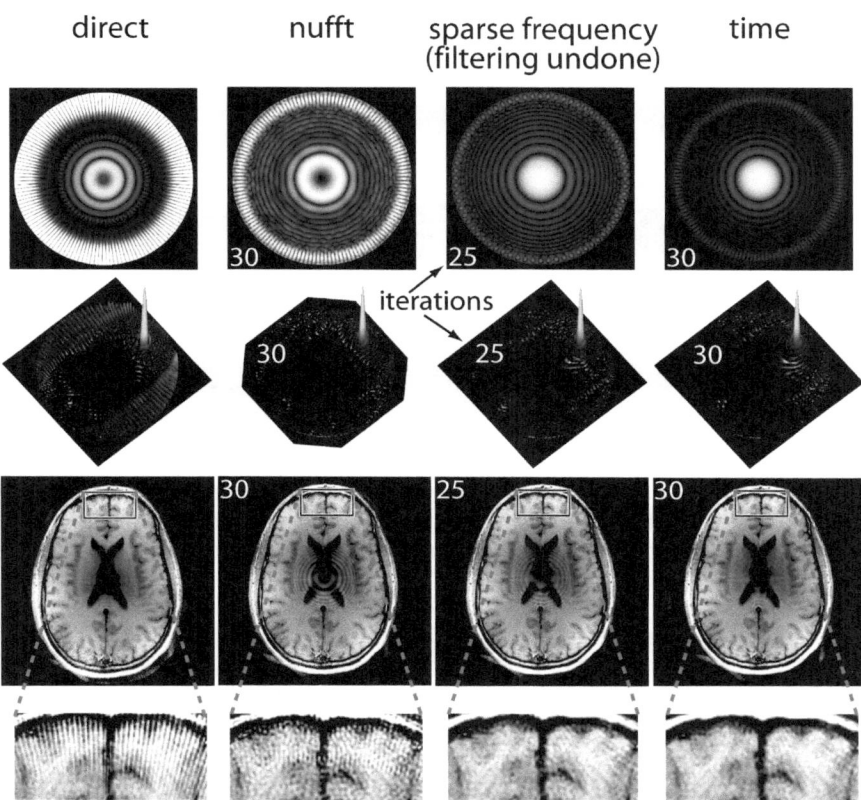

Figure 7.10: PSF analysis and Gibbs ringing; similar to Figure 7.8, but with a $4\times$ subsampled radial trajectory. Top row: For the central PSF, a star-shaped artifact appears along the radial direction. Compared to the direct method, signal contamination is less pronounced, yet still present, for the nuFFT reconstruction, and does almost not occur with the sparse frequency-domain reconstruction and the time-domain method. Middle row: The peripheral PSFs indicate that signal contributions from distant voxels should usually not pose a problem; only direct reconstruction exhibits slight leakage. Bottom row: The star-shaped artifact resulting from the central region corrupts the image for the direct and the iterative nuFFT method. The artifact is almost entirely suppressed with the other two methods. Note that the data were not filtered for the frequency-domain reconstruction as in Fig. 7.8. Consequently, already after 25 iteration, an optimal image resolution is reached; however, a Gibbs ringing artifact appears at the center.

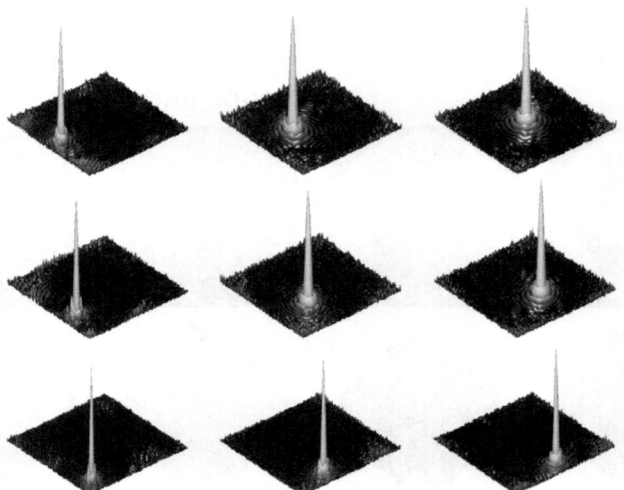

Figure 7.11: PSFs for the time-domain reconstruction simulated with a 4D-RIO PatLoc trajectory. The PSFs indicate that the reconstruction is generally well-behaved; only some minor signal contamination to distant voxels is observed. Shown are PSFs at nine locations from the bottom left quadrant of the FOV. Therefore, the PSF at the top right is actually at the center of the FOV. For the other three quadrants, the PSFs look very similar (not depicted). It is clearly visible that near the center, the PSFs are slightly broader than at the periphery. This is in conformity with the corresponding extent of the local k-space shown in Fig. 3.6c.

the artifact that occurs with the nuFFT reconstruction, yet less pronounced. This ringing is not observed when the signal data are filtered (cf. Fig. 7.8).

c) Multi-Dimensional PatLoc Trajectory

An exciting further development of the PatLoc hardware has been the extension to multiple gradient channels. The 4D-RIO trajectory is an excellent example, which makes full use of the new hardware configuration. The time-domain and the accelerated frequency-domain method are evaluated here using this trajectory.

PSF Analysis Fig. 7.11 represents a PSF analysis of the 4D-RIO trajectory with 24 readouts, each having 24 data points, reconstructed on a 256 × 256-grid with the time-domain method. The PSFs are in conformity with the local k-space of the trajectory, shown in Fig. 3.6c, page 113, with a

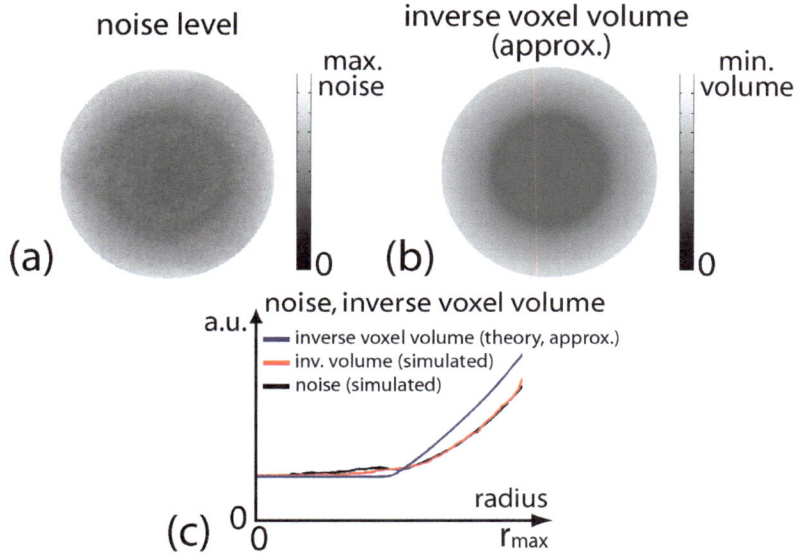

Figure 7.12: Noise distribution for a 4D-RIO trajectory. (a) The noise level in the reconstructed image has a nearly radially symmetric distribution. (b) A similar distribution has the inverse of the voxel volume, estimated from the extent of the local k-space at the corresponding position. (c) The 1D plot illustrates that noise (black) and estimated inverse voxel volume (blue) deviate moderately from each other. Interestingly, there is almost no difference if the voxel volume is determined more exactly by measuring the 2D-FWHM of the 2D-PSFs for locations with different distance from the symmetry center (red). Note that only relative deviations are plotted, normalized at $r = 0$.

nearly constant spatial resolution at the center, and a higher resolution at the periphery. The PSFs are generally well-behaved. The frequency-domain reconstruction yields results that are very similar; a separate figure is therefore not shown. It has to be noted that it would be possible to improve image resolution (width of main peak) with the same amount of data points by moving farther out in PatLoc k-space; this would, however, reduce the sampling density with adverse consequences for the quality of the PSF sidelobes, very similar to conventional PI, but in a more sensitive way than usual.

Noise Analysis Results of an SNR analysis for the 4D-RIO trajectory and the time-domain reconstruction (25 iterations) are illustrated in Fig. 7.12.

The graph shows that - similar to 2D PatLoc (cf. Fig. 7.9) - variations in SNR are dominated by differences in image resolution. According to subfigure 7.12c, almost no difference between the spatial variations of noise and image resolution can be appreciated if the voxel size is measured from the 2D-FWHM of the PSF at the corresponding location. The figure also verifies that the extent of local k-space can serve as a quick (but only rough) estimate of local image resolution, and therefore also of the noise distribution in the image. In the shown example, the extent of the local k-space was estimated by calculating the length of the largest local k-space vector. This approximate method seems to overestimate the spatial resolution once the central regime of constant resolution is abandoned toward the periphery of the FOV.

Experimental Results   Reconstruction results of a phantom consisting of tubes filled with doped water and results of an in vivo slice of a human head are shown in Fig. 7.13. All measurements were performed using 4D-RIO with 256^2 data points and a reconstruction grid with 320×320 lattice points. The images verify the capability of the time-domain and the accelerated frequency-domain method (with filtering of the signal data) to consistently reconstruct a magnetization distribution that has been encoded with a multi-dimensional PatLoc trajectory.[10] In the depicted example, the frequency-domain reconstruction needed about twice as many iterations to reach a comparable image resolution than the time-domain method. As the image could be reconstructed approximately 20-times faster, a total speedup factor of one order of magnitude could be achieved. The images are not higher resolved than typical 256×256 acquisitions performed with linear gradients. Moving out farther in PatLoc k-space would significantly improve image resolution (thereby, however, reducing the sampling density that might negatively affect image quality). In this example, one of the very first 4D-RIO in vivo acquisitions, optimization of image resolution was not the focus. On the contrary, a high sampling density was chosen in order to ensure that no artifacts would be introduced that are caused by insufficient sampling, thereby facilitating the detection of other causes for residual image artifacts.

In fact, the reconstructed phantom images are almost artifact-free. Close inspection of the in vivo image shows some ringing-like artifacts originating

---

[10]For the frequency-domain method, each readout was divided into two segments because, in 4D-RIO, the effective encoding field changes abruptly at the center of the signal readout.

from the center. This artifact shows a problem that seems to be related to multi-dimensional encoding: Already very small differences between the SEM sensitivities that are assumed in the reconstruction and the actual SEMs that are applied during signal encoding cause significant artifacts. The images shown in subfigures 7.13a,b and d have been reconstructed from data, where the SEMs have been calibrated as explained in [[42]]. Subfigure 7.13c demonstrates that severe artifacts indeed occur if SEM calibration is not adequately performed prior to image reconstruction. The effects of miscalibration are currently being investigated.

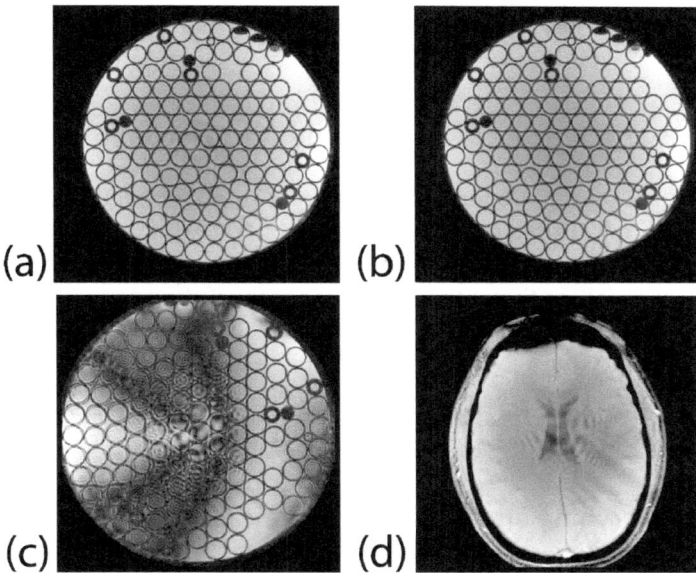

Figure 7.13: Reconstruction from phantom and in vivo measurements using a 4D-RIO PatLoc trajectory. (a) Time-domain reconstruction (30 iterations) of a phantom consisting of parallel tubes filled with doped water. (b) Sparse frequency-domain reconstruction with data filtering (60 iterations) for the same dataset. Almost no difference to the unfiltered reconstruction is visible. The good image quality of the images (a,b) are a result of exact calibration of the SEMs. (c) If the calibration is performed with less care, deterioration of image quality occurs. (d) Time-domain reconstruction for an in vivo brain slice. The brain slice is well depicted. Only some extended Gibbs ringing-like artifacts are visible which may be attributed to non-exact SEM calibration.

7.3 Evaluation

Several image reconstruction methods were tested with a Cartesian, a radial and a 4D-RIO PatLoc encoding trajectory. Results were presented that allow assessment of the methods regarding image resolution, SNR and the capability to suppress aliasing artifacts. In this chapter, the emphasis has been given to a CG-based method that circumvents direct inversion of the encoding process by iterated forward evaluation of a linear signal model. This approach is very general, but also very computation-intensive, and therefore several approaches were investigated to accelerate image reconstruction. These and related topics are further evaluated below, and alternatives beyond linear image reconstruction are briefly discussed.

7.3.1 Image Properties: Encoding and Reconstruction

One may ask to what extent image properties are predetermined by the chosen encoding strategy, and to what extent they can further be influenced by the particular image reconstruction method. Note that the iterative CG reconstruction algorithms, that are the subject of the present chapter, can be treated as linear methods.[11] Therefore, this problem can be approached with the tools of chapter 4.2.2c, page 151f.

Image Resolution   The spatial resolution of the reconstructed images can be analyzed with the SRF; the SRF naturally separates encoding from reconstruction because it is, according to Eq. 2.16, page 50, given by a weighted sum of the encoding functions, and, whereas the encoding functions exclusively depend on the chosen encoding strategy, it is the reconstruction method that determines the weighting.

Note that the encoding functions have spatial oscillations whose frequency varies significantly over the FOV for nonlinear encoding. These frequencies are primarily caused by SEM encoding and are described by the local k-space (cf. paragraph *The Concept of Local k-Space* in chapter 3.2.2, on page 112ff). Image resolution is bounded by the largest spatial frequency of the local k-space, or, correspondingly, by the maximum oscillation frequency of the encoding functions. The encoding strategy therefore defines the maximum resolution that is achievable at a certain location.

---

[11]However, pay attention to fn. 25, page 93.

Depending on the reconstruction method, the weighting of the encoding functions can be more, but also less efficient, and therefore it is decisive to apply a reconstruction method that is capable of recovering the highest of all encoded spatial oscillations. RF-sensitivity variations can even - especially in regions with weak SEM encoding - enhance the oscillation frequency of the encoding functions. Image reconstruction algorithms can make use of this effect that has been termed *superresolution* in chapter 2.3.1e, page 86ff. And indeed, the results show a superresolution effect for the iterative time-domain reconstruction, especially in regions of very weak gradient encoding.

In some situations, it can be useful to low-pass filter the signal data, for example, in order to reduce Gibbs ringing or to accelerate image reconstruction. If, in this case, the reconstruction remains unaltered, high spatial frequencies are disregarded, and some loss of image resolution occurs. This behavior is observed with the filtered direct reconstructions. If, however, also the reconstruction algorithm is appropriately modified, the high spatial frequencies can be recovered. This is achieved with the filtered frequency-domain reconstruction.

SNR The results, especially Fig. 7.12, have shown that SNR is strongly coupled to the local image resolution, and is therefore primarily determined by the chosen encoding strategy. In the previous two chapters, the proportionality of SNR and effective voxel volume could be proven explicitly for the direct Cartesian and radial PatLoc reconstruction (cf. Eq. 5.28 and Eq. 6.14). The results suggest that this is also the case for multi-dimensional PatLoc trajectories, expressing a general law that local image resolution and local SNR are inversely related to each other, a property that is well-known from conventional imaging with linear SEMs (cf. Eq. 2.36).

This relationship between resolution and SNR also explains, at least to some extent, unequal noise levels in images that are reconstructed from the same dataset, but with a different method. For example, consider Fig. 7.8 and Fig. 7.9; there it is shown that, if the iterative algorithms are stopped at an early stage, the time-domain reconstruction has already recovered higher spatial frequencies than the accelerated frequency-domain reconstruction with data filtering. Consequently, also the noise level is higher for the time-domain reconstruction. However, the noise level of the reconstructed images is not uniquely determined by the resulting image resolution. In Fig. 7.9c it is shown that the iterative nuFFT reconstruction, type 1/2, has a high noise level which does not come along with a corresponding increase in image resolution (cf. Fig. 7.8). Fig. 7.9d illustrates that with Tikhonov regularization the expected relationship of image SNR and image resolution can be recovered. As regularization is related to the numerical condition of the encoding matrix, numerical effects seem to have a crucial influence on the noise distribution of the reconstructed images when iterative CG methods are used for reconstruction.

Aliasing   In this chapter, aliasing was only investigated for fourfold sub-sampled radial trajectories. The PSF plots shown in Fig. 7.10 reveal that the star-shaped undersampling artifact exists for all reconstruction methods. However, compared to the direct and type 1/2 nuFFT reconstruction, the artifacts are nearly entirely suppressed by the time- and frequency-domain reconstructions such that no undersampling artifact is visible in the shown in vivo images. The artifact suppression is achieved by a similar mechanism that is also responsible for superresolution: The time-domain method and its frequency-domain analogue efficiently incorporate RF-sensitivity information into the reconstruction. The results show that artifact suppression is typically much more effective than the superresolution effect. This is in conformity with standard PI. The reasons for this behavior are similar for PatLoc and standard PI. Image resolution is a local effect, where (apart from extreme locations) SEM encoding generates much higher spatial frequencies than RF encoding. Aliasing, on the other hand, is a non-local effect, where accrued RF variations can effectively compensate for deficiencies in SEM encoding.

7.3.2   "Gold Standard": Time-Domain Reconstruction

The results have demonstrated that, overall, the time-domain reconstruction outperforms the other reconstruction methods regarding image quality. Image resolution and artifact suppression are highly optimized, and also SNR is near-to-optimal. Only occasionally, other methods perform better (for example, increased SNR and reduced Gibbs ringing by direct reconstruction from radial PatLoc data in Fig. 7.8). Therefore, the time-domain method may be regarded as a sort of "gold standard". Keep in mind, however, that the time-domain method is an iterative method that cannot converge under the presence of noise. This is problematic because the algorithm must be

stopped at the right time to find a good compromise between image resolution and noise/artifact level (cf. Fig. 2.17, page 94). For ill-conditioned
problems, Tikhonov regularization might be required to control the noise.
By far the largest problem with the time-domain method is its unfavorable
numerical complexity of typically about $\mathcal{O}(N^4)$ for each CG iteration and
2D imaging, where $N \approx 256$ for high-resolution anatomical images. As
a result, the reconstruction time can already be prohibitively long for 2D
imaging, not to mention the time required for 3D imaging sequences.

7.3.3 Methods to Accelerate Image Reconstruction

To overcome the problem of long reconstruction times several strategies
were suggested in this chapter to accelerate the time-domain reconstruction.

Brute Force: Parallel Computing Recall that the time-consuming step of
the reconstruction is a matrix-vector multiplication involving the very large
encoding matrix $\mathbf{E}$ and its adjoint $\mathbf{E}^H$. For high-resolution 2D imaging, $\mathbf{E}$
cannot be stored in memory. For example, consider a 256^2 acquisition with
8 receiver coil reconstructed onto a 512^2 lattice. Even with single precision,
explicit storage of $\mathbf{E}$ would require more than 1 TB of memory capacity,
which is currently far beyond from being acceptable for standard image
processing. Therefore, it is useful to break down the matrix-vector multiplication to less than 10^6 vector-vector multiplications with almost no storage
needs. These vector-vector multiplications are ideally performed simultaneously with an enormous potential for the reduction of reconstruction time
through parallel computation. In the last few years CPUs have begun to
being equipped with several cores, thus allowing a small amount of parallelization. Much more useful in this regard are GPUs, which have many
more processing units. Compared to an initial Matlab implementation of
the time-domain method for CPU processing, an acceleration of three orders
of magnitude could already be achieved with an optimized code that has
also been parallelized using CUDA (Compute Unified Device Architecture;
Nvidia, Santa Clara, CA, USA), thereby reducing reconstruction time from
several days to a few minutes only for typical high-resolution 2D datasets.

Sparsification of the Encoding Matrix Parallel computing may reduce
the reconstruction time, however, the number of computed operations
remains the same. All multi-dimensional imaging sequences that have been

discussed so far in the literature form generalized projections, for which the computation load can be reduced by approximating the encoding matrix by a sparser frequency-domain version of it. This approximation leads to artifacts. In this chapter, methods were presented, which reduce these artifacts by applying an appropriate filter function. With the developed methods, computation time becomes independent from the amount of data that is acquired along the signal readout. In fact, the numerical complexity reduces from $\mathcal{O}(N^4)$ to $\mathcal{O}(kN^3)$, $k \ll N$, for each CG loop. This means that the speedup factor scales linearly with the length of the readout. In the shown examples, a readout of length $64, 128, 256$ resulted approximately in a speedup of $10, 20, 40$, respectively. The exact acceleration depends on the used computer hardware and implementation.

It has been shown that data consistency is affected by the filter, and needs to be restored. Two methods were described. One method corrects the filtering in the forward operation after application of the encoding matrix. It could be verified that not more CG iterations are required than if filtering is omitted. The reconstruction has worked very well for the radial PatLoc trajectory, but the ringing artifact at the center was less effectively suppressed compared to the unfiltered reconstruction. The ringing might be further suppressed by using an adaptive threshold level, with a more precise modeling at the center; with a similar method, the artifact power could be reduced for 4D-RIO [[43]].

The ringing did not appear with an alternative method, also discussed in this chapter, where the signal data are filtered to ensure data consistency. It was shown that this method is less sensitive to inconsistencies that are introduced by thresholding, yielding a high image quality also for the Cartesian PatLoc dataset and the 4D-RIO trajectory. The results have shown that this approach requires $2 - 3\times$ more iterations than usual to achieve an optimal image resolution; nevertheless, a speedup factor of 10 to 20 seems realistic also for this method in high-resolution applications, but numerical options should be evaluated in the future to reduce the number of iterations. No image degradation (e.g. higher noise level) by the increased number of iterations was observed. Finally, note that the filtering only affects frequency encoding, not phase encoding. As a consequence, an anisotropic image resolution may occur during the first iterations (for example, for Cartesian trajectories). The anisotropy vanishes with an increasing number of iterations, and is typically not even observable during the first iterations because the spatial direction of frequency encoding typically changes in PatLoc imaging between successive projections (for example, for radial trajectories or for 4D-RIO).

nuFFT For encoding with only two SEMs, image reconstruction can be accelerated by several orders of magnitude because SEM encoding can then be described as a nuDFT for which fast nuFFT implementations exist that reduce the numerical complexity of each CG iteration from $\mathcal{O}(N^4)$ to $\mathcal{O}(k^2 N^2 \log N^2)$, $k \ll N$, thus permitting sub-second calculations for each iteration. For the nuFFT of type 3, k is typically higher than for the nuFFT of the other two types (cf. e.g. [30]). Note that the nuFFT has the same dependency on the problems size as the FFT, however, with a constant $k > 1$ for the nuFFT.

Latest results [[86]] show that acceleration of the iterative time-domain method with the type 3 nuFFT does almost not affect image quality. The examples above have shown that the same is typically true for the type 1/2 nuFFT – with one exception: Problems may occur at locations, where the SEMs have vanishing spatial gradients. Conceptually, type 3 and type 1/2 nuFFT reconstructions differ in that the former uses a regular distribution of image voxels and the latter a non-regular, with larger and fewer image voxels in regions where the SEMs are flat. The type 3 nuFFT therefore has the advantage that a higher voxel density exists in problematic regions. Consequenty, RF encoding is more efficient in those regions, and a superresolution effect with better image quality can be observed. An exact analysis of this effect, and whether other effects are involved, is part of ongoing work.

7.3.4 Beyond Matrix Inversion Approaches

The iterative reconstruction methods that were analyzed in this chapter use the CG method to solve a linear signal model without additional constraints. From a numerical point of view, the two properties - linearity and absence of constraints - make the methods of this chapter some of the most fundamental and also best-behaved reconstruction problems that one may encounter. Nevertheless, experience with conventional imaging has shown that under certain circumstances it can be useful to formulate and solve more complex reconstruction problems. Some approaches that might be useful also in the context of PatLoc imaging are given below.

Nonlinear Reconstruction   Very interesting is the method developed by Uecker et al. [184] to determine the magnetization distribution without the need of having to provide predetermined RF-coil sensitivity profiles as inputs to the iterative reconstruction. In this method, magnetization and RF-coil sensitivity profiles are jointly estimated. Then, the forward operation is not a linear system any more, but a nonlinear problem. Therefore, the linear CG method is not appropriate and other, nonlinear, optimization algorithms must be employed like the (iteratively regularized) Gauss Newton method [184]. This method might be extended in PatLoc to reduce the problem of accurate SEM calibration by estimating additional calibration parameters.

Nonlinear reconstruction has found even more attention when prior knowledge is added. For example, Block et al. [13] have included an l_1-total-variation regularization term into the forward model yielding reduced artifacts for subsampled conventional radial imaging data. Noteworthy is the approach pursued by Knoll et al. [85, 84] who use a generalized total variation regularization term of second order [16], and a primal-dual optimization algorithm [20] to further improve image quality. Initial investigations with this regularization term in combination with radial PatLoc data are very promising [[86]].

Learning from the Fractional Fourier Transform   A very different approach has recently been introduced [127], and was adapted in [179] for O-space imaging [178], where a quadratic field is applied in conjunction with two gradient fields for in-plane encoding. Motivated by the special nature of the used encoding strategy, a reconstruction was proposed that is based on the fractional Fourier transform.

For the three-dimensional O-space trajectory a similar problem occurs with CG-based reconstructions that is also encountered with 4D-RIO: Slight systematic errors between the encoding model and the actual encoding process can lead to signal loss, even signal voids, that destroy the diagnostic usability of the reconstructed images if not adequately accounted for by applying a well-tuned calibration method prior to reconstruction. Stockmann et al. observed in [179] that the fractional Fourier transform can transfer the problem of generating signal voids to mere geometric distortions, which are far more acceptable than signal voids. Unfortunately, the fractional Fourier transform is not suited for a general encoding scheme, and was even not exactly suited for the O-space model (therefore introducing significant artifacts). Nevertheless, the approach points in the right direction and is a first indication that the calibration issue might ultimately be overcome by making use of alternative reconstruction methods beyond simply inverting the encoding matrix directly, or indirectly with the help of iterative solvers. However, adequate methods that can be used for a large class of encoding strategies are still waiting to be discovered.

7.3.5 Conclusions

For 2D encoding with two SEMs, iterative reconstruction offers a valuable alternative to direct image reconstruction, especially for subsampled trajectories. Reconstruction can be performed efficiently because the calculations can be accelerated with nuFFT algorithms. The faster nuFFT type 1/2 reconstruction yields images represented in PatLoc encoding space. While this approach should often be acceptable, problematic encoding strategies (like those with locally very weak SEM encoding) are better handled with a nuFFT of type 3 with reconstruction immediately into the final image space.

For 2D encoding with more than two SEMs, acceleration with the nuFFT is not possible. The time-domain CG reconstruction can be speeded up through parallel processing of the imaging data. Further acceleration is possible for generalized projections, where the encoding process can be modeled with a filtered and sparser frequency-domain version of the encoding matrix. This approach is feasible because the filtering does not affect consistency with the measurement data if appropriately accounted for. For high-resolution 2D imaging, image reconstruction can be performed in the range of seconds with an optimized implementation of the filtered frequency-domain method, which would allow image reconstruction immediately on the imaging hardware while the examination is being carried out.

Further reduction of computing time and lower requirements for the fidelity of the SEM-sensitivity data are two major objectives that should guide the development of alternative ways of signal encoding and image reconstruction in the future.

Chapter 8

Summary and Outlook

T He thesis is summarized in this concluding chapter, and some directions for future research are suggested.

8.1 Summary

The goal of this thesis was to contribute to the research field of encoding with nonlinear magnetic fields in MRI, a topic of increasing interest that has only received scant attention in the past. The conducted work has been part of PatLoc, a research direction that combines nonlinear encoding with parallel imaging, initiated by Prof. Dr. Jürgen Hennig within the INUMAC project. PatLoc offers new options to improve the encoding efficiency, to reduce peripheral nerve stimulation and to develop other interesting applications such as those that arise from advances in shimming methodology with nonlinear phase preparation, with many more applications expected to arise (see chapter 3.2); research in this field is still at the beginning.

During the course of this thesis the theoretical foundations of PatLoc encoding and image reconstruction were elaborated. Efficient reconstruction algorithms were developed, and the effectiveness of several encoding and reconstruction strategies was theoretically discussed and assessed by evaluating imaging results.

The algorithms were applied to simulated data, but also to experimental data. The experimental part resulted from team work, in total conducted by not fewer than ten researchers, mainly members of the Freiburg MR-Physics group, but also employees from industrial partners. The experiments required:

- Design and manufacturing of hardware for the generation of NB-SEMs and integration into existing MR scanner environments.
- Development and implementation of useful encoding strategies.
- Data acquisition and pre-processing.

In this thesis, only those topics were presented with significant own contributions that have resulted (or will result) at least in a co-authorship of a
publication or a co-inventorship of a patent application.

Generalizing Parallel Imaging   For this work, it has been extremely useful to realize that PatLoc generalizes state-of-the-art imaging technology
that makes use of parallel reception devices. Parallel imaging has been the
subject of intensive research activities for more than ten years now, and
therefore mature know-how was available on which this thesis could be
based on, even though not much knowledge had been generated up to that
point on nonlinear encoding. The generalization to nonlinear encoding
favored the adoption of a rather abstract theoretical point of view; this
approach facilitated the detection of principles that are common to conventional imaging and PatLoc imaging, and the analysis of effects which are
specifically caused by the nonlinearities and/or non-bijectiveness of the
encoding fields. While writing this thesis and reviewing existing reconstruction methods, it became apparent that this abstract point of view also
sheds new light onto conventional image reconstruction by revealing connections between established methods like SENSE and GRAPPA or between
gridding reconstruction and the general matrix approach (see chapter 2).

The theoretical background of encoding with nonlinear fields was elaborated in chapter 4. A generalized k-space concept was introduced that loses
its meaning as the Fourier space of the encoded object. The advantage of the
introduced concept is that it leads to a separation of the temporal degrees
of freedom (k-space trajectory) and the spatial degrees of freedom (SEM
geometries). Despite the nonlinearity of the SEMs, the encoding process is
still described as a linear operator that allows application of linear image
reconstruction methods. Image reconstruction reduces therefore to a simple
matrix inversion and image properties can be calculated easily with linear
algebra. Unfortunately, this approach normally only works in 1D. In higher
dimensions, the matrix to be handled is huge, in 2D almost as large as
one million entries along each of the two dimensions. Therefore, it was
essential to develop efficient reconstruction algorithms. Due to the inverse
nature of the reconstruction a high degree of accuracy is required for the
formulation of adequate reconstruction methods. It could be shown that, in
this regard, the requirements can be less demanding for the determination
of fundamental image properties; an acceptable accuracy is often ensured

with approximate methods. For example, image resolution can be predicted well with the concept of local k-space.

In this thesis, the possibilities of PatLoc were explored by analyzing encoding strategies of increasing complexity, thereby developing a number of methods for accurate image reconstruction. To focus on the essentials, only static anatomical imaging was dealt with (thus excluding for example cardiac imaging), where a 2D slice was excited with the standard z-gradient.

Encoding and Reconstruction with Two SEMs The most basic 2D situation one might think of when dealing with NB-SEMs is an experiment where the x- and y-gradients are replaced by a PatLoc coil that generates two orthogonal quadrupolar SEMs. There is evidence (see Appendix A.4) that these fields represent a first natural generalization from linear SEMs toward arbitrarily-shaped NB-SEMs.

Such a setup was put into practice (see chapter 3.3); this had the advantage that conventional sequences could be reused, thus allowing to purely focus on the additional spatial degrees of freedom that come along with PatLoc imaging. Image properties that depend on the time-courses of the applied SEMs, such as image contrast, are not affected compared to conventional imaging as long as the same sequence parameters are used. In standard imaging, the most basic sequence is a Cartesian trajectory. This sequence was adapted for PatLoc imaging. Encoding and reconstruction with this trajectory was analyzed in detail in chapter 5. The same experimental setup was then driven with a non-Cartesian (radial) trajectory and formed the subject matter of chapter 6.

It is remarkable that for the Cartesian trajectory, image resolution and noise propagation can be described by simple analytical expressions, thus allowing a precise analysis of this basic PatLoc experiment. The main result was that the application of NB-SEMs basically leads to a spatial relocalization of the magnetization in the Fourier domain of the signal data. The non-bijectiveness of the encoding has the positive effect of an intrinsic acceleration, however, also aliasing is observed. This artifact is resolved in PatLoc by supplementing SEM encoding with RF-sensitivity encoding. Undersampling typically results in reduced noise amplification in PatLoc compared to Cartesian SENSE because aliased locations are distributed over the image and not along a single direction. It could also be shown that the nonlinearities of the SEMs lead to image distortions and intensity modulations. These SEM-dependent effects are corrected by rewarping the image and multiplying the final image with an intensity correction factor, thus introducing variations in image resolution and SNR.

These effects are therefore directly related to variations of the gradient strength of the SEMs. This property can be exploited to improve the encoding efficiency by increasing the gradient strength in a ROI. Due to the fact that magnetic fields are the strongest near the coil surfaces, the encoding information can be enhanced most efficiently at the periphery of the imaging volume. This could be verified also with the quadrupolar design that showed a higher spatial resolution at the periphery of the imaging volume compared to standard imaging and a lower resolution at the center, which is useful for example in cortical imaging.

Image properties are determined by the SEM geometry to a high degree, but also the trajectory and the chosen reconstruction method can have a significant influence. Three different reconstruction approaches were discussed for Cartesian as well as non-Cartesian trajectories:

1. Direct Reconstruction in the image domain.
2. Direct Reconstruction in the PatLoc k-space domain.
3. Iterative reconstruction using the CG method.

It turned out that all reconstructions could be formulated in a way that is similar to the corresponding counterparts in PI. Methods which are based on k-space, such as GRAPPA, can be applied to subsampled PatLoc data without any modification. In the image domain, Cartesian SENSE must be slightly modified to account for the nonlinearities of the SEMs (intensity-correction, rewarping). An interesting difference between the two methods is that aliasing can be resolved in the image domain, whether resulting from subsampling or from the non-bijectiveness of the SEM encoding. In the k-domain, it is, however, a much more intricate process to resolve the ambiguities that are caused by the non-bijectiveness of the SEMs.

Not much less efficient than those direct methods is iterative CG reconstruction because, with two SEMs, the time-domain reconstruction algorithm can be accelerated by applying the nuFFT in the forward operation. Almost no compromise regarding image quality has to be made with such a nuFFT-based reconstruction. In extreme cases of vanishing gradients, an implementation that uses the nuFFT of type 3 with a homogeneous distribution of image voxels should be preferred to the nuFFT of type 1/2 with an inhomogeneous distribution. This is different for direct reconstruction, which does not profit from using a homogeneous reconstruction grid.

To be precise, the number of required elementary computations is the least for the Cartesian direct method with $\mathcal{O}(N^2 \log N^2)$, where $N \approx 256$ describes the problem size, followed by $\mathcal{O}(k^2 N^2 \log N^2)$, $k \ll N$, for the fastest direct non-Cartesian method to $\mathcal{O}(lk^2 N \log N)$ for iterative nuFFT reconstruction, where l describes the number of iterations and where $k \ll N$ is larger for the nuFFT of type 3 than for the nuFFT of type 1/2. Direct image space reconstruction is therefore faster than any of the presented iterative algorithms. However, the dependency on the problem size N is the same, and even equivalent to the FFT; this ensures that the reconstruction times do not differ by several orders of magnitude and can compete with the fastest image reconstruction algorithms used in standard MRI.

In most situations, the faster methods guarantee a similar image quality than the more computation-intensive methods. Only at locations with heavy SEM-encoding deficiencies (vanishing local gradients) significant differences may occur. It has been shown that radial imaging trajectories are less problematic than Cartesian trajectories because the isotropic shape of the radial PSF reduces pronounced Gibbs ringing artifacts that emanate from regions with vanishing gradients. Iterative reconstruction makes more efficient use of the additional information provided by the RF sensitivities than the direct methods and are therefore superior, especially for subsampled trajectories; for example, a star-shaped undersampling artifact, resulting from radial quadrupolar encoding, could be reduced significantly with iterative reconstruction. With respect to image quality, the unaccelerated iterative time-domain algorithm may serve as a "gold standard" reconstruction technique.

It can be concluded that the presented direct reconstruction methods are typically a good choice, also under strongly nonlinear and non-bijective imaging conditions. They are very fast and do not suffer from the problem of having to define a proper stopping criterion. In extreme cases, however, iterative image reconstruction can be superior to direct reconstruction.

Encoding and Reconstruction with More than Two SEMs The last encoding strategy that was analyzed marked an important step toward more flexible encoding. When only two SEMs are available combinations of those can be formed, but tight restrictions on the achievable field geometry exist.

For example, with pure quadrupolar encoding, the superimposed field still has a quadrupolar geometry. With more than two SEMs, driven to its extreme, the effective magnetic encoding field can take a great variety of shapes and can change from one instant of time to the next almost without restriction.

The experimental setup did not provide such flexible encoding, but it allowed superposition of the two quadrupolar SEMs with the standard linear gradient fields. The resulting field is also a quadrupolar field, whose center, however, is not bound to one location, thus eliminating the problem of extreme encoding deficiencies. Signal encoding and image reconstruction was investigated with 4D-RIO, a particularly efficient sequence.

A problem with multi-dimensional trajectories, such as 4D-RIO, is that direct inversion of the encoding matrix with a complexity of $\mathcal{O}(N^6)$ is intractable, and iterative CG-based reconstruction cannot be accelerated with a nuFFT and therefore requires $\mathcal{O}(lN^4)$ elementary operations. Image reconstruction is therefore a challenging problem for multi-dimensional PatLoc trajectories. Reconstruction time can be reduced significantly by exploiting the highly-parallelizable structure of the reconstruction. Even further acceleration is possible by making the problem sparser. For example, it was shown that a large class of multi-dimensional sequences, among them 4D-RIO, form generalized image projections that are sparse in the frequency domain if adequately filtered, thereby reducing the numerical complexity to $\mathcal{O}(lkN^3)$, with $k \ll N$. With this method, the computation time does not increase for longer signal readouts. For high-resolution 2D-imaging applications, the additional speedup is typically well above one order of magnitude, and reconstruction time is brought down to the range of seconds, fast enough to be applicable during the examination, provided that the imaging hardware is equipped with processing units that are specialized for parallel computing.

With the iterative CG method high-quality images from 4D-RIO phantom and in vivo data could be reconstructed. However, successful reconstruction required extremely well-calibrated data, thus showing a very high sensibility to systematic errors of the used signal model.

The performed analysis has shown that multi-dimensional encoding offers more degrees of freedom for trajectory design than encoding with only two SEMs. At the same time, the imaging problem becomes more complex, but it could be shown that tools are available that help to get the problems under control. Especially helpful in this regard is the local k-space concept, which has proven useful in estimating spatial encoding properties such as local image resolution or in assessing if the encoding strategy ensures that the bulk part of the relevant signal energy is acquired.

Overall Assessment Table 8.1 lists several reconstruction algorithms that were discussed in this thesis and compares their numerical complexity with the range of encoding strategies that are compatible with the corresponding algorithm. The table clearly shows a rule that often appears in practice: The smaller the scope of a method, the more optimization is possible concerning computing time. In practice, this means that the Cartesian reconstruction can be performed in the range of milliseconds whereas the iterative time-domain method requires at least several minutes to reconstruct a single 2D image on a modern desktop PC equipped with a GPU. As a rule of thumb, image reconstruction is fast and also robust as long as only two SEMs are used to encode a 2D slice; the situation becomes much more challenging for multi-dimensional encoding strategies, where some problems could be solved already, yet by far not all.

Within the scope of this thesis, only three encoding strategies could be analyzed in detail. Bringing the results of these three examples together can only explain a small part of what can actually be done with PatLoc. However, the encoding strategies were chosen with care and give an overview of the implications that PatLoc may have on MRI. Nevertheless, caution must be taken when generalizing to other trajectories without a closer analysis. A goal of this thesis was to provide insight and tools for future research in this direction.

The presented material appears to be a good starting point for further generalizations, for example, to nonlinear encoding also during RF transmission, a topic that is part of a separate PhD project that has been termed *ExLoc* by Hans Weber. The general approach taken in this thesis may also serve to quantify further specializations such as the briefly discussed imaging with nonlinear phase-preparation that has generated useful applications already like reduced field-of-view imaging or the elimination of balanced SSFP banding artifacts.

Despite its extent, this thesis has only treated *static* effects; it has largely been disregarded that MRI is a *dynamic* process, where temporal effects play

Table 8.1: Reconstruction algorithms: numerical complexity and scope of applicability ($N \approx 256, k \ll N, l \approx 20 - 40$)

property \ method	direct Cartesian	direct non-Cartesian	iterative nuFFT
operations required $\mathcal{O}(\cdot)$	$N^2 \log N^2$	$k^2 N^2 \log N^2$	$lk^2 N^2 \log N^2$
number of SEMs	2	2	2
direct/iterative	direct	direct	iterative
works with undersampling	+	-	+
trajectory	Cartesian	non-Cartesian	non-Cartesian

property	iterative frequency-domain	iterative time-domain	matrix inversion
operations required $\mathcal{O}(\cdot)$	lkN^3	lN^4	N^6
number of SEMs	arbitrary	arbitrary	arbitrary
direct/iterative	iterative	iterative	direct
works with undersampling	+	+	+
trajectory	generalized projection	arbitrary	arbitrary

a fundamental role. However, a variety of new options also for dynamic encoding become available with PatLoc imaging, especially when multiple magnetic fields are used for signal encoding. As an example may serve a comparison of conventional Fourier imaging with 4D-RIO. The results have shown that static image properties, such as image resolution or SNR, are similar over an extended region; however, the temporal evolution of the applied magnetic fields is very different. Therefore, physiological reactions like PNS will be different. Another example is the separation of signal echoes with a quadratic field that allows dynamic shimming during the acquisition of a single slice. This thesis may have shown the capabilities of PatLoc imaging for spatial encoding; however, these examples illustrate that a great potential also lies in the temporal domain, an aspect that needs to become a focus of future research.

8.2 Ongoing and Future Research

In the course of the PatLoc project, a novel type of gradient hardware has been built, sequences with interesting properties have been realized, adequate reconstruction methods have been implemented and initial medical applications have been developed. This work is currently being continued and future research will also follow these four directions: hardware design, sequence design, image reconstruction and medical applications.

Hardware Design   A high-performance PatLoc coil for in vivo imaging is currently under development. The coil will be similar to the existing PatLoc hardware, but with significantly improved specifications. The industrially manufactured new system will allow a fair comparison with state-of-the-art gradient hardware, and it will be possible to evaluate the imaging results also from a clinical perspective. One drawback will, however, persist: As before, the new system will be equipped with a very limited amount of SEM channels. We have therefore begun to develop also other PatLoc coils with completely different geometries. Sebastian Littin has recently completed construction of a three-channel planar surface coil [[103]]. The next step has to be and will be the development of a much more flexible gradient coil. Christoph Juchem has recently shown that impressive improvements for $B0$-homogeneity can be achieved with a flexible shimming system [79]. Initial steps toward a flexible gradient system have been undertaken by Stefan Wintzheimer [203]. This system has interesting properties, however, there is much room for improvement. The insight we have gained so far in the PatLoc project will enable us to build a gradient system that is as powerful, but much more flexible than our current hardware implementations.

Sequence Design   In this thesis, 2D PatLoc imaging modalities were considered, where slice selection was performed with the linear z-gradient. Very interesting encoding strategies have recently been tested or are being elaborated in the PeXLoc [54, 152] and ExLoc [[191]] projects, where the implications of NB-SEM encoding during RF transmission on the magnetization are explored.

The current PatLoc hardware requires that all developed sequences define time-courses of a maximum of six independent gradient channels. A flexible gradient design will particularly have implications to sequence design. A more flexible system will have many more channels that can all be controlled independently from each other, thus increasing the complexity, most probably to a degree which will be difficult to be handled without the introduction of new concepts.

The local k-space concept [[42]] may help to design appropriate trajectories. In its current form the local k-space distribution only gives a vague estimate of how much aliasing is to be expected, but generally it provides an excellent measure of how the acquired spatial information is distributed over the ROI (thus defining for example image resolution in the ROI). It will be crucial in the future to extend this concept also along the temporal dimension to be able to reliably assess the temporal encoding efficiency and other dynamic properties of the trajectory such as the resulting image contrast or the probability to cause PNS. Novel performance measures also need to be developed that allow one to assess if the trajectory can meet other requirements; for example, the hardware constrains magnetic field amplitudes, as well as spatial and temporal derivatives thereof, and encoding strategies have to be designed such that inevitable calibration errors can be tolerated by the method that is used for image reconstruction. The definition of such performance measures will be essential to facilitate the design of useful PatLoc encoding strategies in the future.

Image Reconstruction   In this thesis, unconstrained linear image reconstruction was shown to be effective in PatLoc imaging. This is especially the case when only two SEMs are involved; in this regard, only occasionally, the presentation has remained vague. For example, evidence still has to be provided that a direct reconstruction is not only partially, but also entirely, feasible in PatLoc k-space, including non-Cartesian trajectories. Also, it is yet not fully clear why iterative reconstruction yields better results with a nuFFT of type 3 than with a nuFFT of type 1/2. These few problems need to be solved in the future, but much more challenging are the unsolved problems of multi-dimensional encoding. It has been shown that the time-domain reconstruction can be applied almost universally, most often resulting in images of high quality. The method can also easily incorporate model refinements. However, the time-domain reconstruction has shown to be problematic with regard to several aspects that need to be tackled in the future.

1. The time-domain algorithm could already be accelerated by more than a factor of 1000 compared to an initial implementation; yet, it is currently still not fast enough to be useful in the clinical routine.

2. Artifacts like Gibbs ringing or those resulting from undersampling, amplified by weak SEM encoding, may not be suppressed sufficiently by linear unconstrained image reconstruction.

3. For multi-dimensional PatLoc trajectories, image reconstruction requires very accurate knowledge of the applied encoding fields in order to yield images of sufficient quality.

It will be an important aspect of future work to further accelerate the computing time by optimizing parallel computing implementations and by further exploiting any encoding sparsity. This thesis has shown that a close analysis of a specific encoding strategy can lead to accelerations of reconstruction time up to several orders of magnitude. For the success of imaging with NB-SEMs, it will be essential to achieve orders-of-magnitude acceleration also under general conditions of imaging with matrix gradient coils that have a multitude of encoding elements.

Problems associated with weak encoding gradients can be circumvented by ensuring sufficient encoding over the whole excited volume. However, this reduces the encoding efficiency, and therefore improvements in this regard are important and are currently being pursued in a collaboration with Dr. Florian Knoll from the University of Graz, where it could be shown that nonlinear image reconstruction with regularization using total generalized variation effectively eliminates the star-shaped artifact that occurs in quadrupolar radial PatLoc imaging up to very high undersampling factors. It will also be tested to what extent nonlinear signal modeling and nonlinear reconstruction will help to reduce the calibration problem, one of the most urgent problems that need to solved in the near future.

Medical Applications The aim of this thesis was not to develop medical applications, but to elaborate fundamental theoretical principles of MR signal encoding with nonlinear magnetic fields, to contribute solutions to technical problems, and to develop practical image reconstruction methods. Up to this point, also the whole PatLoc project was rather technologically-oriented. Notwithstanding, we have already demonstrated that the increased encoding efficiency at the periphery has implications to cortical imaging. Other applications like reduced field-of-view imaging and advantages for dynamic shimming have been evaluated, showing the potential of PatLoc for a variety of medical applications.

With state-of-the-art gradient hardware, magnetic field gradients are generated homogeneously across a large volume, in human systems allowing to faithfully image large portions of the human body. Very often, diagnostic or functional information is required only from small ROIs. With nonlinear fields encoding can be focused onto the location of interest with flexible volume coverage. Thus, organ-specific applications will profit most from the additional degrees of freedom offered by PatLoc imaging. Reduced scan-time, mitigation of problems like acoustic noise or PNS are just a few examples that are noted here. However, it has to be admitted that the range of possibilities that multi-dimensional encoding strategies offer are not yet foreseeable at the current stage of research, and it will be exciting to observe what medical applications will eventually be developed. Undoubtedly, there is work for many future PhD students in this interesting research field that involves nonlinear encoding fields.

I am very happy to see that a new large project, RANGEmri[1], lead by Dr. Maxim Zaitsev, has recently been funded by the European Research Council. This will guarantee that the work performed in PatLoc will be continued in Freiburg for at least five additional years with radically fresh ideas about technological and methodological advancements and prospective diagnostic and functional applications in such different medical areas like neuroscience, neurology and oncology.

---

[1] Acronym for *Rapid Adaptive Nonlinear Gradient Encoding for Magnetic Resonance Imaging*.

Appendix

A.1 Notation and Abbreviations

A.1.1 Notation

Throughout this thesis, scalars and scalar functions are written with non-bold letters; variable quantities or running indices are typically written in lowercase $(a, j, c(\cdot))$, whereas fixed parameters or constants are normally written with capital letters (C, R, L); lowercase letters with an arrow $(\vec{a}, \vec{u}, \vec{\psi}(\cdot))$ describe vectors or vector fields in 2D or 3D; lowercase letters in boldface $(\mathbf{a}, \mathbf{k}_\kappa, \boldsymbol{\psi}(\cdot))$ represent multi-dimensional vectors or multi-dimensional functions, and capital letters in boldface $(\mathbf{A}, \mathbf{B}, \mathbf{C})$ denote matrices.

Standard notation for matrix operations is used. $\mathbf{M}^T, \mathbf{M}^H, \mathbf{M}^+$ denote transpose, conjugate transpose and Moore-Penrose pseudo-inverse, the trace of a matrix is given by $Tr\{\mathbf{M}\}$ and $\mathbf{L} \otimes \mathbf{M}$ describes the Kronecker product (see Appendix A.2 for more details). If not otherwise stated, the norm $v := \|\vec{v}\|$ indicates the standard Euclidian norm (or induced norm for matrices).

Only those symbols that are not necessarily self-explanatory and/or that are used in several chapters are listed below:

Concerning the Measurement

$\vec{B}, \vec{\mathfrak{B}}^{re}$	magnetic field, field generated by the receiver coil per unit current
B_W	bandwidth of the receiver
$c, c_\alpha(\cdot)$	RF-coil sensitivity
$\vec{E}, \vec{\mathcal{E}}$	electric field and field per unit current (electric sensitivity)
$\vec{k}, \vec{k}_\kappa, \mathbf{k}, \mathbf{k}_\kappa$	standard and PatLoc k-space vector
Δk	k-space sampling distance

$\mathcal{K}$	sampled k-space coverage; i.e., the set of all sampled k-space locations
K	effective k-space coverage; i.e., all frequencies which are effectively covered by the acquisition (including the information from the RF-sensitivity profiles)
$\mathrm{enc}_{\alpha,\kappa}(\vec{x})$	the (α, κ)-th encoding function evaluated at location $\vec{x}$
$m(\cdot)$	magnetization
R	acceleration factor
s, s_α	received signal
T_1, T_2	time constants of the longitudinal and transversal relaxation
T_E, T_R	echo time, repetition time
U, I	voltage, current
$\omega, \vec{\omega}$	(angular) frequency

Concerning Image Reconstruction

$\mathbf{B}$	correlation matrix of the encoding functions
$\mathbf{DFT}, \mathbf{iDFT}$	matrices that describe the 2D-DFT and its inverse
$\mathbf{DFT}_t, \mathbf{iDFT}_t$	DFT (and inverse DFT) taken along the readout direction only
$\mathbf{F}, \mathbf{E}$	reconstruction matrix, encoding matrix
$f_\rho(\cdot)$	voxel function (= spatial response function) for voxel location ρ
g_ρ	g-factor for voxel location ρ
$\mathbf{G}$	that part of the encoding matrix that contains the phase information from gradient encoding for non-Cartesian trajectories
$\mathcal{G}, \Sigma_{cart}$	reconstruction grid, Cartesian grid
$\mathbf{s}$	received signal, collected in a vector
$m_\rho, \mathbf{m}$	reconstructed magnetization
N_c	number of RF-receiver coils
N_κ	number of acquired k-space data points
N_ρ	number of reconstructed voxels

N_{pe} number of phase encodes

N_p number of projections for a radial trajectory

N_r number of samples along the readout direction for a radial trajectory

$\tilde{\Psi} := \mathbb{1}_{N_\kappa} \otimes \Psi$ noise covariance matrix of the signal measurements

Miscellaneous

$[a, b] = ab - ba$ commutator of a and b

$f(N) = \mathcal{O}(g(N))$ "big O notation"; means that the function f has the same asymptotic behavior as the function g with respect to N

$\hat{f}, \hat{v}, \hat{\mathbf{F}}$ a hat may indicate a continuous or discrete, forward or inverse Fourier operation

$\mathcal{FT}, \mathcal{FT}^{-1}$ continuous Fourier transform and its inverse

$\gamma\!\!\!\!- = \gamma/(2\pi)$ gyromagnetic ratio of hydrogen ($= 42.58\,\mathrm{MHz/T}$)

$\hbar = h/(2\pi)$ Planck constant ($= 1.05 \times 10^{-34}$ Js)

k_B Boltzmann factor ($= 1.38 \times 10^{-23}$ JK^{-1})

$\mathbb{1}, \mathbb{0}$ unity matrix, zero matrix

$\mathcal{I}_N$ set of N equidistantly spaced locations ($\mathcal{I}_N := [-N/2, N/2 - 1]$)

$\mathbf{I}_q$ square matrix that has a non-zero entry only at location q, q, where it is defined to be unity

$g_N(\cdot)$ a function, defined in Eq. 2.32 on page 61, that is used to describe the truncation window of Cartesian Fourier imaging

$\mathbf{R}(\vec{e}_z, \phi) := \begin{pmatrix} \cos(\phi) & -\sin(\phi) & 0 \\ \sin(\phi) & \cos(\phi) & 0 \\ 0 & 0 & 1 \end{pmatrix}$ 3D rotation around the z-axis by an angle ϕ

$\mathbf{R}(\delta) := \begin{pmatrix} \cos(\delta) & -\sin(\delta) \\ \sin(\delta) & \cos(\delta) \end{pmatrix}$ 2D rotation by an angle δ

A.1.2   Abbreviations

ACS	auto-calibration k-space signal
ADC	analog-to-digital converter
CG	conjugate gradient
(D)FT	(discrete) Fourier transform
FBP	filtered back-projection
FFT	fast Fourier transform
FOV	field-of-view
FWHM	full width at half maximum
MPPI	Moore-Penrose pseudo-inverse
MR(I)	magnetic resonance (imaging)
NB-SEM	nonlinear and non-bijective SEM
NMR	nuclear magnetic resonance
nuFFT	non-uniform fast Fourier transform
PI	parallel imaging
PSF	point spread function
RF	radio frequency
ROI	region of interest
SEM	spatial encoding magnetic field
SNR	signal-to-noise ratio
SRF	spatial response function
SSFP	steady-state free precession
SVD	singular value decomposition

A.2   Kronecker Product

Here, only those aspects of the Kronecker product are presented which are relevant to this thesis. Definitions are introduced and some properties of the Kronecker product are listed. Consult, for example, the textbook [91], chapter 13, for more information on this topic.

Definition of the Kronecker product   The Kronecker product of an $m \times p$ matrix $\mathbf{A}$ and an $n \times q$ matrix $\mathbf{B}$ is an $mn \times pq$ matrix $\mathbf{A} \otimes \mathbf{B}$ with entries:

$$\mathbf{A} \otimes \mathbf{B} = \begin{pmatrix} A_{11}\mathbf{B} & \cdots & A_{1p}\mathbf{B} \\ \vdots & \ddots & \vdots \\ A_{n1}\mathbf{B} & \cdots & A_{np}\mathbf{B} \end{pmatrix}. \tag{A.1}$$

Definition of a block-diagonal matrix   A block-diagonal matrix $\mathbf{D}$ is a diagonal matrix where the diagonal elements $\mathbf{D}^{(1)}, \ldots, \mathbf{D}^{(n)}$ are block matrices. Such a matrix is typically written as the direct sum of the individual matrices $\mathbf{D}^{(j)}$, $j = 1, \ldots, n$. In the context of this thesis, the sub-matrices $\mathbf{D}^{(j)}$ are all equal in size; in this case, it can be useful to write the block-diagonal matrix with the help of the Kronecker product:

$$\mathbf{D} = \begin{pmatrix} \mathbf{D}^{(1)} & 0 & \cdots & 0 \\ 0 & \mathbf{D}^{(2)} & & \vdots \\ \vdots & & \ddots & 0 \\ 0 & \cdots & 0 & \mathbf{D}^{(n)} \end{pmatrix} = \sum_{j=1}^{n} \mathbf{I}_j \otimes \mathbf{D}^{(j)}. \tag{A.2}$$

In this definition, $\mathbf{I}_j$ represents a square matrix of size $n \times n$ that is unity at index j,j and otherwise zero. If the blocks $\mathbf{D}^{(j)}$ are all equal, i.e., if $\mathbf{D}^{(j)} := \mathbf{D}^{(1)}$ for all j, the expression of the block-diagonal matrix can be simplified considering that the sum of all matrices $\mathbf{I}_j$ is just the unity matrix:

$$\mathbf{D} = \sum_{j=1}^{n} \left(\mathbf{I}_j \otimes \mathbf{D}^{(1)} \right) = \left(\sum_{j=1}^{n} \mathbf{I}_j \right) \otimes \mathbf{D}^{(1)} = \mathbb{1}_n \otimes \mathbf{D}^{(1)}. \tag{A.3}$$

Definition of a block-circulant matrix   A block-circulant matrix is a circulant matrix where the elements are block matrices. Such a matrix can also be written with the help of the Kronecker product involving a circulant matrix $\mathbf{\Pi}$ and the individual blocks $\mathbf{A}^{(j)}$:

$$\begin{pmatrix} \mathbf{A}^{(1)} & \mathbf{A}^{(2)} & \cdots & \mathbf{A}^{(n)} \\ \mathbf{A}^{(n)} & \mathbf{A}^{(1)} & \cdots & \mathbf{A}^{(n-1)} \\ \vdots & & \ddots & \vdots \\ \mathbf{A}^{(2)} & \mathbf{A}^{(3)} & \cdots & \mathbf{A}^{(1)} \end{pmatrix} = \sum_{j=1}^{n} \mathbf{\Pi}^{j} \otimes \mathbf{A}^{(j)}; \ \mathbf{\Pi} = \begin{pmatrix} 0 & 1 & 0 & \cdots & \\ \vdots & 0 & 1 & 0 & \cdots \\ & & & \ddots & \\ 1 & 0 & \cdots & & \end{pmatrix}.$$
(A.4)

Properties of the Kronecker Product The following properties are important in the context of this thesis:

- The Kronecker product is bilinear and associative:

$$\mathbf{A} \otimes \mathbf{B} + \mathbf{A} \otimes \mathbf{C} = \mathbf{A} \otimes (\mathbf{B} + \mathbf{C}),$$
$$\mathbf{A} \otimes \mathbf{C} + \mathbf{B} \otimes \mathbf{C} = (\mathbf{A} + \mathbf{B}) \otimes \mathbf{C},$$
$$(k\mathbf{A}) \otimes \mathbf{B} = \mathbf{A} \otimes (k\mathbf{B}) = k(\mathbf{A} \otimes \mathbf{B}), \ \text{where } k \text{ is a scalar,}$$
$$(\mathbf{A} \otimes \mathbf{B}) \otimes \mathbf{C} = \mathbf{A} \otimes (\mathbf{B} \otimes \mathbf{C}).$$

- The Kronecker product is not commutative. In general $\mathbf{A} \otimes \mathbf{B} \neq \mathbf{B} \otimes \mathbf{A}$. However, there exist permutation matrices $\mathbf{P}$ and $\mathbf{Q}$ such that $\mathbf{A} \otimes \mathbf{B} = \mathbf{P}(\mathbf{B} \otimes \mathbf{A})\mathbf{Q}$. If $\mathbf{A}$ and $\mathbf{B}$ are square, then $\mathbf{P} = \mathbf{Q}^{T}$.

- $(\mathbf{A} \otimes \mathbf{B})(\mathbf{C} \otimes \mathbf{D}) = (\mathbf{A}\mathbf{C} \otimes \mathbf{B}\mathbf{D})$.

- $(\mathbf{A} \otimes \mathbf{B})^{-1} = \mathbf{A}^{-1} \otimes \mathbf{B}^{-1}$.

- $(\mathbf{A} \otimes \mathbf{B})^{+} = \mathbf{A}^{+} \otimes \mathbf{B}^{+}$.

A.3 On the Relationship Between GRAPPA and SENSE

In chapter 2.3.2b, page 99ff, the relationship between GRAPPA and SENSE is reviewed. In this appendix, two aspects are covered in greater detail; the main conclusions of this appendix are used in chapter 2.3.2b. The first issue is an equivalent formulation of the weak reconstruction condition.

The second issue concerns the property of the encoding matrix that it can be truncated without causing significant reconstruction errors. The presentation is very detailed because these issues are not sufficiently discussed in the reviewed literature (particularly [135, 49, 209, 147, 136, 104]). In order to avoid confusion by extensive notation, the mathematical treatment only considers explicitly one variable along the accelerated dimension. Keep in mind, however, that GRAPPA and SENSE actually deal with 2D datasets.

A.3.1 Equivalent Formulation of the Weak Reconstruction Condition

It is proven here that the weak condition $\mathbf{FE} = \mathbb{1}$, from which the SENSE algorithm is derived, is equivalent to the expression $\hat{c}_{\alpha'} = \mathbf{w}_{\alpha'}^{(m)} \hat{\mathbf{E}}^{(m)}$, where $\hat{\mathbf{E}}_{(\alpha',b),l}^{(m)} = (\hat{c}_{\alpha'})_{l-(Rb-m)}$. This equivalence is used in chapter 2.3.2b, page 99ff, to establish a relationship between GRAPPA and SENSE.

The proof starts with representing the weak condition $\mathbf{FE} = \mathbb{1}$ in k-space by defining $\hat{\mathbf{F}} := \mathbf{DFT} \cdot \mathbf{F}$ and $\hat{\mathbf{E}} := \mathbf{E} \cdot \mathbf{iDFT}$. Then, the weak condition reads $\hat{\mathbf{F}}\hat{\mathbf{E}} = \mathbb{1}$. Define the diagonal matrix $\mathbf{C}_{\alpha'}$ with the coil sensitivity values on the diagonal evaluated at the center of the image voxels and $\hat{\mathbf{C}}_{\alpha'}$ as the k-space analogue: $\hat{\mathbf{C}}_{\alpha'} := \mathbf{DFT} \cdot \mathbf{C}_{\alpha'} \cdot \mathbf{iDFT}$ with $(\hat{C}_{\alpha'})_{l,l'} = (\hat{c}_{\alpha'})_{l'-l}$. Multiplication of $\hat{\mathbf{F}}\hat{\mathbf{E}} = \mathbb{1}$ from left with $\hat{\mathbf{C}}_{\alpha'}$ yields:

$$\hat{\mathbf{F}}^{\alpha'}\hat{\mathbf{E}} = \hat{\mathbf{C}}_{\alpha'}, \tag{A.5}$$

where $\hat{\mathbf{F}}^{\alpha'} := \hat{\mathbf{C}}_{\alpha'}\hat{\mathbf{F}} = \mathbf{DFT} \cdot \mathbf{C}_{\alpha'}\mathbf{F}.$[2] Recall from the main text that $\hat{\mathbf{E}}$ has a block-circulant structure. Liu et al. show in [104] that $\hat{\mathbf{F}}$ has the same block-circulant structure. It is straightforward to show that also $\hat{\mathbf{C}}_{\alpha'}$ and $\hat{\mathbf{F}}^{\alpha'}$ are block-circulant. With definition (A.4) the transformed weak condition (Eq. A.5) has the following explicit form:

$$\underbrace{\left[\sum_{b'} \mathbf{\Pi}_{N/R}^{b'} \otimes (\mathbf{W}^{\alpha'})_{R,N_c}^{(b')}\right]}_{\hat{\mathbf{F}}^{\alpha'}} \cdot \underbrace{\left[\sum_{b'} \mathbf{\Pi}_{N/R}^{b'} \otimes \hat{\mathbf{C}}_{N_c,R}^{(b')}\right]}_{\hat{\mathbf{E}}} = \underbrace{\left[\sum_{b'} \mathbf{\Pi}_{N/R}^{b'} \otimes (\hat{\mathbf{C}}^{\alpha'})_{R,R}^{(b')}\right]}_{\hat{\mathbf{C}}_{\alpha'}} \cdot$$

$$\tag{A.6}$$

---

[2] The matrix $\hat{\mathbf{F}}^{\alpha'}$ represents the MPPI reconstruction corresponding to the GRAPPA k-space filling operation because, with the signal data $\mathbf{s}$, one finds that $\mathbf{s}_{\alpha'} = \hat{\mathbf{F}}^{\alpha'}\mathbf{s}$ is the k-space of the reconstructed image weighted with the corresponding RF-coil sensitivity map.

The blocks $(\mathbf{W}^{\alpha'})_{R,N_c}^{(b')}$ represent analogues of the GRAPPA weights. Resorting the double summation and making use of the fact that $\mathbf{\Pi}^{b'}\mathbf{\Pi}^{k} = \mathbf{\Pi}^{[(b'+k) \bmod N/R]}$ the above expression can be simplified to:

$$\sum_{b'} \mathbf{\Pi}_{N/R}^{b'} \otimes \left[\sum_{b}(\mathbf{W}^{\alpha'})_{R,N_c}^{(b)} \, \hat{\mathbf{C}}_{N_c,R}^{(b'-b)} - (\hat{\mathbf{C}}^{\alpha'})_{R,R}^{(b')}\right] = 0, \qquad (A.7)$$

where all superscripts are evaluated modulo N/R; i.e., $(b' - b) := (b' - b) \bmod N/R$. This equation is valid if and only if the expression in the brackets is zero for all b'. This equivalence therefore results in:

$$\sum_{b}(\mathbf{W}^{\alpha'})_{R,N_c}^{(b)} \, \hat{\mathbf{C}}_{N_c,R}^{(b'-b)} = (\hat{\mathbf{C}}^{\alpha'})_{R,R}^{(b')}. \qquad (A.8)$$

This is a decisive result: It states that the number of reconstruction weights, which actually need to be determined, can be vastly reduced (compare Eq. A.8 with Eq. A.5). Explicitly evaluating this equation at matrix element (m, m') results in:

$$\sum_{\alpha,b}(w_{\alpha'}^{(m)})_{\alpha,b}(\hat{c}_\alpha)_{R(b'-b)+m'} = (\hat{c}_{\alpha'})_{Rb'+m'-m}, \qquad (A.9)$$

with $(w_{\alpha'}^{(m)})_{\alpha,b} := (W^{\alpha'})_{m,\alpha}^{(b)}$. Set $l = Rb' + m'$.[3] The latter equation then yields:

$$\sum_{\alpha,b}(w_{\alpha'}^{(m)})_{\alpha,b}(\hat{c}_\alpha)_{l-Rb} = (\hat{c}_{\alpha'})_{l-m}$$

or, equivalently

$$\sum_{\alpha,b}(w_{\alpha'}^{(m)})_{\alpha,b}(\hat{c}_\alpha)_{l-(Rb-m)} = (\hat{c}_{\alpha'})_l.$$

The sought expression is finally found by writing the two latter equations in matrix form with right and left swapped:

$$\hat{\mathbf{c}}_{\alpha'}^{(m)} = \mathbf{w}_{\alpha'}^{(m)}\hat{\mathbf{E}} \quad \text{or, equivalently,} \quad \hat{\mathbf{c}}_{\alpha'} = \mathbf{w}_{\alpha'}^{(m)}\hat{\mathbf{E}}^{(m)}. \qquad (A.10)$$

---

[3]Note that this definition is well-defined: The assignment $(b', m') \mapsto l = Rb' + m'$ is bijective.

A.3.2 Truncation of the Encoding Matrix

It is shown here that it is possible to truncate the encoding matrix without introducing significant reconstruction errors. This property justifies the usage of small GRAPPA kernels and the acquisition of a limited amount of ACS-lines.

Limited kernel size Reconsider the untruncated problem, represented by Eq. A.10. Here, the version on the left hand side, $\hat{c}_{\alpha'}^{(m)} = w_{\alpha'}^{(m)}\hat{E}$, is used. This equation can be satisfied exactly. Therefore, no residual error is produced:

$$(r_{\alpha'}^{(m)})^2 = \left\| w_{\alpha'}^{(m)}\hat{E} - \hat{c}_{\alpha'}^{(m)} \right\|^2 = \sum_l \left| (\hat{c}_{\alpha'})_{l-m'} - \sum_{\alpha,b}(w_{\alpha'}^{(m')})_{\alpha,b}(\hat{c}_{\alpha})_{l-Rb} \right|^2 = 0.$$

(A.11)

For limited kernel sizes, not all values of b are considered, but only the smallest. What residual error is produced with limited kernel sizes? In this regard, it is important that the k-space footprint of the RF-coil sensitivity profiles is typically very localized with $\hat{c}_l$ vanishing rapidly with increasing l. The residual error for large values of l is therefore almost negligible. But also for small values of l, the residual error is low: As shown at the end of this appendix, also the weights $(w_{\alpha'}^{(m')})_{\alpha,b}$ quickly vanish with increasing values of b. Therefore, for small l, the product in Eq. A.11 of the weights with the sensitivities is mainly determined by the smallest values of b. Altogether, it can be concluded that the residual error is low if the sum is truncated to a few values of b only.[4] The amount of how much the solution can be truncated depends on the k-space extent of the RF-sensitivity profiles, but also on the k-space extent of the reconstruction weights.

Restricted amount of ACS-lines In GRAPPA, only a restricted amount of ACS-lines is acquired. Correspondingly, the encoding matrix is further truncated. In particular, this means that in Eq. A.11, not only fewer values of b are considered, but also fewer values of l. This is not problematic because the k-space extent of the sensitivities is restricted and - as mentioned

---

[4]As shown here, this is true if weights are used that are determined from the *untruncated* encoding matrix. Note that the reconstruction weights are actually determined by minimizing the residual error for the *truncated* encoding matrix. The weights determined via this minimization will result in a residuum, which is even smaller. Thus, the solution to the truncated problem will lead to even better data consistency.

above - large values of l do not contribute significant information for the determination of optimal weights. On the contrary; note that the ACS-lines are typically acquired at the k-space center, where the highest SNR is available. The inclusion of additional ACS-lines with low SNR does therefore not always ensure higher image quality. Significant deterioration of image quality is not expected, if the encoding matrix is truncated to the smallest values of l.

k-space extent of the reconstruction weights   It remains to be shown that the k-space extent of the reconstruction weights is restricted. This is the case if the weights inherit this property from the RF-coil sensitivity profiles. According to Eq. A.10, the weights of the untruncated problem are determined via $\mathbf{w}_{\alpha'}^{(m)} = \hat{\mathbf{c}}_{\alpha'}^{(m)} [\hat{\mathbf{E}}^H \hat{\mathbf{E}}]^{-1} \hat{\mathbf{E}}^H$. The weights are therefore found by first multiplying the k-space coil sensitivities with the inverse of $\hat{\mathbf{R}} = \hat{\mathbf{E}}^H \hat{\mathbf{E}}$ and then with $\hat{\mathbf{E}}^H$. The encoding matrix $\hat{\mathbf{E}}$ has a restricted k-space extent because it is formed from the RF sensitivities; also, it is straightforward to show (cf. e.g. [104]) that the k-space support remains restricted, if two quantities of limited k-space extent are multiplied with each other. The weights are therefore limited in k-space if the inversion of the correlation matrix $\hat{\mathbf{R}}$ does not significantly increase its own k-space support. Such a conservative property is not usual for a matrix inversion and therefore thorough justification must be established.

The problem can also be tackled in the image domain, where limited k-space extent manifests as smooth spatial variations. According to Eq. 2.39, page 75, the image-domain analogue of the correlation matrix is given by $\mathbf{R} = \mathbf{iDFT} \cdot \hat{\mathbf{R}} \cdot \mathbf{DFT} = \mathbf{E}^H \mathbf{E} = \widetilde{\mathbf{C}}^H \cdot \widetilde{\mathbf{iDFT}} \cdot \widetilde{\mathbf{DFT}} \cdot \widetilde{\mathbf{C}} = \widetilde{\mathbf{C}}^H \widetilde{\mathbf{C}}$. The inverse of $\mathbf{R}$ then has the explicit form:[5]

$$\mathbf{R}^{-1} = \sum_q \mathbf{I}_q \otimes \left[\mathbf{A}^{(q)} \right]^{-1}, \text{ with } \mathbf{A}^{(q)} = (\mathbf{C}^{(q)})^H \mathbf{C}^{(q)}. \tag{A.12}$$

The inverse of $\mathbf{R}$ varies smoothly along the spatial dimension q if each component $[\mathbf{A}^{(q)}]^{-1}$ does not jump heavily from one location q to the next location $\tilde{q}$. Typical reconstruction grids are dense enough such that the finite difference $[\mathbf{A}^{(\tilde{q})}]^{-1} - [\mathbf{A}^{(q)}]^{-1}$ can be approximated by the derivative $\frac{d\mathbf{A}^{-1}}{dq}$. Matrix theory shows that the derivative of a matrix can be expressed by its

---

[5]In order to simplify the notation, (q, q') is simply written as q.

inverse: $\frac{d\mathbf{A}^{-1}}{dq} = -\mathbf{A}^{-1}\frac{d\mathbf{A}}{dq}\mathbf{A}^{-1}$. With this relation, it is possible to calculate an upper bound for the derivative of each component of $[\mathbf{A}^{(q)}]^{-1}$:

$$\left|\left(\frac{d\mathbf{A}^{-1}}{dq}\right)_{l,l'}\right| \leq \left\|\frac{d\mathbf{A}^{-1}}{dq}\right\| \leq \left\|[\mathbf{A}^{(q)}]^{-1}\right\|^2 \left\|\frac{d\mathbf{A}}{dq}\right\| = \dots$$
$$\dots = \lambda_{max}^2([\mathbf{A}^{(q)}]^{-1}) \left\|\frac{d\mathbf{A}}{dq}\right\| = \lambda_{min}^{-2}(\mathbf{A}^{(q)}) \left\|\frac{d\mathbf{A}}{dq}\right\|.$$

(A.13)

The variations of the correlation matrix $\mathbf{R}^{-1}$ are therefore bound by the square-inverse of the minimum eigenvalue of $\mathbf{A}^{(q)}$ multiplied with the variations of $\mathbf{A}^{(q)}$. According to Eq. A.12, these variations correspond to the spatial variations of the RF coils, which are typically very low in image space. These variations are enhanced by the inversion. However, the enhancement should often be moderate because the eigenvalues are closely related to the g-factor,[6] and the g-factor has proven to be fairly well-behaved as long as acceleration is not driven to its limit.

It can therefore be concluded that the reconstruction weights $\mathbf{w}_{\alpha'}^{(m)}$ of the untruncated problem have a limited k-space extent that is often not much higher than the extent of the RF-coil sensitivities. Examples for acceleration factors 2 and 4, simulated with sensitivity data of a head coil with eight channels (Siemens Healthcare, Erlangen, Germany) are depicted in Fig. A.1.

A.4 Significance of Multipolar Magnetic Fields for Spatial Encoding

The following statement is proven: The orthogonal multipolar SEMs ($r^L \cos(L\varphi)$ and $r^L \sin(L\varphi)$, with multipolarity $L = 1, \dots, \infty$) form a set of encoding fields which can be combined to generate *each possible* set of two

---

[6]The relationship is the following: Consider w. l. o. g. that the sum-of-squares of the RF sensitivities is constant and that the noise in the receiver channels is uncorrelated; then, it follows from Eq. 2.50, page 82, that the square of the g-factor at location $\rho = (q, l)$ is given by $(A^{(q)})_{l,l}^{-1}$. The matrix $(\mathbf{A}^{(q)})^{-1}$ is Hermitian and therefore it is diagonalizable and has only positive eigenvalues λ_i. Also consider that the trace of a diagonalizable matrix equals the sum of the eigenvalues. If $\bar{g}$ is defined to be the average g-factor for the voxel group at the locations $(q, l), l = 1, \dots, R$, it follows that $\lambda_{max} < \sum_i \lambda_i = R \cdot \bar{g}^2$. The average g-factor squared (and multiplied with the acceleration factor) is therefore an upper bound for the maximum eigenvalue of the matrix $(\mathbf{A}^{(q)})^{-1}$.

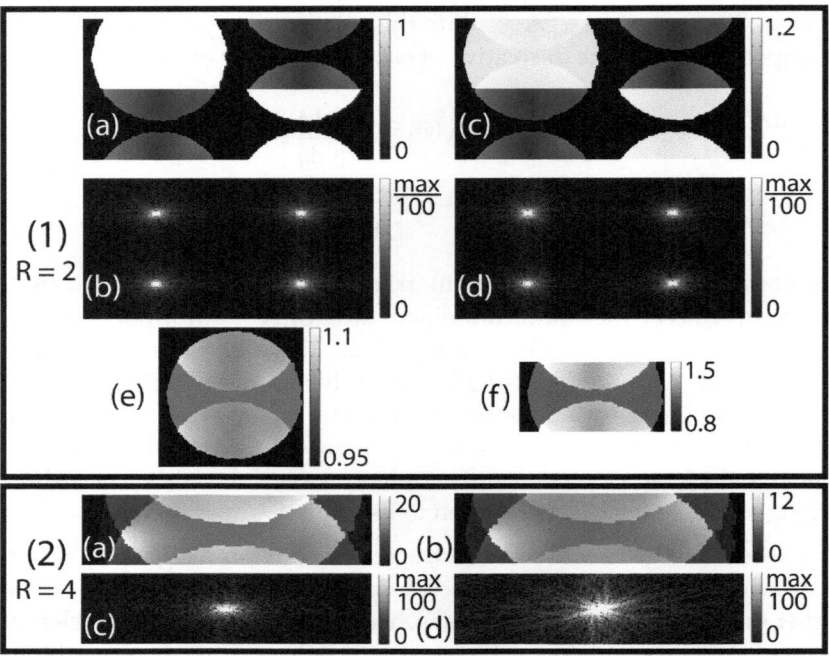

Figure A.1: The purpose of this figure is to illustrate the limited k-space extent of the reconstruction weights. This extent is mainly determined by the k-space footprint of the inverse of the correlation matrix $\mathbf{R}^{-1}$. The k-space extent of the correlation matrix $\mathbf{R}$ and its inverse $\mathbf{R}^{-1}$ are compared in this figure for two different acceleration factors. (1) Acceleration factor 2. (2) Acceleration factor 4. (1a) The four components of the block-diagonal matrix $\mathbf{R}$ only have low spatial frequencies. (1b) Correspondingly, the k-space footprint of the Fourier-domain analogue $\hat{\mathbf{R}}$ is narrow. (1c) Also the inverse $\mathbf{R}^{-1}$ only has low spatial frequency components. (1d) Correspondingly, $\hat{\mathbf{R}}^{-1}$ is not more spread out in k-space than $\hat{\mathbf{R}}$. (1e) The g-factor of the reconstruction. (1f) The distribution of the maximum eigenvalue of the diagonal blocks of $\mathbf{R}$ is similar to the distribution of the corresponding g-factor. For this acceleration of only two the maximum eigenvalues are all below 1.5. As a consequence, the k-space extent of the correlation matrix is not broadened by the inversion. (2a) For an acceleration of 4, the maximum eigenvalues rise up to 20. (2b) However, the spatial variations of the inverse of the correlation matrix are still fairly smooth (Shown is one of the $16 = 4 \times 4$ components of $\mathbf{R}^{-1}$). (2c,d) For this acceleration, the k-space footprint of the inverse correlation matrix is slightly broadened, but its extent is still limited. (Fig. (2c) shows the component with maximum k-space extent of $\hat{\mathbf{R}}$, whereas Fig. (2d) shows the component with maximum extent of $\hat{\mathbf{R}}^{-1}$).

magnetic encoding fields where the local gradient fields of the two SEMs and the z-gradient are orthogonal to each other at all spatial locations. This proof has been published previously in the appendix of [[158]].

1. For three-dimensional imaging, exactly three encoding fields are needed to fulfill the requirement of mutual orthogonality. Two fields must be orthogonal to the z-gradient. This means that they cannot have a gradient along the z-direction. They must therefore necessarily be constant along the z-axis and the problem can be reduced to 2D.

2. Basic complex analysis can be used to solve the 2D problem. First it is shown that the real and imaginary part of a holomorphic function can be interpreted as magnetic fields which have the desired properties. Consider an arbitrary holomorphic function $f(s)$ with $s \in \mathbb{C}$ and $f(s) \in \mathbb{C}$. This function can then be decomposed into its real and imaginary part:

$$f(s) = u(s) + iv(s) = u(x, y) + iv(x, y), \quad \text{with} \quad s = x + iy. \quad (A.14)$$

The real and imaginary components of s can therefore be interpreted as spatial components x, y in two-dimensional Euclidian space. As $f(s)$ is holomorphic, the functions u and v satisfy the Cauchy-Riemann differential equations. Two important properties can be derived directly from those differential equations:

a) u and v satisfy Laplace's equation $\Delta u(x, y) = 0$ and $\Delta v(x, y) = 0$.

b) The gradient fields of u and v are orthogonal everywhere; i.e., $(\nabla u(x, y)) \cdot (\nabla v(x, y)) = 0$.

With the definition of $B_1(x, y, z) := \text{real}\,(f(s)) = u(x, y)$, $B_2(x, y, z) := \text{imag}\,(f(s)) = v(x, y)$ and $B_z(x, y, z) := z$ a set of three magnetic fields is constructed, which are all mutually orthogonal and which are feasible magnetic fields as they fulfill Laplace's equation.

3. It remains to be proven that there is no set of fields which cannot be represented by a holomorphic function. This is ensured by a well-known mathematical theorem stating: *An arbitrary function satisfying Laplace's equation on a simply-connected region (that is an arbitrary magnetic encoding field) can be written as the real or imaginary part of a*

holomorphic function (cf. e.g. [14], page 585). Therefore all mutually orthogonal encoding fields can be found by just analyzing holomorphic functions.

4. Around the location of expansion, a holomorphic function $f(s)$ is represented by its Taylor series. If $f(s)$ is expanded about the origin, $f(s)$ can be written as:

$$f(s) = \sum_L a_L s^L. \tag{A.15}$$

The important observation is that the monomials s^L generate the orthogonal multipolar encoding fields:

$$\begin{aligned}
\text{real } s^L &= \text{real}\left(r^L e^{iL\varphi}\right) = r^L \cos(L\varphi), \\
\text{imag } s^L &= \text{imag}\left(r^L e^{iL\varphi}\right) = r^L \sin(L\varphi).
\end{aligned} \tag{A.16}$$

5. In order to prove the original statement, it is therefore sufficient to show that the real and imaginary parts of any holormophic function can be generated using the real and the imaginary parts of the monomials. This is shown here for the real part of $f(s)$. The same also applies to the imaginary part.

$$\begin{aligned}
\text{real}\left(f(s)\right) &= \text{real}\left(\sum_L a_L s^L\right) = \sum_L \text{real}\left(a_L s^L\right) = \dots \\
\dots &= \sum_L \text{real}\left(a_L\right)\text{real}\left(s^L\right) - \text{imag}\left(a_L\right)\text{imag}\left(s^L\right).
\end{aligned} \tag{A.17}$$

The multipolar SEMs along with the z-gradient are therefore sufficient to generate arbitrary encoding fields which have the desired properties. The magnitude of the complex-valued weighting factor a_L corresponds to the magnetic field strength to be applied and the angular part of a_L represents a rotation of a multipolar field, which is achieved by adequately superimposing the two orthogonal fields of order L.

6. The monomials of lowest order generate the most basic fields. The two lowest orders are discussed here. For low orders of L, Cartesian and

polar coordinates can both be used just as easily to do the calculations. For $L = 1$, one finds:

$$s^1 = (x + \mathrm{i}y), \tag{A.18}$$

and therefore $B_1(x, y, z) = x$ and $B_2(x, y, z) = y$; i.e., the monomial s generates the linear gradient fields. For $L = 2$, one finds:

$$s^2 = (x + \mathrm{i}y)^2 = (x^2 - y^2) + \mathrm{i}(2xy), \tag{A.19}$$

and therefore $B_1(x, y, z) = x^2 - y^2 \; (= r^2 \cos(2\varphi))$ and $B_2(x, y, z) = 2xy \; (= r^2 \sin(2\varphi))$; i.e., the monomial s^2 generates the quadrupolar SEMs used for the experimental realizations. Some practical consequences of the proven statement are presented in [159].

A.5   Local k-Space: Image Resolution and Relation to PatLoc k-Space

This appendix supplements the paragraph *The concept of local k-space* in chapter 3.2.2, page 112ff. Two separate topics are treated here. The first topic substantiates the claim that local image resolution is described by the extent of local k-space. The second topic concerns the relationship between local k-space and the "global" PatLoc k-space trajectory.

A.5.1   Theoretical Background Concerning Image Resolution

Here, a relationship between local k-space and reconstructed image voxels is established and some conclusions are drawn. Suppose the magnetization m_ρ is reconstructed at location $\vec{x}_\rho$. Then, according to Eq. 2.6, the reconstructed magnetization is related to the true magnetization via a weighting with the SRF. Note that the SRF is spatially highly localized for faithful reconstructions, where the image is not corrupted by aliasing. Therefore, the reconstructed magnetization is well described by restricting the integration to a local region W_ρ which contains $\vec{x}_\rho$:

$$
\begin{aligned}
m_\rho &= \int_V m(\vec{x}) f_\rho(\vec{x}) \, d\vec{x} \approx \int_{W_\rho} m(\vec{x}) f_\rho(\vec{x}) \, d\vec{x} = \dots \\
&\dots \stackrel{(2.7)}{=} \sum_{\alpha,\kappa} F_{\rho,(\alpha,\kappa)} \int_{W_\rho} m(\vec{x}) c_\alpha(\vec{x}) e^{-i\phi(\vec{x};\mathbf{k}_\kappa)} \, d\vec{x}.
\end{aligned}
\tag{A.20}
$$

Here, the temporal variable t has been replaced by the PatLoc k-space variable $\mathbf{k}_\kappa$ (defined by Eq. 4.5, page 137). Consider now the Taylor series expansion of the phase distribution $\phi(\cdot)$ about $\vec{x}_\rho$:

$$
\phi(\vec{x}, \mathbf{k}_\kappa) = \phi(\vec{x}_\rho, \mathbf{k}_\kappa) + \vec{k}_{loc}(\vec{x}_\rho, \mathbf{k}_\kappa)(\vec{x} - \vec{x}_\rho) + \mathcal{O}(\|\vec{x} - \vec{x}_\rho\|^2).
\tag{A.21}
$$

The restriction of the region of integration on W_ρ allows the truncation of this series after the first order term with minor influence for the voxel of interest as long as the voxel is small enough, which is typically the case for high-resolution imaging apart from degenerate locations. Then, the reconstructed magnetization is well approximated by:

$$
m_\rho \approx \sum_{\alpha,\kappa} \tilde{F}_{\rho,(\alpha,\kappa)} \int_{W_\rho} m(\vec{x}) c_\alpha(\vec{x}) e^{-i\vec{k}_{loc}(\vec{x}_\rho,\mathbf{k}_\kappa)\vec{x}} \, d\vec{x},
\tag{A.22}
$$

where $\tilde{F}_{\rho,(\alpha,\kappa)} = F_{\rho,(\alpha,\kappa)} e^{-i(\phi(\vec{x}_\rho,\mathbf{k}_\kappa) - \vec{k}_{loc}(\vec{x}_\rho,\mathbf{k}_\kappa)\vec{x}_\rho)}$. According to Eq. A.23, local k-space patterns cannot vary abruptly on a local scale. It can be followed that the local k-space variable $\vec{k}_{loc}$ plays a similar role in PatLoc imaging as the standard k-space variable in conventional imaging with linear SEMs.

Some concrete conclusions may be drawn from this result. First, *local* image resolution is described approximately by the extent of the *local* k-space sampling grid (cf. e.g. Fig. 7.12, page 265). Second, signal voids will occur in regions, where the local k-space center is not acquired. This behavior has been observed for a variant of the 4D-RIO trajectory [42] and is the basic principle that underlies GradLoc (cf. chapter 3.2.4a, page 117ff).

Note that Eq. A.22 has been derived based on the assumption that aliasing does not pose a problem for the reconstruction. Therefore, it would not be correct to draw a conclusion with respect to aliasing. In fact, ambiguous locations from non-unique SEM encoding cannot be detected and, especially for multi-dimensional PatLoc trajectories, the relationship between aliasing and sampling density is more complicated than in conventional imaging.

A.5.2   Relation to PatLoc k-Space

The relationship between local ($\vec{k}_{loc}$) and "global" ($\mathbf{k}_\kappa$) k-space is established and illustrated with examples.

Theory   Recall from Eq. 3.1, page 113, that the local k-space variable is given by $\vec{k}_{loc}(\vec{x}_\rho, t) := (\nabla\phi)(\vec{x}_\rho, t)$, where $\phi(\cdot)$ represents the encoded phase distribution. In PatLoc imaging, the temporal dependency is described by the k-space variable $\mathbf{k}_\kappa$, and, with Eq. 4.9, the phase distribution is given by $\phi(\vec{x}_\rho, \mathbf{k}_\kappa) = \mathbf{k}_\kappa^T \psi(\vec{x}_\rho)$. Therefore the local k-space can be specified:

$$\vec{k}_{loc}(\vec{x}_\rho, \mathbf{k}_\kappa) \overset{(3.1)}{=} \nabla_{\vec{x}}(\mathbf{k}_\kappa^T \psi(\vec{x}_\rho)) = \mathbf{J}^T(\vec{x}_\rho)\mathbf{k}_\kappa, \qquad (A.23)$$

where $\mathbf{J}$ is the Jacobian matrix $\partial\psi/\partial\vec{x}$. This equation illustrates that the spatial derivates of the SEMs links the encoding trajectory with its local k-space distribution.

2D examples   Consider first conventional imaging with two linear gradient fields. In this case $\vec{\psi}(\vec{x}) = (x, y)^T$ and therefore $\mathbf{J} = \mathbb{1}$. It follows that $\vec{k}_{loc} = \vec{k}$. In conformity with the results from conventional imaging, the local k-space variable is therefore independent from the spatial location. Conventional k-space, PatLoc k-space and local k-space are equivalent. An illustration of this example (and the following two examples) is found on page 113 in chapter 3.2.2, Fig. 3.6. The local k-space of a Cartesian trajectory is depicted in Fig. 3.6a. A reconstructed numerical example is shown in Fig. 3.6d.

Next, consider two orthogonal quadrupolar fields. According to chapter 3.3.1, page 122ff (also cf. Eq. 6.8, page 215), the encoding function is described by $\psi_1(\vec{x}) = x^2 - y^2$ and $\psi_2(\vec{x}) = 2xy$. By defining the 2D rotation matrix $\mathbf{R}(\delta)$ in conformity with Appendix A.1, page 291, local k-space is calculated as $\vec{k}_{loc} = 2r\mathbf{R}(\delta)$, where r is the distance from the rotation center of the SEMs and δ the angle in relation to the x-axis. The local k-space is therefore broad at the periphery of the image and reduces to a point at the center. Correspondingly, image resolution is high at the periphery and very low at the center. The angle δ means that the main axes of the local k-space are rotated according to the angular location of the position of interest. The local k-space of a Cartesian PatLoc trajectory is depicted in Fig. 3.6b with a reconstruction shown in Fig. 3.6e.

As last example, consider 4D encoding with linear and quadrupolar SEMs. Then, it is easy to show that $\vec{k}_{loc} = \vec{k}_{lin} + 2r\mathbf{R}(\delta)\vec{k}_{quad}$, where $\vec{k}_{lin}$ describes the two components of the linear PatLoc k-space variables and $\vec{k}_{quad}$ the corresponding components of the quadrupolar SEMs. The local k-space of a complex four-dimensional PatLoc trajectory is depicted in Fig. 3.6c with a reconstruction shown in Fig. 3.6f.

Bibliography

[1] J. ASSLÄNDER, M. BLAIMER, F. A. BREUER, M. ZAITSEV, AND P. M. JAKOB, *Combination of arbitrary gradient encoding fields using SPACE RIP for reconstruction (COGNAC)*, in Proc. of the ISMRM, Montreal, Canada, 2011, p. 2870.

[2] F. AURENHAMMER, *Voronoi diagrams - A survey of a fundamental geometric data structure*, ACM Comput. Surv., 23 (1991), pp. 345–405.

[3] A. V. BARGER, W. F. BLOCK, Y. TOROPOV, T. M. GRIST, AND C. A. MISTRETTA, *Time-resolved contrast-enhanced imaging with isotropic resolution and broad coverage using an undersampled 3D projection trajectory*, Magn. Reson. Med., 48 (2002), pp. 297–305.

[4] C. BARMET, N. DE ZANCHE, AND K. P. PRÜSSMANN, *Spatiotemporal magnetic field monitoring for MR*, Magn. Reson. Med., 60 (2008), pp. 187–197.

[5] S. BAUER, *Entwicklung und Analyse von Beschleunigungsmethoden für die funktionelle Untersuchung des kardiovaskulären Systems mit Magnetresonanztomographie*, PhD thesis, University of Freiburg, Germany, 2011.

[6] S. BAUER, M. MARKL, M. HONAL, AND B. A. JUNG, *The effect of reconstruction and acquisition parameters for GRAPPA-based parallel imaging on the image quality*, Magn. Reson. Med., 66 (2011), pp. 402–409.

[7] P. J. BEATTY, *Reconstruction Methods for Fast Magnetic Resonance Imaging*, PhD thesis, Stanford University, CA, USA, 2006.

[8] P. J. BEATTY, D. NISHIMURA, AND J. M. PAULY, *Rapid gridding reconstruction with a minimal oversampling ratio*, IEEE Trans. Med. Imaging, 24 (2005), pp. 799–808.

[9] M. BENCSIK, R. BOWTELL, AND R. M. BOWLEY, *Using the vector potential in evaluating the likelihood of peripheral nerve stimulation due to*

switched magnetic field gradients, Magn. Reson. Med., 50 (2003), pp. 405–410.

[10] M. A. BERNSTEIN, K. F. KING, AND X. J. ZHOU, *Handbook of MRI Pulse Sequences*, Elsevier, 2004.

[11] F. BLOCH, *Nuclear induction*, Phys. Rev., 70 (1946), pp. 460–474.

[12] K. T. BLOCK, *Advanced Methods for Radial Data Sampling in Magnetic Resonance Imaging*, PhD thesis, University of Göttingen, Germany, 2008.

[13] K. T. BLOCK, M. UECKER, AND J. FRAHM, *Undersampled radial MRI with multiple coils. Iterative image reconstruction using a total variation constraint*, Magn. Reson. Med., 57 (2007), pp. 1086–1098.

[14] M. L. BOAS, *Mathematical Methods in the Physical Sciences*, Wiley, 2 ed., 1983.

[15] S. BOYD AND L. VANDENBERGHE, *Convex Optimization*, Cambridge University Press, 2009.

[16] K. BREDIES, K. KUNISCH, AND T. POCK, *Total generalized variation*, SIAM J. Imaging Sci., 3 (2010), pp. 492–526.

[17] T. R. BROWN, B. M. KINCAID, AND K. UGURBIL, *NMR chemical shift imaging in three dimensions*, Proc. Natl. Acad. Sci. USA, 79 (1982), pp. 3523–3526.

[18] J. W. CARLSON, *An algorithm for NMR imaging reconstruction based on multiple RF receiver coils*, J. Magn. Reson., 74 (1987), pp. 376–380.

[19] Y. CENSOR, *Row-action methods for huge and sparse systems and their applications*, SIAM Rev., 23 (1981), pp. 444–466.

[20] A. CHAMBOLLE AND T. POCK, *A first-order primal-dual algorithm for convex problems with applications to imaging*, J. Math. Imaging Vis., 40 (2010), pp. 120–145.

[21] Z. H. CHO AND J. H. YI, *A novel type of surface gradient coil*, J. Magn. Reson., 94 (1991), pp. 471–485.

[22] P. A. CIRIS, J. P. STOCKMANN, L.-K. TAM, AND R. T. CONSTABLE, *O-space imaging: Tailoring encoding gradients to coil profiles for highly accelerated imaging*, in Proc. of the ISMRM, Honolulu, HI, USA, 2009, p. 4556.

[23] A. C. CLARKE, *Clarke's Three Laws.* http://en.wikipedia.org/wiki/Clarke%27s_three_laws. March 26th, 2012.

[24] C. A. COCOSCO, A. DEWDNEY, P. DIETZ, M. SEMMLER, A. M. WELZ, D. GALLICHAN, H. WEBER, G. SCHULTZ, J. HENNIG, AND M. ZAIT-SEV, *Safety considerations for a PatLoc gradient insert coil for human head imaging*, in Proc. of the ISMRM, Stockholm, Sweden, 2010, p. 3946.

[25] C. A. COCOSCO, D. GALLICHAN, A. DEWDNEY, G. SCHULTZ, A. M. WELZ, W. R. WITSCHEY, H. WEBER, J. HENNIG, AND M. ZAITSEV, *First in-vivo results with a PatLoc gradient insert coil for human head imaging*, in Proc. of the ISMRM, Montreal, Canada, 2011, p. 714.

[26] S. CONOLLY, D. NISHIMURA, AND A. MACOVSKI, *Optimal control solutions to the magnetic resonance selective excitation problem*, IEEE Trans. Med. Imaging, 5 (1986), pp. 106–115.

[27] G. DAHLQUIST AND A. BJÖRCK, *Numerical Methods in Scientific Computing - Volume I*, SIAM, 2008.

[28] D. L. DONOHO, *For most large underdetermined systems of linear equations the minimal L1-norm near-solution is also the sparsest near-solution*, Comm. Pure Appl. Math., 59 (2006), pp. 797–829.

[29] S. J. DORAN, L. CHARLES-EDWARDS, S. A. REINSBERG, AND M. O. LEACH, *A complete distortion correction for MR images: I. Gradient warp correction*, Phys. Med. Biol., 50 (2005), pp. 1343–1361.

[30] A. DUTT, *Fast Fourier Transforms for Nonequispaced Data*, PhD thesis, Yale University, New Haven, CT, USA, 1993.

[31] H. EGGER, *Preconditioning CGNE-iterations for inverse problems*, Numer. Linear Algebra Appl., 14 (2007), pp. 183–196.

[32] C. L. EPSTEIN, *Mathematics of Medical Imaging*, Prentice Hall, 2003.

[33] S. C. FABER, *Stimulation peripherer Nerven durch zeitlich veränderliche Magnetfeldgradienten in der Magnetresonanztomographie*, Radiologie, 38 (1998), pp. 743–749.

[34] H.-P. FAUTZ, M. VOGEL, P. GROSS, A. KERR, AND Y. ZHU, *B1 mapping of coil arrays for parallel transmission*, in Proc. of the ISMRM, Toronto, Canada, 2008, p. 1247.

[35] J. A. FESSLER, *Image reconstruction toolbox containing a NUFFT Matlab toolbox.* http://www.eecs.umich.edu/~fessler/. March 26th, 2012.

[36] J. A. FESSLER AND B. P. SUTTON, *Nonuniform fast Fourier transforms using min-max interpolation*, IEEE Trans. Signal Process., 51 (2003), pp. 560–574.

[37] O. FORSTER, *Lectures on Riemann Surfaces*, Springer, 1981.

[38] G. FRESE, F. X. HEBRANK, W. RENZ, AND T. STORCH, *Physikalische Parameter bei der Anwendung der MRT*, Radiologie, 38 (1998), pp. 750–758.

[39] A. FRYDRYCHOWICZ, B. LANDGRAF, O. WIEBEN, AND C. J. FRANÇOIS, *Scimitar syndrome: Added value by isotropic flow-sensitive four-dimensional magnetic resonance imaging with PC-VIPR*, Circulation, 121 (2010), pp. e434–e436.

[40] W. FULTON, *Algebraic Topology - A first course*, Springer, 1995.

[41] G. GALIANA, J. P. STOCKMANN, L. TAM, AND R. T. CONSTABLE, *Spin dephasing under nonlinear gradients: Implications for imaging and field mapping*, Magn. Reson. Med., (Published online, July 2011).

[42] D. GALLICHAN, C. COCOSCO, A. DEWDNEY, G. SCHULTZ, A. WELZ, J. HENNIG, AND M. ZAITSEV, *Simultaneously driven linear and nonlinear spatial encoding fields in MRI*, Magn. Reson. Med., 65 (2011), pp. 702–714.

[43] D. GALLICHAN, C. COCOSCO, G. SCHULTZ, H. WEBER, A. M. WELZ, J. HENNIG, AND M. ZAITSEV, *Practical considerations for in-vivo MRI with higher dimensional spatial encoding*, Magn. Reson. Mater. Phy., (Accepted, March 2012).

[44] D. GALLICHAN, G. SCHULTZ, J. HENNIG, AND M. ZAITSEV, *Designing k-space trajectories for simultaneous encoding with linear and PatLoc gradients*, in Proc. of the ISMRM, Stockholm, Sweden, 2010, p. 547.

[45] W. GERLACH AND O. STERN, *Der experimentelle Nachweis der Richtungsquantelung im Magnetfeld*, Z. Phys. A - Hadron. Nucl., 9 (1922), pp. 349–352.

[46] P. M. GLOVER, *Interaction of MRI field gradients with the human body*, Phys. Med. Biol., 54 (2009), pp. R99–R115.

[47] A. F. GMITRO, M. KONO, R. J. THEILMANN, M. I. ALTBACH, Z. LI, AND T. P. TROUARD, *Radial GRASE: Implementation and applications*, Magn. Reson. Med., 53 (2005), pp. 1363–1371.

[48] M. A. GRISWOLD, R. M. HEIDEMANN, AND P. M. JAKOB, *Direct parallel imaging reconstruction of radially sampled data using GRAPPA with relative shifts*, in Proc. of the ISMRM, Toronto, Canada, 2003, p. 2349.

[49] M. A. GRISWOLD, P. M. JAKOB, R. M. HEIDEMANN, M. NITTKA, V. JELLUS, J. WANG, B. KIEFER, AND A. HAASE, *Generalized autocalibrating partially parallel acquisitions (GRAPPA)*, Magn. Reson. Med., 47 (2002), pp. 1202–1210.

[50] M. A. GRISWOLD, P. M. JAKOB, M. NITTKA, J. W. GOLDFARB, AND A. HAASE, *Partially parallel imaging with localized sensitivities (PILS)*, Magn. Reson. Med., 44 (2000), pp. 602–609.

[51] T. GROTZ, B. ZAHNEISEN, A. ELLA, M. ZAITSEV, AND J. HENNIG, *Fast functional brain imaging using constrained reconstruction based on regularization using arbitrary projections*, Magn. Reson. Med., 62 (2009), pp. 394–405.

[52] T. GU, F. R. KOROSEC, W. F. BLOCK, S. B. FAIN, Q. TURK, D. LUM, Y. ZHOU, T. M. GRIST, V. HAUGHTON, AND C. A. MISTRETTA, *PC VIPR: a high-speed 3D phase-contrast method for flow quantification and high-resolution angiography*, Am. J. Neuroradiol., 26 (2005), pp. 743–749.

[53] M. HAACKE, R. W. BROWN, M. R. THOMPSON, AND R. VENKATESAN, *Magnetic Resonance Imaging: Physical Principles and Sequence Design*, Wiley, 1999.

[54] M. HAAS, P. ULLMANN, J. T. SCHNEIDER, W. RUHM, J. HENNIG, AND M. ZAITSEV, *Large tip angle parallel excitation using nonlinear non-bijective PatLoc encoding fields*, in Proc. of the ISMRM, Stockholm, Sweden, 2010, p. 4929.

[55] A. HAASE, F. ODOL, M. VON KIENLIN, J. WARNKING, F. FIDLER, A. WEISSER, M. NITTKA, E. ROMMEL, T. LANZ, B. KALUSCHE, AND M. GRISWOLD, *NMR probeheads for in vivo applications*, Concepts Magn. Reson., 12 (2000), pp. 361–388.

[56] E. L. HAHN, *Spin echoes*, Phys. Rev., 80 (1950), pp. 580–594.

[57] F. HARRIS, *On the use of windows for harmonic analysis with the discrete Fourier transform*, Proc. IEEE, 66 (1978), pp. 51–83.

[58] R. M. HEIDEMANN, M. A. GRISWOLD, A. HAASE, AND P. M. JAKOB, *VD-AUTO-SMASH imaging*, Magn. Reson. Med., 45 (2001), pp. 1066–1074.

[59] J. HENNIG, *Echoes – How to generate, recognize, use or avoid them in MR-imaging sequences. Part I: Fundamental and not so fundamental properties of spin echoes*, Concepts Magn. Reson., 3 (1991), pp. 125–143.

[60] J. HENNIG, A. NAUERTH, AND H. FRIEDBURG, *RARE imaging: A fast imaging method for clinical MR*, Magn. Reson. Med., 3 (1986), pp. 823–833.

[61] J. HENNIG, A. M. WELZ, G. SCHULTZ, J. KORVINK, Z. LIU, O. SPECK, AND M. ZAITSEV, *PatLoc: Imaging in non-bijective, curvilinear magnetic field gradients. A concept study*, Magn. Reson. Mater. Phy., 21 (2008), pp. 5–14.

[62] J. HENNIG, M. ZAITSEV, AND O. SPECK, *PatLoc: Imaging in non-bijective, curvilinear magnetic field gradients*, in Proc. of the ISMRM, Berlin, Germany, 2007, p. 453.

[63] J. HENNIG, M. ZAITSEV, A. M. WELZ, AND G. SCHULTZ, *NMR tomography method based on NBSEM with 2D spatial encoding by two mutually rotated multipole gradient fields*, DE102007054744B4, EP2060927A3, US7906968B2, 2007.

[64] J. HENNIG, K. ZHONG, AND O. SPECK, *MR-Encephalography: Fast multi-channel monitoring of brain physiology with magnetic resonance*, NeuroImage, 34 (2007), pp. 212–219.

[65] M. R. HESTENES AND E. STIEFEL, *Methods of conjugate gradients for solving linear systems*, J. Res. Natl. Bur. Stand., 49 (1952), pp. 409–436.

[66] D. I. HOULT, *The principle of reciprocity in signal strength calculations – a mathematical guide*, Concepts Magn. Reson., 12 (2000), pp. 173–187.

[67] D. I. HOULT AND B. BHAKAR, *NMR signal reception: Virtual photons and coherent spontaneous emission*, Concepts Magn. Reson., 9 (1997), pp. 277–297.

[68] D. I. HOULT AND R. E. RICHARDS, *The signal-to-noise ratio of the nuclear magnetic resonance experiment*, J. Magn. Reson., 24 (1976), pp. 71–85.

[69] T. HUGGER, *Mehrkanal-Bildrekonstruktion bei Unterabtastung in der funktionellen Magnetresonanztomographie*, PhD thesis, University of Freiburg, Germany, 2011.

[70] M. HUTCHINSON AND U. RAFF, *Fast MRI data acquisition using multiple detectors*, Magn. Reson. Med., 6 (1988), pp. 87–91.

[71] W. IRNICH AND F. SCHMITT, *Magnetostimulation in MRI*, Magn. Reson. Med., 33 (1995), pp. 619–623.

[72] S. ITO AND Y. YAMADA, *Alias-free image reconstruction using Fresnel transform in the phase-scrambling Fourier imaging technique*, Magn. Reson. Med., 60 (2008), pp. 422–430.

[73] J. I. JACKSON, C. H. MEYER, AND D. G. NISHIMURA, *Selection of a convolution function for Fourier inversion using gridding*, IEEE Trans. Med. Imaging, 10 (1991), pp. 473–478.

[74] A. K. JAIN, *Fundamentals of Digital Image Processing*, Prentice Hall, New Delhi, India, 2005.

[75] P. M. JAKOB, M. A. GRISWOLD, R. R. EDELMAN, AND D. K. SODICKSON, *AUTO-SMASH: A self-calibrating technique for SMASH imaging. SiMultaneous Acquisition of Spatial Harmonics*, Magn. Reson. Mater. Phy., 7 (1998), pp. 42–54.

[76] F. JIA, *Design Optimization of MRI Gradient Coils*, PhD thesis, University of Freiburg, Germany, 2010.

[77] J. B. JOHNSON, *Thermal agitation of electricity in conductors*, Phys. Rev., 32 (1928), pp. 97–109.

[78] K. O. JOHNSON AND J. G. PIPE, *Convolution kernel design and efficient algorithm for sampling density correction*, Magn. Reson. Med., 61 (2009), pp. 439–447.

[79] C. JUCHEM, T. W. NIXON, S. MCINTYRE, V. O. BOER, D. L. ROTHMANN, AND R. A. DE GRAAF, *Dynamic multi-coil shimming of the human brain at 7T*, in Proc. of the ISMRM, Montreal, Canada, 2011, p. 716.

[80] C. JUCHEM, T. W. NIXON, S. MCINTYRE, D. L. ROTHMANN, AND R. A. DE GRAAF, *Magnetic field modeling with a set of individual localized coils*, J. Magn. Reson., 204 (2010), pp. 281–289.

[81] U. KATSCHER, P. BÖRNERT, C. LEUSSLER, AND J. S. VAN DEN BRINK, *Transmit SENSE*, Magn. Reson. Med., 49 (2003), pp. 144–150.

[82] J. KELTON, R. MAGIN, AND S. WRIGHT, *An algorithm for rapid image acquisition using multiple receiver coils*, in Proc. of the SMRM, Amsterdam, 1989, p. 1172.

[83] F. KNOLL, *Constrained MR Image Reconstruction of Undersampled Data from Multiple Coils*, PhD thesis, Graz University of Technology, Austria, 2011.

[84] F. KNOLL, K. BREDIES, T. POCK, AND R. STOLLBERGER, *Second order total generalized variation (TGV) for MRI*, Magn. Reson. Med., 65 (2011), pp. 480–491.

[85] F. KNOLL, C. CLASON, K. BREDIES, M. UECKER, AND R. STOLLBERGER, *Parallel imaging with nonlinear reconstruction using variational penalties*, Magn. Reson. Med., 67 (2012), pp. 34–41.

[86] F. KNOLL, G. SCHULTZ, K. BREDIES, D. GALLICHAN, M. ZAITSEV, J. HENNIG, AND R. STOLLBERGER, *Reconstruction of undersampled radial PatLoc imaging using Total Generalized Variation*, Magn. Reson. Med., (Submitted, January 2012).

[87] E. KOPANOGLU, B. AKIN, V. B. ERTURK, AND E. ATALAR, *SAR reduction using non-linear gradients*, in Proc. of the ISMRM, Montreal, Canada, 2011, p. 1848.

[88] D. KWIAT, S. EINAV, AND G. NAVON, *A decoupled coil detector array for fast image acquisition in magnetic resonance imaging*, Med. Phys., 18 (1991), pp. 251–265.

[89] L. LAPICQUE, *Définition expérimentale de l'excitabilité*, C. R. Hébd. Séances Mém. Soc. Biol., 67 (1909), pp. 280–283.

[90] D. J. LARKMAN AND R. G. NUNES, *Parallel magnetic resonance imaging*, Phys. Med. Biol., 52 (2007), pp. R15–R55.

[91] A. J. LAUB, *Matrix Analysis for Scientists and Engineers*, SIAM, 2005.

[92] P. C. LAUTERBUR, *Image formation by induced local interactions: Examples employing nuclear magnetic resonance*, Nature, 242 (1973), pp. 190–191.

[93] K. J. LAYTON, P. M. MORELANDE, M.AND FARRELL, B. MORAN, AND L. A. JOHNSTON, *Performance analysis for magnetic resonance imaging with nonlinear encoding fields*, Magn. Reson. Med., 31 (2012), pp. 391–404.

[94] S. LEE, G. WOLBERG, AND S. Y. SHIN, *Scattered data interpolation with multilevel B-splines.*, IEEE Trans. Vis. Comput. Graphics, 3 (1997), pp. 228–244.

[95] M. H. LEVITT, *Spin Dynamics - Basics of Nuclear Magnetic Resonance*, Wiley, 2 ed., 2008.

[96] Z.-P. LIANG AND P. C. LAUTERBUR, *Principles of Magnetic Resonance Imaging*, IEEE Press, 2000.

[97] F.-H. LIN, T. W. A. NUMMENMAA, P. VESANEN, R. J. ILMONIEMI, AND J. W. BELLIVEAU, *Multi-dimensional encoded (MDE) magnetic resonance imaging*, in Proc. of the ISMRM, Montreal, Canada 2011, p. 480.

[98] F.-H. LIN, P. VESANEN, T. W. R. ILMONIEMI, AND J. HENNIG, *Parallel imaging technique using localized gradients (PatLoc) reconstruction using*

compressed sensing (CS), in Proc. of the ISMRM, Stockholm, Sweden 2010, p. 546.

[99] F.-H. LIN, L. L. WALD, S. P. AHLFORS, M. S. HÄMÄLÄINEN, K. K. KWONG, AND J. W. BELLIVEAU, *Dynamic magnetic resonance inverse imaging of human brain function*, Magn. Reson. Med., 56 (2006), pp. 787–802.

[100] F.-H. LIN, T. WITZEL, J. POLIMENI, J. HENNIG, G. SCHULTZ, J. W. BELLIVEAU, AND L. L. WALD, *Parallel imaging technique using localized gradients (PatLoc) reconstruction using orthogonal mode decomposition*, in Proc. of the ISMRM, Honolulu, HI, USA, 2009, p. 4557.

[101] F.-H. LIN, T. WITZEL, G. SCHULTZ, D. GALLICHAN, W.-J. JUI, F.-N. WANG, J. HENNIG, M. ZAITSEV, AND J. W. BELLIVEAU, *Reconstruction of MRI data encoded by multiple non-bijective curvilinear magnetic fields*, Magn. Reson. Med., (Published online, January 2012).

[102] S. LITTIN, A. WELZ, D. GALLICHAN, F. JIA, G. SCHULTZ, C. CO-COSCO, J. HENNIG, AND M. ZAITSEV, *Optimization of a planar gradient system for imaging with non-linear gradients*, in Proc. of the ESMRMB, Leipzig, Germany, 2011, p. 529.

[103] S. LITTIN, A. M. WELZ, D. GALLICHAN, G. SCHULTZ, C. COCOSCO, J. HENNIG, W. DE BOER, AND M. ZAITSEV, *Planar gradient system for imaging with non-linear gradients*, in Proc. of the ISMRM, Montreal, Canada, 2011, p. 1837.

[104] T. LIU, B. KRESSLER, K. WANG, AND Y. WANG, *Block circulant quasi-band matrix property for the SENSE unfolding in k-space and justification for GRAPPA*, in Conf. Proc. IEEE Eng. Med. Biol. Soc., 2008, pp. 1659–1662.

[105] Z. LIU, F. JIA, M. ZAITSEV, A. M. WELZ, G. SCHULTZ, J. G. KORVINK, AND J. HENNIG, *Parametrical optimization of a PatLoc gradient coil*, in Proc. of the ISMRM, Toronto, Canada, 2008, p. 1164.

[106] M. LUSTIG, D. DONOHO, AND J. M. PAULY, *Sparse MRI: The application of compressed sensing for rapid MR imaging*, Magn. Reson. Med., 58 (2007), pp. 1182–1195.

[107] J. MACLAREN, K. J. LEE, C. LUENGVIRIYA, O. SPECK, AND M. ZA-ITSEV, *Combined prospective and retrospective motion correction to relax navigator requirements*, Magn. Reson. Med., 65 (2011), pp. 1724–1732.

[108] P. MANSFIELD AND P. K. GRANNELL, *NMR "diffraction" in solids?*, J. Phys. C: Solid State Phys., 6 (1973), pp. L422–L426.

[109] P. MANSFIELD AND A. A. MAUDSLEY, *Planar spin imaging by NMR*, J. Phys. C: Solid State Phys., 9 (1976), pp. 409–412.

[110] A. A. MAUDSLEY, *Dynamic range improvement in NMR imaging using phase scrambling*, J. Magn. Reson., 76 (1988), pp. 287–305.

[111] J. MISPELTER, M. LUPU, AND A. BRIGUET, *NMR Probeheads: For Biophysical and Biomedical Experiments*, Imperial College Press, 2006.

[112] C. A. MISTRETTA, O. WIEBEN, J. VELIKINA, W. BLOCK, J. PERRY, Y. WU, K. JOHNSON, AND Y. WU, *Highly constrained backprojection for time-resolved MRI*, Magn. Reson. Med., 55 (2006), pp. 30–40.

[113] C. T. W. MOONEN AND P. A. BANDETTINI, eds., *Functional MRI*, Springer, 1999.

[114] R. NANA, *On Optimality and Efficiency of Parallel Magnetic Reconance Imaging Reconstruction: Challenges and Solutions*, PhD thesis, Georgia Institute of Technology, Atlanta, GA, USA, 2008.

[115] J. NOCEDAL AND S. J. WRIGHT, *Numerical Optimization*, Springer, 1999.

[116] H. NYQUIST, *Thermal agitation of electric charge in conductors*, Phys. Rev., 32 (1928), pp. 110–113.

[117] O. OCALI AND E. ATALAR, *Ultimate intrinsic signal-to-noise ratio in MRI*, Magn. Reson. Med., 39 (1998), pp. 462–473.

[118] M. A. OHLIGER, *Fundamental and Practical Limits to Image Acceleration in Parallel Magnetic Resonance Imaging*, PhD thesis, Massachusetts Institute of Technology, Cambridge, MA, USA, 2005.

[119] M. A. OHLIGER, A. K. GRANT, AND D. K. SODICKSON, *Ultimate intrinsic signal-to-noise ratio for parallel MRI: electromagnetic field considerations*, Magn. Reson. Med., 50 (2003), pp. 1018–1030.

[120] S. OHREL, H. LEHR, F. JASPARD, P. ULLMANN, AND H. POST, *Development of a new high-performance PatLoc gradient system for small-animal imaging*, in Proc. of the ISMRM, Stockholm, Sweden, 2010, p. 3936.

[121] S. OHREL, H. LEHR, G. SCHULTZ, M. BERBERICH, D. SCHINKO, J. T. SCHNEIDER, A. M. WELZ, J. HENNIG, H. POST, AND P. ULLMANN, *PatLoc imaging in small animals - first in vivo results*, in Proc. of the ESMRMB, Antalya, Turkey, 2009, p. 192.

[122] N. OHYAMA, S. OHKI, S. INOUE, J. TSUJIUCHI, AND T. HONDA, *Discrete Radon transform in a continuous space*, J. Opt. Soc. Am. A, 4 (1987), pp. 318–324.

[123] A. E. OPPELT, *Imaging Systems for Medical Diagnostics*, Publicis Corporate Publishing, Erlangen, Germany, 2005.

[124] J. D. O'SULLIVAN, *A fast sinc function gridding algorithm for Fourier inversion in computer tomography*, IEEE Trans. Med. Imaging, 4 (1985), pp. 200–207.

[125] R. OTAZO, F.-H. LIN, G. WIGGINS, R. JORDAN, D. SODICKSON, AND S. POSSE, *Superresolution parallel magnetic resonance imaging: Application to functional and spectroscopic imaging*, NeuroImage, 47 (2009), pp. 220–230.

[126] D. L. PARKER AND J. R. HADLEY, *Multiple-region gradient arrays for extended field of view, increased performance, and reduced nerve stimulation in magnetic resonance imaging*, Magn. Reson. Med., 56 (2006), pp. 1251–1260.

[127] V. PAROT, C. SING-LONG, C. LIZAMA, C. TEJOS, S. URIBE, AND P. IRARRAZAVAL, *Application of the fractional fourier transform to image reconstruction in MRI*, Magn. Reson. Med., (Published online, October 2011).

[128] S. PATZ, M. I. HROVAT, Y. M. PULYER, AND F. J. RYBICKI, *Novel encoding technology for ultrafast MRI in a limited spatial region*, Int. J. Imaging Syst. Technol., 10 (1999), pp. 216–224.

[129] J. PAULY, P. L. ROUX, D. NISHIMURA, AND A. MACOVSKI, *Parameter relations for the Shinnar-Le Roux selective excitation pulse design algorithm [NMR imaging]*, IEEE Trans. Med. Imaging, 10 (1991), pp. 53–65.

[130] D. C. PETERS, J. A. DERBYSHIRE, AND E. R. MCVEIGH, *Centering the projection reconstruction trajectory: Reducing gradient delay errors*, Magn. Reson. Med., 50 (2003), pp. 1–6.

[131] J. G. PIPE, *Spatial encoding and reconstruction in MRI with quadratic phase profiles*, Magn. Reson. Med., 33 (1995), pp. 24–33.

[132] J. G. PIPE AND P. MENON, *Sampling density compensation in MRI: Rationale and an iterative numerical solution*, Magn. Reson. Med., 41 (1999), pp. 179–186.

[133] D. POTTS, G. STEIDL, AND M. TASCHE, *Fast Fourier transforms for nonequispaced data: A tutorial*, in Modern Sampling Theory: Mathematics and Application, J. J. Benedetto and P. J. S. G. Ferreira, eds., Birkhäuser, 2000, pp. 251–274.

[134] K. PRÜSSMANN, M. WEIGER, P. BÖRNERT, AND P. BÖSIGER, *Advances in sensitivity encoding with arbitrary k-space trajectories*, Magn. Reson. Med., 46 (2001), pp. 638–651.

[135] K. PRÜSSMANN, M. WEIGER, M. SCHEIDEGGER, AND P. BÖSIGER, *SENSE: Sensitivity encoding for fast MRI*, Magn. Reson. Med., 42 (1999), pp. 952–962.

[136] K. P. PRÜSSMANN, *Encoding and reconstruction in parallel MRI*, NMR Biomed., 19 (2006), pp. 288–299.

[137] E. M. PURCELL, H. C. TORREY, AND R. V. POUND, *Resonance absorption by nuclear magnetic moments in a solid*, Phys. Rev., 69 (1946), pp. 37–38.

[138] P. QU, K. ZHONG, B. ZHANG, J. WANG, AND G. X. SHEN, *Convergence behavior of iterative SENSE reconstruction with non-Cartesian trajectories*, Magn. Reson. Med., 54 (2005), pp. 1040–1045.

[139] J. B. RA AND C. Y. RIM, *Fast imaging using subencoding data sets from multiple detectors*, Magn. Reson. Med., 30 (1993), pp. 142–145.

[140] I. I. RABI, J. R. ZACHARIAS, S. MILLMANN, AND P. KUSCH, *A new method of measuring nuclear magnetic moment*, Phys. Rev., 53 (1938), p. 318.

[141] J. RAHMER, P. BÖRNERT, J. GROEN, AND C. BOS, *Three-dimensional radial ultrashort echo-time imaging with T2 adapted sampling*, Magn. Reson. Med., 55 (2006), pp. 1075–1082.

[142] V. RASCHE, R. PROSKA, R. SINKUS, P. BORNERT, AND H. EGGERS, *Resampling of data between arbitrary grids using convolution interpolation*, IEEE Trans. Med. Imaging, 18 (1999), pp. 385–392.

[143] I. L. H. REICHERT, M. BENJAMIN, P. D. GATEHOUSE, K. E. CHAPPELL, J. HOLMES, T. HE, AND G. M. BYDDER, *Magnetic resonance imaging of periosteum with ultrashort TE pulse sequences*, J. Magn. Reson. Imaging, 19 (2004), pp. 99–107.

[144] J. P. REILLY, *Peripheral nerve stimulation by induced electric currents: Exposure to time-varying magnetic fields*, Med. Biol. Eng. Comput., 27 (1989), pp. 101–110.

[145] P. B. ROEMER, W. A. EDELSTEIN, C. E. HAYES, S. P. SOUZA, AND O. M. MUELLER, *The NMR phased array*, Magn. Reson. Med., 16 (1990), pp. 192–225.

[146] J. B. T. M. ROERDINK AND M. A. WESTENBERG, *Data-parallel tomographic reconstruction: A comparison of filtered backprojection and direct Fourier reconstruction*, Parallel Comput., 24 (1998), pp. 2129–2142.

[147] A. A. SAMSONOV, W. F. BLOCK, A. ARUNACHALAM, AND A. S. FIELD, *Advances in locally constrained k-space-based parallel MRI*, Magn. Reson. Med., 55 (2006), pp. 431–438.

[148] G. E. SARTY, *Single trajectory radial (STAR) imaging*, Magn. Reson. Med., 51 (2004), pp. 445–451.

[149] L. SCHAD, S. LOTT, F. SCHMITT, V. STURM, AND W. J. LORENZ, *Correction of spatial distortion in MR imaging: A prerequisite for accurate stereotaxy*, J. Comput. Assist. Tomogr., 11 (1987), pp. 499–505.

[150] K. SCHEFFLER, *Spin Zoo*. http://www.kyb.tuebingen.mpg.de/de/forschung/abt/ks/spinzoo.html. March 26th, 2012.

[151] K. SCHEFFLER AND J. HENNIG, *Reduced circular field-of-view imaging*, Magn. Reson. Med., 40 (1998), pp. 474–480.

[152] J. T. SCHNEIDER, M. HAAS, S. OHREL, H. LEHR, W. RUHM, H. POST, J. HENNIG, AND P. ULLMANN, *Parallel spatially selective excitation using nonlinear non-bijective PatLoc encoding fields: Experimental realization and first results*, in Proc. of the ISMRM, Montreal, Canada, 2011, p. 211.

[153] G. SCHULTZ, D. GALLICHAN, M. REISERT, J. HENNIG, AND M. ZAIT-SEV, *Fast image reconstruction for generalized projection imaging*, in Proc. of the ISMRM, Montreal, Canada, 2011, p. 2868.

[154] G. SCHULTZ, D. GALLICHAN, H. WEBER, W. R. WITSCHEY, M. HONAL, J. HENNIG, AND M. ZAITSEV, *K-space based image reconstruction of MRI data encoded with ambiguous gradient fields*, in Proc. of the ISMRM, Montreal, Canada, 2011, p. 481.

[155] G. SCHULTZ, J. HENNIG, AND M. ZAITSEV, *Image reconstruction from ambiguous PatLoc-encoded MR data*, in Proc. of the ISMRM, Toronto, Canada, 2008, p. 786.

[156] G. SCHULTZ, P. ULLMANN, H. LEHR, A. M. WELZ, J. HENNIG, AND M. ZAITSEV, *Reconstruction of MRI data encoded with arbitrarily shaped, curvilinear, nonbijective magnetic fields*, Magn. Reson. Med., 64 (2010), pp. 1390–1403.

[157] G. SCHULTZ, H. WEBER, D. GALLICHAN, J. HENNIG, AND M. ZA-ITSEV, *Image reconstruction from radially acquired data using multipolar encoding fields*, in Proc. of the ISMRM, Stockholm, Sweden, 2010, p. 82.

[158] G. SCHULTZ, H. WEBER, D. GALLICHAN, W. R. WITSCHEY, A. M. WELZ, C. A. COCOSCO, J. HENNIG, AND M. ZAITSEV, *Radial imaging with multipolar magnetic encoding fields*, IEEE Trans. Med. Imaging, 30 (2011), pp. 2134–2145.

[159] G. SCHULTZ, A. M. WELZ, J. HENNIG, AND M. ZAITSEV, *Generalized two-dimensional orthogonal spatial encoding fields*, in Proc. of the ISMRM, Toronto, Canada, 2008, p. 2992.

[160] G. SCHULTZ AND M. ZAITSEV, *Estimation of superresolution performance*, in Proc. of the ISMRM, Stockholm, Sweden, 2010, p. 2935.

[161] G. SCHULTZ, M. ZAITSEV, AND J. HENNIG, *Effects of discrete and finite sampling in PatLoc imaging*, in Proc. of the ISMRM, Honolulu, HI, USA, 2009, p. 563.

[162] G. SCHULTZ, M. ZAITSEV, P. ULLMANN, H. LEHR, AND J. HENNIG, *Noise behavior of Cartesian PatLoc reconstruction*, in Proc. of the ISMRM, Honolulu, HI, USA, 2009, p. 762.

[163] G. C. SCOTT, *NMR Imaging of Current Density and Magnetic Fields*, PhD thesis, University of Toronto, Canada, 1993.

[164] H. SEDARAT AND D. G. NISHIMURA, *On the optimality of the gridding reconstruction algorithm*, IEEE Trans. Med. Imaging, 19 (2000), pp. 306–317.

[165] N. SEIBERLICH, F. BREUER, R. HEIDEMANN, M. BLAIMER, M. GRISWOLD, AND P. M. JAKOB, *Reconstruction of undersampled non-Cartesian data sets using pseudo-Cartesian GRAPPA in conjunction with GROG*, Magn. Reson. Med., 59 (2008), pp. 1127–1137.

[166] N. SEIBERLICH, F. A. BREUER, M. BLAIMER, K. BARKAUSKAS, P. M. JAKOB, AND M. A. GRISWOLD, *Non-Cartesian data reconstruction using GRAPPA operator gridding (GROG)*, Magn. Reson. Med., 58 (2007), pp. 1257–1265.

[167] N. SEIBERLICH, F. A. BREUER, P. EHSES, H. MORIGUCHI, M. BLAIMER, P. M. JAKOB, AND M. A. GRISWOLD, *Using the GRAPPA operator and the generalized sampling theorem to reconstruct undersampled non-Cartesian data*, Magn. Reson. Med., 61 (2009), pp. 705–715.

[168] C. E. SHANNON, *Communication in the presence of noise*, Proc. IEEE, 86 (1998), pp. 447–457.

[169] J. R. SHEWCHUK, *An introduction to the conjugate gradient method without the agonizing pain.* http://www.cs.cmu.edu/~quake-papers/painless-conjugate-gradient.pdf. March 26th, 2012.

[170] J. SÁNCHEZ-GONZÁLEZ, J. TSAO, U. DYDAK, M. DESCO, P. BÖSIGER, AND K. P. PRÜSSMANN, *Minimum-norm reconstruction for sensitivity-encoded magnetic resonance spectroscopic imaging*, Magn. Reson. Med., 55 (2006), pp. 287–295.

[171] D. K. SODICKSON, *Tailored SMASH image reconstructions for robust in vivo parallel MR imaging*, Magn. Reson. Med., 44 (2000), pp. 243–251.

[172] D. K. SODICKSON, *The many guises of tomography – personal history of parallel imaging*, Enc. Magn. Reson., (Published online, June 15th, 2011).

[173] D. K. SODICKSON AND W. J. MANNING, *Simultaneous acquisition of spatial harmonics (SMASH): Fast imaging with radiofrequency coil arrays*, Magn. Reson. Med., 38 (1997), pp. 591–603.

[174] D. N. SPLITTHOFF, *SENSE Shimming (SSH) – Fast Detection of B0 Field Inhomogeneities in Magnetic Resonance Imaging*, PhD thesis, University of Freiburg, Germany, 2011.

[175] D. N. SPLITTHOFF AND M. ZAITSEV, *SENSE shimming (SSH): A fast approach for determining B0 field inhomogeneities using sensitivity coding*, Magn. Reson. Med., 62 (2009), pp. 1319–1325.

[176] A. STALDER, *Quantitative Analysis of Blood Flow and Vessel Wall Parameters Using 4D Flow-Sensitive MRI*, PhD thesis, University of Freiburg, Germany, 2009.

[177] J. P. STOCKMANN, P. A. CIRIS, AND R. T. CONSTABLE, *Efficient "O-space" parallel imaging with higher-order encoding gradients and no phase encoding*, in Proc. of the ISMRM, Honolulu, HI, USA, 2009, p. 761.

[178] J. P. STOCKMANN, P. A. CIRIS, G. GALIANA, L. TAM, AND R. T. CONSTABLE, *O-space imaging: Highly efficient parallel imaging using second-order nonlinear fields as encoding gradients with no phase encoding*, Magn. Reson. Med., 64 (2010), pp. 447–456.

[179] J. P. STOCKMANN, G. GALIANA, V. PAROT, L. TAM, AND R. T. CONSTABLE, *The variable-order fractional Fourier transform: A new tool for efficient reconstruction of images encoded by linear and quadratic gradients with reduced sensitivity to calibration errors*, in Proc. of the ISMRM, Montreal, Canada, 2011, p. 744.

[180] J. SUNNEGARDH, *Iterative Filtered Backprojection Methods for Helical Cone-Beam CT*, PhD thesis, Linköping University, 2009.

[181] L. K. TAM, J. P. STOCKMANN, G. GALIANA, AND R. T. CONSTABLE, *Null space imaging: Nonlinear magnetic encoding fields designed complementary to receiver coil sensitivities for improved acceleration in parallel imaging*, Magn. Reson. Med., (Published online, December 2011).

[182] H. C. TORREY, *Bloch equations with diffusion terms*, Phys. Rev., 104 (1956), pp. 563–565.

[183] J. TSAO, K. P. PRÜSSMANN, AND P. BÖSIGER, *Feedback regularization for SENSE reconstruction*, in Proc. of the ISMRM, Honolulu, HI, USA, 2002, p. 739.

[184] M. UECKER, T. HOHAGE, K. T. BLOCK, AND J. FRAHM, *Image reconstruction by regularized nonlinear inversion–joint estimation of coil sensitivities and image content*, Magn. Reson. Med., 60 (2008), pp. 674–682.

[185] P. ULLMANN, *Parallele Sendetechniken in der Kernspintomographie. Experimentelle Realisierung, Anwendung und Perspektiven*, PhD thesis, University of Freiburg, Germany, 2007.

[186] S. VANDENBERGHE, Y. D'ASSELER, R. V. DE WALLE, T. KAUPPINEN, M. KOOLE, L. BOUWENS, K. V. LAERE, I. LEMAHIEU, AND R. A. DIERCKX, *Iterative reconstruction algorithms in nuclear medicine*, Comput. Med. Imaging Graphics, 25 (2001), pp. 105–111.

[187] P. VEDRINE, W. A. MAKSOUD, G. AUBERT, F. BEAUDET, J. BELORGEY, S. BERMOND, C. BERRIAUD, P. BREDY, D. BRESSON, A. DONATI, O. DUBOIS, G. GILGRASS, F. JUSTER, H. LANNOU, C. MEURIS, F. MOLINIÉ, M. NUSBAUM, F. NUNIO, A. PAYN, T. SCHILD, L. SCOLA, AND A. SINANNA, *Latest progress on the Iseult/INUMAC whole body 11.7 T MRI magnet*, IEEE Trans. Appl. Supercond., (Early access, received September 2011).

[188] D. O. WALSH, A. F. GMITRO, AND M. W. MARCELLIN, *Adaptive reconstruction of phased array MR imagery*, Magn. Reson. Med., 43 (2000), pp. 682–690.

[189] H. WEBER, D. GALLICHAN, G. SCHULTZ, C. COCOSCO, S. LITTIN, W. REICHARDT, A. M. WELZ, W. R. WITSCHEY, J. HENNIG, AND M. ZAITSEV, *Excitation and geometrically matched local encoding of curved slices*, Magn. Reson. Med., (Submitted, March 2012).

[190] H. WEBER, D. GALLICHAN, G. SCHULTZ, J. HENNIG, AND M. ZAITSEV, *A time-efficient sub-sampling strategy to homogenise resolution in PatLoc imaging*, in Proc. of the ISMRM, Stockholm, Sweden, 2010, p. 548.

[191] H. WEBER, D. GALLICHAN, G. SCHULTZ, W. R. WITSCHEY, A. M. WELZ, C. A. COCOSCO, J. HENNIG, AND M. ZAITSEV, *ExLoc: Excitation and encoding of curved slices*, in Proc. of the ISMRM, Montreal, Canada, 2011, p. 2806.

[192] H. WEBER, M. ZAITSEV, D. GALLICHAN, AND G. SCHULTZ, *Method for homogenising resolution in magnetic resonance tomography recordings using non-linear encoding fields*, DE102010003552B4, EP2378308A1, US20110241678A1, 2010.

[193] V. J. WEDEEN, Y. S. CHAO, AND J. L. ACKERMAN, *Dynamic range compression in MRI by means of a nonlinear gradient pulse*, Magn. Reson. Med., 6 (1988), pp. 287–295.

[194] M. WEIGER, K. P. PRÜSSMANN, AND P. BÖSIGER, *Cardiac real-time imaging using SENSE. SENSitivity Encoding scheme*, Magn. Reson. Med., 43 (2000), pp. 177–184.

[195] G. WEISS, *La loi de l'excitation électrique des nerfs*, C. R. Hébd. Séances Mém. Soc. Biol., 53 (1901), pp. 466–468.

[196] A. M. WELZ, C. COCOSCO, A. DEWDNEY, H. SCHMIDT, H. JIA, J. G. KORVINK, J. HENNIG, AND M. ZAITSEV, *PatLoc gradient insert coil for human imaging at 3T*, in Proc. of the ESMRMB, Antalya, Turkey, 2009, p. 316.

[197] A. M. WELZ, D. GALLICHAN, C. COCOSCO, R. KUMAR, F. JIA, J. SNYDER, A. DEWDNEY, J. G. KORVINK, J. HENNIG, AND M. ZAITSEV, *Characterization of a PatLoc gradient coil*, in Proc. of the ISMRM, Stockholm, Sweden, 2010, p. 1527.

[198] A. M. WELZ, M. ZAITSEV, F. JIA, Z. LIU, J. G. KORVINK, H. SCHMIDT, H. LEHR, H. POST, A. DEWDNEY, AND J. HENNIG, *Development of a non-shielded PatLoc gradient insert for human head imaging*, in Proc. of the ISMRM, Honolulu, HI, USA, 2009, p. 762.

[199] A. M. WELZ, M. ZAITSEV, H. LEHR, G. SCHULTZ, Z. LIU, F. JIA, H. POST, J. KORVINK, AND J. HENNIG, *Initial realisation of a multichannel, non-linear PatLoc gradient coil*, in Proc. of the ISMRM, Toronto, Canada, 2008, p. 1164.

[200] F. WIESINGER, P. BÖSIGER, AND K. P. PRÜSSMANN, *Electrodynamics and ultimate SNR in parallel MR imaging*, Magn. Reson. Med., 52 (2004), pp. 376–390.

[201] F. WIESINGER, P.-F. VAN DE MOORTELE, G. ADRIANY, N. DE ZAN-CHE, K. UGURBIL, AND K. P. PRÜSSMANN, *Parallel imaging performance as a function of field strength–an experimental investigation using electrodynamic scaling*, Magn. Reson. Med., 52 (2004), pp. 953–964.

[202] WIKIPEDIA, *Main Article: Wilhelm Röntgen.* http://de.wikipedia. org/wiki/Wilhelm_Conrad_R%C3%B6ntgen. March 26th, 2012.

[203] S. WINTZHEIMER, T. DRIESSLE, M. LEDWIG, P. M. JAKOB, AND F. FIDLER, *A 50-channel matrix gradient system: A feasibility study*, in Proc. of the ISMRM, Stockholm, Sweden, 2010, p. 3937.

[204] S. WINTZHEIMER, F. FIDLER, M. LEDWIG, T. DRIESSLE, D. GENSLER, AND P. M. JAKOB, *A novel gradient design: Simultaneous generation of fast switchable linear and high order field gradient for MR imaging*, in Proc. of the ISMRM, Honolulu, HI, USA, 2009, p. 3059.

[205] W. R. WITSCHEY, C. A. COCOSCO, D. GALLICHAN, G. SCHULTZ, H. WEBER, A. M. WELZ, J. HENNIG, AND M. ZAITSEV, *Localization by nonlinear phase preparation and k-space trajectory design (GradLoc)*, in Proc. of the ISMRM, Montreal, Canada, 2011, p. 2805.

[206] W. R. WITSCHEY, C. A. COCOSCO, D. GALLICHAN, G. SCHULTZ, H. WEBER, A. M. WELZ, J. HENNIG, AND M. ZAITSEV, *STAGES: Dynamic shimming by nonlinear phase preparation and k-space parcellation in steady-state MRI*, in Proc. of the ISMRM, Montreal, Canada, 2011, p. 4583.

[207] W. R. WITSCHEY, C. A. COCOSCO, D. GALLICHAN, G. SCHULTZ, H. WEBER, A. M. WELZ, J. HENNIG, AND M. ZAITSEV, *Localization by nonlinear phase preperation and k-space trajectory design*, Magn. Reson. Med., (Published online, November 2011).

[208] Y. YAMADA, K. TANAKA, AND Z. ABE, *NMR Fresnel transform imaging technique using a quadratic nonlinear field gradient*, Rev. Sci. Instrum., 63 (1992), pp. 5348–5358.

[209] E. N. YEH, C. A. MCKENZIE, M. A. OHLIGER, AND D. K. SODICK-SON, *Parallel magnetic resonance imaging with adaptive radius in k-space (PARS): Constrained image reconstruction using k-space locality in radiofrequency coil encoded data*, Magn. Reson. Med., 53 (2005), pp. 1383–1392.

[210] B. ZAHNEISEN, *Funktionelle Magnetresonanztomographie mit stark unterabgetasteten Trajektorien*, PhD thesis, University of Freiburg, Germany, 2011.

[211] B. ZAHNEISEN, T. GROTZ, K. J. LEE, S. OHLENDORF, M. REISERT, M. ZAITSEV, AND J. HENNIG, *Three-dimensional MR-encephalography: Fast volumetric brain imaging using rosette trajectories*, Magn. Reson. Med., 65 (2011), pp. 1260–1268.

[212] M. ZAITSEV, *Development of Methods for functional magnetic resonance imaging and relaxation time mapping*, PhD thesis, University of Cologne, Germany, 2002.

[213] M. ZAITSEV, G. SCHULTZ, AND J. HENNIG, *Extended anti-aliasing reconstruction for phase-scrambed MRI with quadratic phase modulation*, in Proc. of the ISMRM, Honolulu, HI, USA, 2009, p. 1425.

[214] X. ZHAO, R. PRATT, AND J. WANSAPURA, *Quantification of aortic compliance in mice using radial phase contrast MRI*, J. Magn. Reson. Imaging, 30 (2009), pp. 286–291.

[215] Y. ZHU, *Parallel excitation with an array of transmit coils*, Magn. Reson. Med., 51 (2004), pp. 775–784.

Publications

Journal Publications

As First Author

- **G. Schultz**, H. Weber, D. Gallichan, W. R. Witschey, A. M. Welz, C. A. Cocosco, J. Hennig, and M. Zaitsev. Radial imaging with multipolar magnetic encoding fields. *IEEE Trans. Med. Imaging*, 30(12):2134–2145, 2011.

- **G. Schultz**, P. Ullmann, H. Lehr, A. M. Welz, J. Hennig, and M. Zaitsev. Reconstruction of MRI data encoded with arbitrarily shaped, curvilinear, nonbijective magnetic fields. *Magn. Reson. Med.*, 64(5):1390–1403, 2010.

As Co-Author

- D. Gallichan, C. Cocosco, **G. Schultz**, H. Weber, A. M. Welz, J. Hennig, and M. Zaitsev. Practical considerations for in-vivo MRI with higher dimensional spatial encoding. *Magn. Reson. Mater. Phy.*, Accepted, March 2012.

- H. Weber, D. Gallichan, **G. Schultz**, C. Cocosco, S. Littin, W. Reichardt, A. M. Welz, W. R. Witschey, J. Hennig, and M. Zaitsev. Excitation and geometrically matched local encoding of curved slices. *Magn. Reson. Med.*, Submitted, March 2012.

- F. Knoll, **G. Schultz**, K. Bredies, D. Gallichan, M. Zaitsev, J. Hennig, and R. Stollberger. Reconstruction of undersampled radial PatLoc imaging using total generalized variation. *Magn. Reson. Med.*, Submitted, January 2012.

- F.-H. Lin, T. Witzel, **G. Schultz**, D. Gallichan, W.-J. Jui, F.-N. Wang, J. Hennig, M. Zaitsev, and J. W. Belliveau. Reconstruction of MRI data encoded by multiple non-bijective curvilinear magnetic fields. *Magn. Reson. Med.*, Published online, January 2012.

- W. R. Witschey, C. A. Cocosco, D. Gallichan, **G. Schultz**, H. Weber, A. M. Welz, J. Hennig, and M. Zaitsev. Localization by nonlinear phase preperation and k-space trajectory design. *Magn. Reson. Med.*, Published online, November 2011.

- D. Gallichan, C. Cocosco, A. Dewdney, **G. Schultz**, A. Welz, J. Hennig, and M. Zaitsev. Simultaneously driven linear and nonlinear spatial encoding fields in MRI. *Magn. Reson. Med.*, 65(3):702–714, 2011.

- J. Hennig, A. M. Welz, **G. Schultz**, J. Korvink, Z. Liu, O. Speck, and M. Zaitsev. PatLoc: Imaging in non-bijective, curvilinear magnetic field gradients. A concept study. *Magn. Reson. Mater. Phy.*, 21(1-2):5–14, 2008.

Publications in Conference Proceedings

2011

- **G. Schultz**, D. Gallichan, H. Weber, W. R. Witschey, M. Honal, J. Hennig, and M. Zaitsev. K-space based image reconstruction of MRI data encoded with ambiguous gradient fields. In *Proc. of the ISMRM*, page 481, Montreal, Canada, 2011.

- **G. Schultz**, D. Gallichan, M. Reisert, J. Hennig, and M. Zaitsev. Fast image reconstruction for generalized projection imaging. In *Proc. of the ISMRM*, page 2868, Montreal, Canada, 2011.

- H. Weber, D. Gallichan, **G. Schultz**, W. R. Witschey, A. M. Welz, C. A. Cocosco, J. Hennig, and M. Zaitsev. ExLoc: Excitation and encoding of curved slices. In *Proc. of the ISMRM*, page 2806, Montreal, Canada, 2011.

- S. Littin, A. M. Welz, D. Gallichan, **G. Schultz**, C. Cocosco, J. Hennig, W. de Boer, and M. Zaitsev. Planar gradient system for imaging with non-linear gradients. In *Proc. of the ISMRM*, page 1837, Montreal, Canada, 2011.

- C. A. Cocosco, D. Gallichan, A. Dewdney, **G. Schultz**, A. M. Welz, W. R. Witschey, H. Weber, J. Hennig, and M. Zaitsev. First in-vivo results with a PatLoc gradient insert coil for human head imaging. In *Proc. of the ISMRM*, page 714, Montreal, Canada, 2011.

- W. R. Witschey, C. A. Cocosco, D. Gallichan, **G. Schultz**, H. Weber, A. M. Welz, J. Hennig, and M. Zaitsev. Localization by nonlinear phase preparation and k-space trajectory design (GradLoc). In *Proc. of the ISMRM*, page 2805, Montreal, Canada, 2011.

- W. R. Witschey, C. A. Cocosco, D. Gallichan, **G. Schultz**, H. Weber, A. M. Welz, J. Hennig, and M. Zaitsev. STAGES: Dynamic shimming by nonlinear phase preparation and k-space parcellation in steady-state MRI. In *Proc. of the ISMRM*, page 4583, Montreal, Canada, 2011.

- S. Littin, A. Welz, D. Gallichan, F. Jia, **G. Schultz**, C. Cocosco, J. Hennig, and M. Zaitsev. Optimization of a planar gradient system for imaging with non-linear gradients. In *Proc. of the ESMRMB*, page 529, Leipzig, Germany, 2011.

2010

- **G. Schultz** and M. Zaitsev. Estimation of superresolution performance. In *Proc. of the ISMRM*, page 2935, Stockholm, Sweden, 2010.

- **G. Schultz**, H. Weber, D. Gallichan, J. Hennig, and M. Zaitsev. Image reconstruction from radially acquired data using multipolar encoding fields. In *Proc. of the ISMRM*, page 82, Stockholm, Sweden, 2010.

- D. Gallichan, **G. Schultz**, J. Hennig, and M. Zaitsev. Designing k-space trajectories for simultaneous encoding with linear and PatLoc gradients. In *Proc. of the ISMRM*, page 547, Stockholm, Sweden, 2010.

- C. A. Cocosco, A.J. Dewdney, P. Dietz, M. Semmler, A. M. Welz, D. Gallichan, H. Weber, **G. Schultz**, J. Hennig, and M. Zaitsev. Safety considerations for a PatLoc gradient insert coil for human head imaging. In *Proc. of the ISMRM*, page 3946, Stockholm, Sweden, 2010.

- H. Weber, D. Gallichan, **G. Schultz**, J. Hennig, and M. Zaitsev. A time-efficient sub-sampling strategy to homogenise resolution in PatLoc imaging. In *Proc. of the ISMRM*, page 548, Stockholm, Sweden, 2010.

2009

- **G. Schultz**, M. Zaitsev, and J. Hennig.   Effects of discrete and finite sampling in PatLoc imaging. In *Proc. of the ISMRM*, page 563, Honolulu, HI, USA, 2009.

- **G. Schultz**, M. Zaitsev, P. Ullmann, H. Lehr, and J. Hennig.   Noise behavior of Cartesian PatLoc reconstruction. In *Proc. of the ISMRM*, page 762, Honolulu, HI, USA, 2009.

- F.-H. Lin, T. Witzel, J. Polimeni, J. Hennig, **G. Schultz**, J. W. Belliveau, and L. L. Wald. Parallel imaging technique using localized gradients (PatLoc) reconstruction using orthogonal mode decomposition. In *Proc. of the ISMRM*, page 4557, Honolulu, HI, USA, 2009.

- M. Zaitsev, **G. Schultz**, and J. Hennig. Extended anti-aliasing reconstruction for phase-scrambed MRI with quadratic phase modulation. In *Proc. of the ISMRM*, page 1425, Honolulu, HI, USA, 2009.

- S. Ohrel, H. Lehr, **G. Schultz**, M. Berberich, D. Schinko, J. T. Schneider, A. M. Welz, J. Hennig, H. Post, and P. Ullmann. PatLoc imaging in small animals - first in vivo results. In *Proc. of the ESMRMB*, page 192, Antalya, Turkey, 2009.

2008

- **G. Schultz**, J. Hennig, and M. Zaitsev.   Image reconstruction from ambiguous PatLoc-encoded MR data. In *Proc. of the ISMRM*, page 786, Toronto, Canada, 2008.

- **G. Schultz**, A. M. Welz, J. Hennig, and M. Zaitsev. Generalized two-dimensional orthogonal spatial encoding fields. In *Proc. of the ISMRM*, page 2992, Toronto, Canada, 2008.

- A. M. Welz, M. Zaitsev, H. Lehr, **G. Schultz**, Z. Liu, F. Jia, H. Post, J. Korvink, and J. Hennig. Initial realisation of a multichannel, nonlinear PatLoc gradient coil. In *Proc. of the ISMRM*, page 1164, Toronto, Canada, 2008.

- Z. Liu, F. Jia, M. Zaitsev, A. M. Welz, **G. Schultz**, J. G. Korvink, and J. Hennig. Parametrical optimization of a PatLoc gradient coil. In *Proc. of the ISMRM*, page 1164, Toronto, Canada, 2008.

Patents and Published Patent Applications

- J. Hennig, M. Zaitsev, A. M. Welz, and **G. Schultz**. NMR tomography method based on NBSEM with 2D spatial encoding by two mutually rotated multipole gradient fields, DE102007054744B4, EP2060927A3, US7906968B2, 2007.

- H. Weber, M. Zaitsev, D. Gallichan, and **G. Schultz**. Method for homogenising resolution in magnetic resonance tomography recordings using non-linear encoding fields, DE102010003552B4, EP2378308A1, US20110241678A1, 2010.

Patents and Published Patent Applications